The Neural Simulation Language

A System for Brain Modeling

The Neural Simulation Language

A System for Brain Modeling

Alfredo Weitzenfeld

Michael Arbib

Amanda Alexander

The MIT Press

Cambridge, Massachusetts

London, England

This book was printed and bound in the United States of America.

Library of Congress Cataloging-in-Publication Data

Weitzenfeld, Alfredo.
   The neural simulation language : a system for brain modeling / Alfredo Weitzenfeld,
Michael Arbib, Amanda Alexander.
        p. cm.
   Includes bibliographical references and index.
   ISBN 0-262-73149-5 (pbk. : alk. Paper)
  1. Neural networks (Neurobiology) 2. Neural networks (Computer science)
  3. Brain—Computr simulation. I. Arbib, Michael A. II. Alexander, Amanda. III. Title.
QP363.3 . W45 2002
006.3'2–dc21

                                                2001056253

Contents

Preface

Since 1985 more than a hundred neurosimulators have been developed (see Murre (1995) for a list of many of the most important ones). These neurosimulators can be generally described as software packages intended to reduce the time and effort in simulating neural networks, ranging from the most rudimentary unsupported systems provided at no cost by academia, to the very expensive ones provided by industry for commercial use with technological applications in mind. Academia neurosimulators tend to be used for exploring new biological and artificial neural architectures while commercial packages are primarily used in non-biological areas such as credit-assessment, signal analysis, time-series prediction, pattern recognition and process control. These particular commercial systems tend to support a predefined set of artificial neural networks. Most existing neurosimulators are useful when using and extending standard paradigms but not so much when developing new ones, a phenomenon marked by the proliferation of the large number of simulators developed by researchers to experiment with specific new neural architectures.

During the last decade our group has worked to overcome the shortcoming of "one group, one neurosimulator" by designing a general-purpose simulator known as the Neural Simulation Language NSL, now in its third major release. NSL is neural network simulator that is both general and powerful, designed for users with diverse interests and programming abilities. As opposed to commercial neurosimulators, we provide NSL at no cost yet with extensive documentation.

We address the needs of a wide range of users. For novice users interested only in an introduction to neural networks, we provide user-friendly interfaces and a set of predefined artificial and biological neural models. For more advanced users well acquainted with the area, who require more sophistication, we provide evolved visualization tools together with extensibility and scalability. We provide support for varying levels in neuron model detail, which is particularly important for biological neural modeling. In artificial neural modeling the neuron model is very simple, with network models varying primarily in their network architectures and learning paradigms. While NSL is not particularly intended to support detailed single neuron modeling, NSL does provide sufficient expressiveness to support this level of modeling.

In general, NSL has the following characteristics:

- provides a powerful neural development environment supporting the efficient creation and execution of scalable neural networks;
- is designed to run on a large number of platforms;
- is built exclusively using object-oriented technology;
- offers rich graphics and a full mouse-driven window interface supporting creation of new models as well as their control and visualization;
- incorporates a compiled language NSLM for model development and a scripting language NSLS for model interaction and simulation control;
- provides extensibility with Java and C++ for users who want to develop applications under specific programming environments or to integrate with other software or hardware;
- offers free download of the complete NSL system, including full source code as well as forthcoming new versions;

- offers free and extensive support for downloading new models from our Web sites, where users may contribute with their own models and may criticize existing ones.

In summary NSL is especially suitable for the following tasks:

- Use in an academic environment where NSL simulation and model development can complement theoretical courses in both biological and artificial neural networks. Models included in the second part of the book are examples of models that can be used for this purpose. Students are able to run these models and change their behavior by modifying input in general or specific network parameters.

- Use in a research environment where scientists require rapid model prototyping and efficient execution. NSL may easily be linked to other software tools, such as additional numerical libraries, or hardware, such as robotics, by doing direct programming in either Java or C++.

- In the book we describe how to design modular neural networks in order to simplify modeling and simulation while providing better model extensibility. We provide extensive examples on how neural models should be built in general and in particular with NSL.

The book is divided in two major parts, the first part is required reading for NSL users, while the second part provides additional model examples for those interested in more specific modeling domains. We define three levels of user expertise:

- **low level** for running existing models—requiring no previous knowledge of software programming;

- **medium level** for developing simple models—requiring the user to learn only the NSL high level programming language;

- **high level** for developing complex models or linkage to other systems—requiring the user to have a basic understanding of Java or C++.

Part I An Overview of NSL Modeling and Simulation

The following table gives a brief description of each chapter in Part I of this book in its order of occurrence and the level of complexity involved (low, medium, high).

Chapter	Complexity	Description
1	Low	Introduction to neural network modeling and simulation
2	Low	Simulation Overview—using computers to explore the behavior of neural networks: Examples of biological and artificial neural network simulation in NSL.
3	Medium	Modeling Overview—developing a neural network to describe a biological system or serve a technological application: Examples of biological and artificial neural networks model in NSL.
4	Medium	Describes the Schematic Capture System for designing neural models and libraries.
5	Medium	Describes the User Interface and Graphical Windows.
6	Medium	Describes the NSLM high level modeling language for writing models.
7	Medium	Describes the NSLS scripting language for specifying simulation interaction.

Part II Neural Modeling and Simulation Examples Using NSL

The following table gives a brief description of each chapter in Part II of this book in its order of occurrence and level of model complexity involved.

Chapter	Complexity	Description
8	Medium	Adaptive Resonance Theory by T. Tanaka and A. Weitzenfeld
9	Medium	Depth Perception by A. Weitzenfeld and M. Arbib
10	Medium	Retina by R. Corbacho and A. Weitzenfeld
11	Medium	Receptive Fields by F. Moran, J. Chacón, M.A. Andrade and A. Weitzenfeld
12	Medium	The Associative Search Network: Landmark Learning and Hill Climbing by M. Bota and A. Guazzelli
13	High	A Model of Primate Visual-Motor Conditional Learning by A. Fagg and A. Weitzenfeld
14	High	The Modular Design of the Oculomotor System in Monkeys by P. Dominey, M. Arbib and A. Alexander
15	High	Crowley-Arbib Saccade Model by M. Crowley, E. Oztop and S. Marmol
16	High	A Cerebellar Model of Sensorimotor Adaptation by Jacob Spoelstra
17	High	Learning to Detour by F. Corbacho and A. Weitzenfeld
18	High	Face Recognition based on Dynamic Link Matching by L. Wiskott and C. von der Malsburg and A. Weitzenfeld

We end the book with a discussion on current work and future directions, such as distributed simulation and robotics, together with appendices containing information on how to download from our web sites (in Los Angeles and in Mexico City) the software described in the book as well as model overviews, FAQs, emails and other relevant information.

Alfredo Weitzenfeld
  Mexico City

Michael A. Arbib
Amanda Alexander
  Los Angeles

Acknowledgments

We acknowledge the support of the Human Brain Project (Grant 5-P20-52194), the NSF-CONACyT collaboration project (NSF grant #IRI-9522999 and CONACyT grant #546500-5-C018-A), CONACyT REDII (Information Research Network by its spanish acronym) the "Asociación Mexicana de Cultura, A.C.," as well as all the people involved in the development of NSL and SCS throughout the past years.

We would especially like to thank the following research assistants at USC: Isaac Ta-yan Siu, Danjie Pan, Erhan Oztop, George Kardaras, Nikunj Mehta, Tejas Rajkotia, Salvador Marmol (previously at ITAM), Weifanf Xie and Nitin Gupta; together with the following research assistants at ITAM: Claudia Calderas, Oscar Peguero, Francisco Peniche, Sebastián Gutiérrez, Francisco Otero, Rafael Ramos, Munir Estevane, Eric Galicia, and Mirlette Islas.

In addition we would like to thank the following individuals for allowing us to use their public domain software: Jacl TCL interpreter: Ioi Lam, Cornell University, 1996; Java preprocessor: David Engberg, Effective Edge, 1995 and Dennis Heimbigner, University of Colorado, 1996; and Display tree: Sandip Chitale, 1996.

And, finally, we would especially like to thank our families for their patience: Tica, Jonathan, Gabriela, Ariel, Prue, Steven, David, and Thomas.

1 Introduction

The NSL Neural Simulation Language provides a platform for building neural architectures (modeling) and for executing them (simulation). NSL is based on object-oriented technology, extended to provide modularity at the application level as well. In this chapter we discuss these basic concepts and how NSL takes advantage of them.

1.1 Neural Networks

Neural network simulation is an important research and development area extending from biological studies to artificial applications. Biological neural networks are designed to model the brain in a faithful way while artificial neural networks are designed to take advantage of various "semi-neural" computing techniques, especially the use of different learning algorithms in distributed networks, in various technological domains. Challenges vary depending on the respective areas although common basic tasks are involved when working with neural networks: *modeling* and *simulation*.

Modeling

Modeling or development of a neural network or neural architecture depends on the type of network being constructed. In the case of artificial neural modeling, neural architectures are created to solve the application problem at hand, while in the case of biological modeling neural architectures are specified to reproduce anatomical and physiological experimental data. Both types of network development involve choosing appropriate data representations for neural components, neurons and their interconnections, as well as network input, control parameters and network dynamics specified in terms of a set of mathematical equations.

For biological modeling, the neuron model varies depending on the details being described. Neuron models can be very sophisticated biophysical models, such as compartmental models (Rall 1959) in turn based on the Hodgkin-Huxley model (Hodgkin and Huxley 1952). When behavioral analysis is desired, the neural network as a whole may often be adequately analyzed using simpler neuron models such as the analog *leaky integrator* model. And sometimes even simpler neural models are enough, in particular for artificial networks, as with discrete binary models where the neuron is either on or off at each time step, as in the McCulloch-Pitts model (McCulloch and Pitts 1943).

The particular neuron model chosen defines the dynamics for each neuron, yet a complete network architecture also involves specifying interconnections among neurons as well as specifying input to the network and choosing appropriate parameters for different tasks using the neural model specified. Moreover, artificial neural networks—as do many biological models—involve learning, requiring an additional training phase in the model architecture.

To generate a neural architecture the network developer requires a modeling language sufficiently expressive to support their representation. On the other hand, the language should be extensible enough to integrate with other software systems, such as to obtain or send data. In general, a neural network modeling or development environment should support a set of basic structures and functions to simplify the task of building new models as well as interacting with them.

Clearly, the user's background plays an important role in the sophistication of the development environment. Novice users depend almost completely on the interactivity provided through window interfaces, while more sophisticated users usually desire extensibility in the form of programming languages.

Simulation

Simulation of neural network architectures also varies depending on whether it relates to artificial or biological networks. Artificial neural networks particularly those involving learning usually require a two-stage simulation process: an initial training phase and a subsequent processing or running phase. Biological networks usually require a single running phase (in which behavior and learning may be intertwined).

Simulation consists of using the computer to see how the model behaves for a variety of input patterns and parameter settings. A simulation may use values pre-specified in the original formulation of the model, but will in general involve specifying one or more aspects of the neural architecture that may be modified by the user. Simulation then involves analyzing the results, both visual and numerical, generated by the simulation; on the basis of these results one can decide if any modifications are necessary in the network input or parameters. If changes are required these may be interactively specified or may require more structural modifications at the neural architecture level going back to the development phase. Otherwise the model is simulated again with newly specified input. Simulation also involves selecting one of the many approximation methods used to solve neural dynamics specified through differential equations.

In addition, the environment requirements can change when moving a model from development phase to test phase. When models are initially simulated, good interactivity is necessary to let the user modify inputs and parameters as necessary. As the model becomes more stable, simulation efficiency is a primary concern where model processing may take considerable time possibly hours or even days for the largest networks to process. Parallelism and distributed computing will increasingly play key roles in speeding up computation.

1.2 Modularity, Object-Oriented Programming, and Concurrency

Modularity, object-oriented programming and concurrency play an important part in building neural networks in NSL as well as in their execution. Furthermore, the actual NSL system is built based on object-oriented technology.

Modularity in Neural Networks

Modularity is today widely accepted as a requirement for structuring software systems. As software becomes larger and more complex, being able to break a system into separate modules enables the software developer to better manage the inherent complexity of the overall system. As neural networks become larger and more complex, they too may become hard to read, modify, test and extend. Moreover, when building biological neural networks, modularization is further motivated by taking into consideration the way we analyze the brain as a set of different brain regions. The general methodology for making a complex neural model of brain function is to combine different modules corresponding to different brain regions. To model a particular brain region, we divide it anatomically or physiologically into different neural arrays. Each brain region is then modeled as a set of neuron arrays, where each neuron is described for example by the leaky integrator, a single-compartment model of membrane potential and firing rate. (However, one can implement other, possibly far more detailed, neural models.) For example, figure 1.1 shows the basic components in a model describing the interaction of the *Superior Colliculus* (*SC*) and the saccade generator of the *Brainstem* involved in the control of eye movements. In this model, each component or module represents a single brain region.

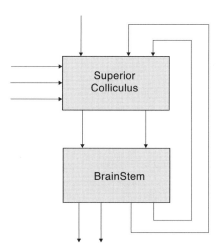

Figure 1.1
The diagram above shows two interconnected modules, the Superior Colliculus (SC) and the Brainstem. Each module is decomposed into several submodules (not shown here) each imple-mented as an array of neurons identified by their different physiological response when a monkey makes rapid eye movements.

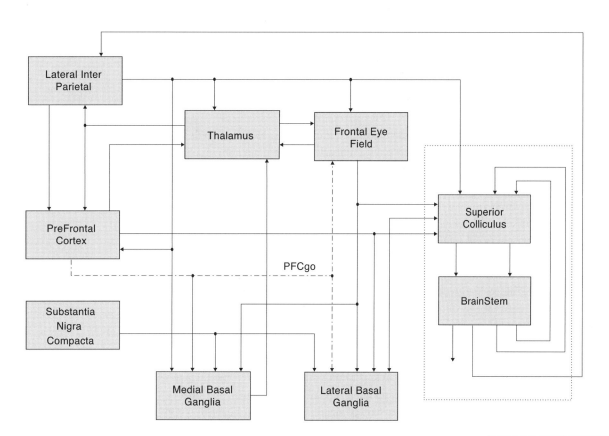

Structured models provide two benefits. The first is that it makes them easier to understand, and the second is that modules can be reused in other models. For example, figure 1.2 shows the two previous *SC* and *BrainStem* modules embedded into a far more complex model, the *Crowley-Arbib* model of basal ganglia. Each of these modules can be further broken down into submodules, eventually reaching modules that take the form of neural arrays. For example, figure 1.3 shows how the single *Prefrontal Cortex* module (*PFC*) can be further broken down into four submodules, each a crucial brain region involved in the control of movement.

There are, basically, two ways to understand a complex system. One is to focus in on some particular subsystem, some module, and carry out studies of that in detail. The other is to step back and look at higher levels of organization in which the details of particular

Figure 1.2
The diagram shows the SC and BrainStem modules from figure 1.1 embedded in a much larger model of interacting brain regions.

modules are hidden. Full understanding comes as we cycle back and forth between different levels of detail in analyzing different subsystems, sometimes simulating modules in isolation, at other times designing computer experiments that help us follow the dynamics of the interactions between the various modules.

Thus, it is important for a neural network simulator to support modularization of models. This concept of modularity is best supported today by object-oriented languages and the underlying modeling concepts described next.

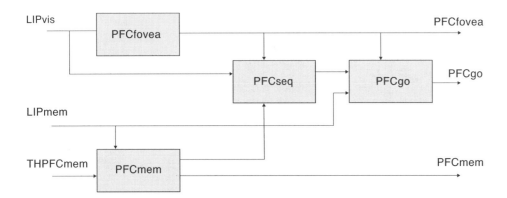

Figure 1.3
The *Prefrontal Cortex* (PFC) model is further decomposed into 4 submodules.

Object-Oriented Programming

Object-oriented technology has existed for more than thirty years. However, only in this past decade have we seen it applied in so many industries. What makes this technology special is the concept of the *object* as the basic modularization abstraction in a program. Prior to object-orientation, a complete application would be written at the data and function level of abstraction. Since data and functions are global to a program any changes to them could potentially affect the complete system, an undesired effect when large and complex systems are being modified. To avoid this problem an additional level of abstraction is added—the object. At the highest level, programs are made exclusively out of objects interacting with each other through pre-defined object interfaces. At the lowest level, objects are individually defined in terms of local data and functions, avoiding global conflicts that make systems so hard to manage and understand. Changes inside objects do not affect other objects in the system so long as the external behavior of the object remains the same. Since there is usually a smaller number of objects in a program than the total number of data or functions, software development becomes more manageable. Objects also provide abstraction and extensibility and contribute to modularity and code reuse. These seemingly simple concepts have great repercussion in the quality of systems being built and its introduction as part of neural modeling reflects this. Obviously, the use of object-orientation is only part of writing better software as well as neural models. How the user designs the software or neural architectures with this technology has an important effect on the system, an aspect which becomes more accessible by providing a simple to follow yet powerful modeling architecture such as that provided by NSL.

Concurrency in Neural Networks

Concurrency can play an important role in neural network simulation, both in order to model neurons more faithfully and to increase processing throughput (Weitzenfeld and Arbib 1991). We have incorporated concurrent processing capabilities in the general design of NSL for this purpose. The computational model on which NSL is based has been inspired by the work on the *Abstract Schema Language ASL* (Weitzenfeld 1992), where *schemas* (Arbib 1992) are *active* or concurrent objects (Yonezawa and Tokoro 1987) resulting in the ability to concurrently process modules. The NSL software supplied with this book is implemented on serial computers, *emulating* concurrency. Extensions to NSL and its underlying software architecture will implement genuine concurrency to permit parallel and distributed processing of modules in the near future. We will discuss this more in the Future Directions chapter.

1.3 Modeling and Simulation in NSL

As an object-oriented system, NSL is built with modularization in mind. As a neural network development platform, NSL provides a modeling and simulation environment for large-scale general-purpose neural networks by the use of modules that can be hierarchically interconnected to enable the construction of very complex models. NSL provides a modeling language NSLM to build/code the model and a scripting language NSLS to specify how the simulation is to be executed and controlled.

Modeling

Modeling in NSL is carried out at two levels of abstraction, *modules* and *neural networks*, somewhat analogous to object-orientation in its different abstraction levels when building applications. Modules define the top-level view of a model, hiding its internal complexity. This complexity is only viewed at the bottom-level corresponding to the actual neural networks. A complete model in NSL requires the following components: (1) a set of modules defining the entire model; (2) neurons comprised in each neural module; (3) neural interconnections; (4) neural dynamics; and (5) numerical methods to solve the differential equations.

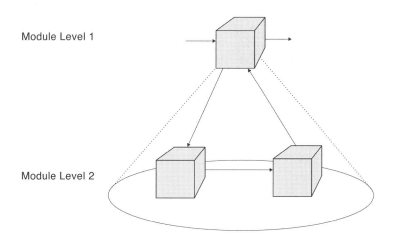

Module Level 1

Module Level 2

Figure 1.4
The NSL computational model is based on hierarchi-cal modules. A module at a higher level (level 1) is decomposed into submod-ules (level 2). These sub-modules are themselves modules that may be further decomposed. Arrows show data communication among modules.

Modules

Modules in NSL correspond to objects in object orientation in that they specify the underlying computational model. These entities are hierarchically organized as shown in figure 1.4.

Thus a given module may either be decomposed into a set of smaller modules or maybe a "leaf module" that may be implemented in different ways, where neural networks are of particular interest here. The hierarchical module decomposition results in what is known as *module assemblages*—a network of *submodules* that can be seen in their entirety in terms of a single higher-level module. These hierarchies enable the development of modular systems where modules may be designed and implemented independently of each other following both top-down and bottom-up development.

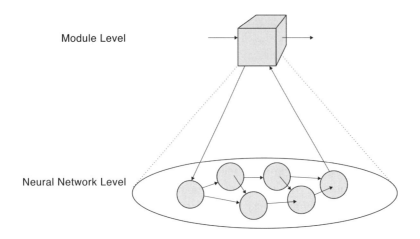

Neural Networks

Some modules will be implemented as neural networks where every neuron becomes an element or attribute of a module, as shown in figure 1.5. (Note that although neurons also may be treated as modules, they are often treated as elements inside a single module—e.g., one representing an array of neurons—in NSL. We thus draw neurons as spheres instead of cubes to highlight the latter possibility.)

There are many ways to characterize a neuron. The complexity of the neuron depends on the accuracy needed by the larger model network and on the computational power of the computer being used. The GENESIS (Bower and Beeman 1998) and NEURON (Hines 1997) systems were designed specifically to support the type of modeling of a single neuron which takes account of the detailed morphology of the neuron in relation to different types of input. The NSL system was designed to let the user represent neurons at any level of desired detail; however, this book will focus on the simulation of large-scale properties of neural networks modeled with relatively simple neurons.

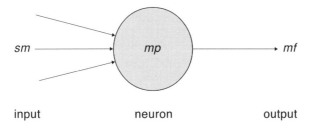

input   neuron   output

Figure 1.6
Single compartment neural model represented by a value *mp* corresponding to its membrane potential, and a value *mf* corresponding to its firing, the only output from the neuron. *sm* represents the set of inputs to the neuron.

We consider the neuron shown in figure 1.6 to be "simple" since its internal state is described by a single scalar quantity, membrane potential *mp*, its input is *sm* and its output is *mf*, specified by some nonlinear function of *mf*.

The neuron may receive input from many different neurons, while it has only a single output (which may "branch" to affect many other neurons or drive the network's outputs). The choice of transformation from *sm* to *mp* defines the particular neural model utilized, including the dependence of *mp* on the neuron's previous history. The membrane potential *mp* is described by a simple first-order differential equation,

$$\tau \frac{dmp(t)}{dt} = f(sm, mp, t) \tag{1.1}$$

depending on its input *s*. The choice of *f* defines the particular neural model utilized, including the dependence of *mp* on the neuron's previous history. In this example we present the leaky integrator. The *leaky integrator* model is described by

$$f(sm, mp, t) = -mp(t) + sm(t) \qquad (1.2)$$

while the *average firing rate* or output of the neuron, *mf*, is obtained by applying some "activation function" to the neuron's membrane potential,

$$mf(t) = \sigma(mp(t)) \qquad (1.3)$$

where σ usually is described by a non-linear function also known as *threshold* functions such as *ramp*, *step*, *saturation* or *sigmoid*. The general idea is that the higher the neuron membrane potential, the higher the firing rate, and thus the greater its effect on other neurons to which it provides input.

The neural network itself is made of any number of interconnected neurons where the most common formula for the input sm_j to a neuron m_j from the output of a neuron m_i as shown in figure 1.7 is given by,

$$sv_j = \sum_{i=0}^{n-1} w_{ij} uf_i \qquad (1.4)$$

where $uf_i(t)$ is the firing rate of the neuron whose output is connected to the *i*th input line of neuron v_j, and w_{ij} is the corresponding weight on that connection (*up* and *vp* are analogous to *mp*, while *uf* and *vf* are analogous to *mf*). These interconnections are called *excitatory* or *inhibitory* depending on whether the weight w_{ij} is positive or negative.

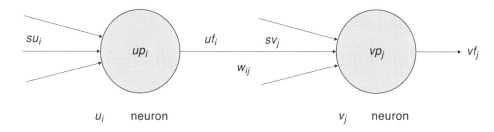

When modeling a large number of neurons it becomes extremely tedious to individually name each one of the neurons. In the brain as well as in many neural engineering applications, we often find neural networks structured into two-dimensional arrays, with regular connection patterns between various arrays. For this reason, as part of our modeling primitives, we extend a simple single neuron into neuron arrays and single neuron-to-neuron links into connection masks, describing spatial arrangements among homogeneous neurons and their connections, respectively. If mask w_k (for $-d \leq k \leq d$) represents the synaptic weight from the uf_{j+k} (for $-d \leq k \leq d$) elements to v_j element for each *j*, we then have

$$sv_j = \sum_{k=-d}^{d} w_k uf_{j+k} \qquad (1.5)$$

The computational advantage of introducing such concepts when describing a "regular" neural network, as shall be seen in chapter 3, is that neuron arrays and interconnection masks can then be more concisely represented. Interconnections among neurons would then be processed by a spatial convolution between a mask and an array. Once interconnections are specified between neurons or neural arrays, we only need to specify network input; weights and any additional parameter before simulation can take place.

Simulation

The simulation process starts with a model already developed. Simulation involves interactively specifying aspects of the model that tend to change often, in particular parameter values and input patterns. Also, this process involves specifying simulation control and visualization aspects.

For example, figure 1.8 shows five snapshots of the Buildup Cell activity after the simulation of one of the submodules in the Superior Colliculus of the Crowley and Arbib model shown in figure 1.1. We observe the activity of single neurons, classes of neurons or outputs in response to different input patterns as the cortical command triggers a movement up and to the right. We see that the cortical command builds up a peak of activity on the Buildup Cell array. This peak moves towards the center of the array where it then disappears (this corresponds to the command for the eye moving towards the target, after which the command is no longer required).

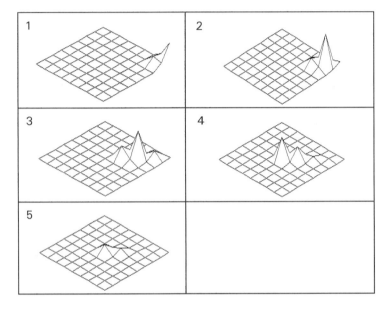

Figure 1.8
An example of Buildup Cell activity in the Superior Colliculus model of figure 1.1.

It is not only important to design a good model, it is also important to design different kinds of graphical output to make clear how the model behaves. Additionally, an experiment may examine the effects of changing parameters in a model, just as much as changing the inputs. One of the reasons for studying the basal ganglia is to understand Parkinson's disease, in which the basal ganglia are depleted of a substance called dopamine, whose depletion is a prime correlate of Parkinson's disease. The model of figure 1.2 (at a level of detail not shown) includes a parameter that represents the level of dopamine. The "normal" model, yields two saccades, one each in turn to the positions at which the two targets appeared; the "low-dopamine" model only shows a response to the first target, a result which gives insight into some of the motor disorders of Parkinson's disease patients. The actual model is described in detail in chapter 15. We shall describe the simulation process in more detail in chapter 2.

1.4 The NSL System

The Neural Simulation Language (NSL) has evolved for over a decade. The original system was written in C (NSL 1) in 1989, with a second version written in C++ (NSL 2) in 1991 and based on object-oriented technology. Both versions were developed at USC by Alfredo Weitzenfeld, with Michael Arbib involved in the overall design. The present version NSL 3 is a major release completely restructured over former versions both as a system as well as the supported modeling and simulation, including modularity and concurrency. NSL 3 includes two different environments, one in Java (NSLJ, developed at USC by Amanda Alexander's team) and the other in C++ (NSLC, developed at ITAM in

Mexico by Alfredo Weitzenfeld's team), again with Arbib involved in the overall design. Both environments support similar modeling and simulation, where each one offers different advantages to the user.

The advantages with Java are

- *portability*: Code written in Java runs without changes "everywhere";
- *maintainability*: Java code requires maintaining one single software version for different operating systems, compilers and other software on different platforms.
- *web-oriented*: Java code runs on the client side of the web, simplifying exchange of models without the owner of the model having to provide a large server on which other people can run simulations.

The advantages with C++ are

- *efficiency*: Since C++ is an extension to C, C++ models get simulated on top of one of the most efficient execution languages;
- *integration*: C++ code may be directly integrated with a large number of software packages already in existence written in C++;
- *linkage to hardware*: Currently most linkages to robots are done through C and C++; however, more and more of these systems are moving to Java.

The great advantage on having support for both environments is the ability to switch between the two of them to get the best of each world with minimum effort.

The complete NSL system is made of three components: the **Simulation System**, the **Schematic Capture System** and the **Model/Module Libraries**, as shown in figure 1.9. Three file types are used as communication between the three modules:

- **mod** files describing NSL models, executed by the Simulation System, stored in the Model Library and optionally generated from SCS,
- **nsl** files describing NSL model simulation, executed by the Simulation System and stored in the Model/Module Libraries,
- **sif** files storing schematic information about the model stored in the Model/Module Libraries as well.

Main Components of the NSL System

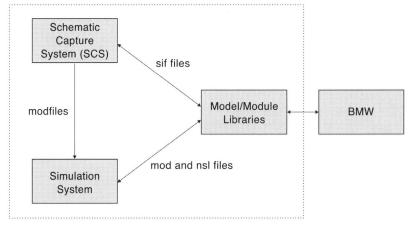

Figure 1.9
Schematic Capture System and its relation to the NSL System.[1]

Simulation System

The NSL Simulation System comprises several subsystems: the **Simulation subsystem** where model interaction and processing takes place and the **Window Interface subsystem** where all graphics interaction takes place, as shown in figure 1.10. Note that we are now discussing the subsystems or modules that comprise the overall simulation system, not the modules of a specific neural model programmed with NSL. But in either case, we take advantage of the methodology of object-oriented programming.

The subsystems of the **Simulation System** are:

- I/O **Control** where external aspects of the simulation are controlled by the *Script Interpreter* and the Window Interface;

- **Scheduler** which executes the model and modules in a specific sequence.

- **Model Compiler** where NSLM code is compiled and linked with NSL libraries to generate an executable file;

- **Script Interpreter** that can be used to specify parameters and to control the simulation.

- The subsystems of the **Window Interface** are:

- **Graphics Output**, consists of all NSL graphic libraries for instantiating display frames, canvases and graphs;

- **Graphics Input** consists of NSL window controllers to interact with the simulation and control its execution and parameters.

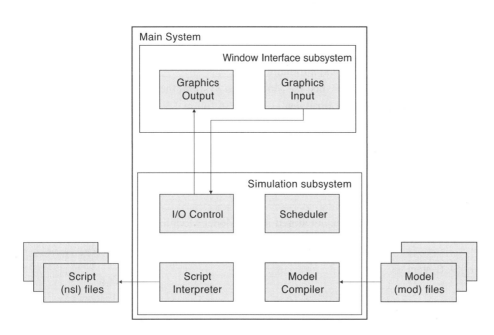

Figure 1.10
NSL Simulation System composed of the Simulation and Window Interface subsystems.

Schematic Capture System

NSL supports development of models by explicitly programming the code for each module as well as visual modeling by using the *Schematic Capture System* (*SCS*). The Schematic Capture System facilitates the creation of modular and hierarchical neural networks. SCS provides graphical tools to build hierarchical models following a top-down or bottom-up methodology. In SCS the user graphically connects icons representing modules, into what we call a *schematic*. Each icon can then be decomposed further into a schematic of its own. The benefit of having a schematic capture system is that modules can be stored in libraries and easily accessed by the schematic capture system. As more modules are added to the NSL Model/Module Libraries, users will benefit by being able to create a rich variety of new models without having to write new code. When coming to view an existing model, the schematics make the relationship between modules much easier to visualize; besides simplifying the model creation process. To create a new model, the user places icons on the screen representing modules already available and connects them to provide a high level view of a model or module. As modules are summoned to the screen and interconnected, the system automatically generates the corresponding NSL module code. The success of this will obviously depend on having good modules and documentation.

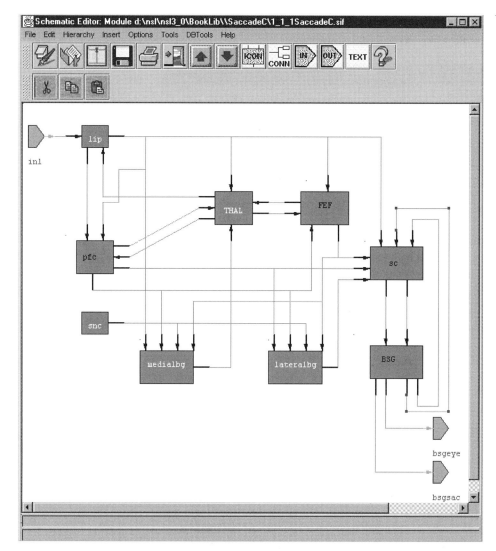

Figure 1.11
Schematic Editor showing the Crowley Top Level Saccade Module. Thin lines describe connections among sub-modules while thick lines describe entry (with arrows) and exit points to and from modules.

Figure 1.11 shows a schematic of the top level of a model. The complete schematic describes a single higher-level module, where rectangular boxes represent lower-level modules or sub-modules. These modules can be newly defined modules or already existing ones. Thin lines describe connections among sub-modules while thick lines describe entry (with arrows) and exit points to and from modules. Pentagon shaped boxes represent input ports (when lines come out from a vertex) and output ports (when lines point to a side) for the higher-level module whose schematics is being described.

SCS also provides many of the library functions that are necessary to organize and manage the modules including model and module version management as overviewed in the following section. More details of the Schematic Capture System are described in chapter 4.

Model/Module Libraries
Models and modules developed under NSL are hierarchically organized in libraries. NSL supports two library structures. The first is called the basic hierarchy while the second

structure is known as the extended hierarchy built and maintained by the Schematic Capture System (SCS). Both are shown in table 1.2. The difference between the two is how modules are managed. The basic organization does not give a version number to modules only models. The extended one gives version numbers to both models and modules, and contains an extra directory, called the **exe** directory, for executables specific to different operating systems for the C++ version of the software.

Library Organization						
Basic Hierarchy			**Extended Hierarchy**			
nsl3_0			nsl3_0			
Library Name			Library Name			
Model Name			Model or Module Name			
Version Number			Version Number			
io	src	doc	io	src	exe	doc

Table 1.1
NSL model library hierarchy organization for the Basic Hierarchy on the left and the Extended Hierarchy on the right.

There are several reasons for maintaining both systems. In the extended one, the user can experiment with different versions of a module shared among a number of models. Typically, larger models will share modules thus needing management by the SCS system. For the basic structure (not using SCS) it is easier to manage all of the module files in one directory, **src**. Additionally, if the modules are not intended to be shared or contributed to Brain Models on the Web (BMW), then they do not necessarily need to be versioned.

Basic Hierarchy

In the general organization of the basic hierarchy levels in the tree correspond to directories. The root of the hierarchy trees is "nsl3_0", the current system version. A library name is defined to distinguish between libraries. Obviously there may be multiple model libraries. Each library may contain multiple *models* identified by their corresponding name. Each model is then associated with different implementations identified each by its corresponding numerical *version*; (version numbers start at 1_1_1). At the end of the directory hierarchy, the last level down contains the directories where the actual model or module files are stored: input/output files (**io**), source module files (**src**) and documentation (**doc**). The **io** directory stores input and output files usually in the form of NSLS script files. The **src** directory contains source code that needs to be compiled written in the NSLM modeling language; this directory also includes files produced from the compilation including executables. The **doc** directory contains any documentation relevant to the model including theoretical background, why certain values were chosen for certain parameters, what is special about each of the protocols, how to perform more sophisticated experiments, relevant papers, etc. All models given in this book where originally developed using the basic system. table 1.2 illustrates the directory hierarchy for the basic book models described in chapters 2 and 3 in the book. Note that we actually have two versions of the Hopfield model; one where we illustrate the use of scripts for input, and another for illustrating the use of input and output modules.

Basic BookLib											
MaxSelectorModel			HopfieldModel						BackPropModel		
1_1_1			1_1_1			1_2_1			1_1_1		
io	src	doc	io	src	doc	io	src	doc	io	src	doc

Extended Hierarchy

In the extended hierarchy, the directory structure for the library is almost identical to the basic one except for the fact that each module is versioned, and there is an extra **exe** directory. There may be multiple libraries, and it is up to the model builder to decide what modules and models will go into each. Also, each library may contain multiple *models* and *modules*, identified by their corresponding name. Each model and module must have a unique name. Also, each model and module is then associated with different implementations identified by its corresponding numerical *version*, (version numbers start at 1_1_1). Obviously, many versions of a model or module may exist in a library, thus we identify versions using a version identification number composed of three digits denoting the model or module release number, revision number, and modification number, respectively. All numbers are initialized to 1. At the end of the directory hier-archy, the last level down contains the directories where the actual model or module files are stored: input/output files (**io**), source module files (**src**), documentation (**doc**), and the executable files (**exe**). Typically the **io** and **exe** directories are empty except for model directories. In table 1.3, we illustrate the MaxSelectorModel hierarchy previously shown in table 1.2 in the basic architecture and now shown with modules in the extended library.

Table 1.2
The basic hierarchy organization for the book models.

Extended BookLib																							
MaxSelectorModel				MaxSelector				MaxSelectorStimuli				MaxSelectorOutput				ULayer				VLayer			
1_1_1				1_1_1				1_1_1				1_1_1				1_1_1				1_1_1			
io	src	doc	exe	io	src	doc	exe	io	src	doc	exe	io	src	doc	exe	io	src	doc	exe	io	src	doc	exe

SCS manipulates the model and module library allowing the user to create new libraries as well as add new revisions to existing models and modules. The user can browse and search the libraries for particular models or modules. When building a schematic, the user has the choice of choosing the most recent modification of a model or module, or sticking with a fixed version of that model or module. If the user chooses a specific version this is called "using the **fixed** version." If the user specifies "0_0_0" the most current version of the module would be used instead and whenever there is a more recent version of the module, that version will be used. This is called "using the **floating** version." Each individual library file stores *metadata* describing the software used to create the corresponding model/module.

Table 1.3
The extended library structure for the basic book library showing one of its models, the MaxSelector, and its children.

1.5 Summary

In this first chapter we have introduced modeling and simulation of neural networks in general and in relation to NSL. We also gave an overview of the NSL system components including a description of the technology used to build the system as well as simulate models using NSL.

Notes

1. Figure 1.9 also shows BMW (Brain Models on the Web). This is not part of NSL, but is a model repository under development by the USC Brain Project in which model assump-tions and simulation results can be explicitly compared with the empirical data gathered by neuroscientists.

2 Simulation in NSL

We will concentrate in this chapter primarily on how to run already existing models and leave new model development for the next chapter. Three neural networks simulated in NSL will be overviewed in this chapter: *Maximum Selector*, *Hopfield* and *Backpropaga-tion*. Simulation in NSL requires a basic level of understanding of neural networks. The models chosen here will help the novice gain that understanding because of their simpli-city and importance in the area of neural networks.

2.1 Selecting a Model

The simulation process begins with the selection of an already developed model; the modeling process which creates such models will be described in chapter 4, the Schematic Capture System.

However, if you do not have SCS, then to select a model from the **BookLib** models, simply change directories to where the desired model is located following the path *<installation-site>*/nsl3_0/BookLib/<modelname>. (Note that if you are working on a PC, you will want to specify the path using backward slashes "\" instead.) From there you will want to change directories to the first version, 1_1_1, and then to the **src** directory. From there either type:

```
nslj model_name
```

or

```
nslc model_name
```

These commands will invoke NSL and load the model specified. Make sure that your system administrator has set up your environment correctly. There are several environment variables we use for both NSL implemented in C++ and Java. These are discussed in chapter 5, The User Interface and Graphical Windows. See Appendix V for further details on executing models for the different platforms.

To select a model from the SCS archive of **BookLib** models, we must first open the library by calling the *Schematic Capture System* (SCS) responsible for model management (see Appendix IV for platform particulars). We execute from a shell (or by double clicking).

```
prompt> scs
```

The system initially presents the *Schematic Editor* (*SE*) window as shown in figure 2.1.

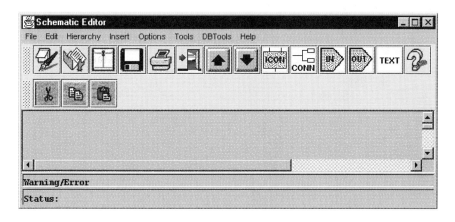

Figure 2.1
Schematic Editor Window. The different menu and button options control the creation and modification of model schematics.

To execute an existing model we select "Simulate Using Java" (or "Simulate Using C++") from the "Tools"menu, as shown in figure 2.2.

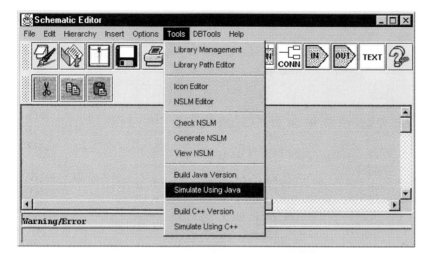

Figure 2.2
Select "Simulate Using Java" from the "Tools" menu to bring a listing of models available in the library of models and modules which are available for use in Java.

SCS then presents a list of available models, as shown in figure 2.3.

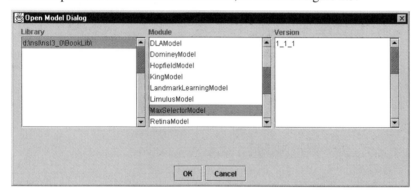

Figure 2.3
Open Model for Execution Window

For example, to choose the *MaxSelectorModel*, we select the model and version found under "nsl3_0/BookLib/ /MaxSelectorModel/1_1_1/".

Once we chose the particular model, the system brings up the NSL Executive window presented in figure 2.4 together with an additional output display window particular to this model shown in figure 2.5. At this point we are ready to simulate the selected model. Yet, before we do that, we will quickly introduce the NSL Simulation Interface.

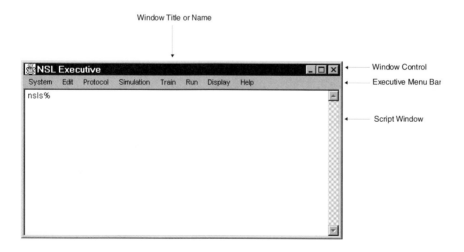

Figure 2.4
The NSL Executive window. The top part of the window contains the title and underneath the title is the Executive Menu Bar. The larger section of the window contains the NSL Script Window or shell.

2.2 Simulation Interface

The NSL **Executive** window, shown in figure 2.4, is used to control the complete simulation process such as visualization of model behavior. Control is handled either via mouse-driven menu selections or by explicitly typing textual commands in the NSL Script (NSLS) window. Since not all possible commands are available from the menus, the "NSLS" window/shell is offered for more elaborate scripts.

The top part of the window (or header) contains the window name, NSL Executive, and the Window Control (right upper corner) used for *iconizing*, enlarging and closing the window. Underneath the header immediately follows the **Executive Menu Bar**, containing the menus for controlling the different aspects involved in a simulation. The lower portion of the window contains the **Script Window**, a scrollable window used for script command entry, recording and editing. The NSL Script Language is a superset of the pull down menus in that any command that can be executed from one of the pull-down menus can also be typed in the Script window, while the opposite is not necessarily so. Furthermore, commands can also be stored in files and then loaded into the Script window at a later time. The NSLS language supports two levels of commands. The basic level allows *Tool Command Language* commands (TCL) (Ousterhout 94) while the second level allows NSL commands. The NSL commands have a special "nsl" prefix to distinguish them from TCL commands. These commands are overviewed later in the chapter and are discussed thoroughly in chapter 7, the NSL Scripting Language.

While there is a single **NSL Executive/Script** window per simulation there may be any number of additional output and input windows containing different displays. For example, the *Maximum Selector* model brings up the additional output frame shown in figure 2.5.

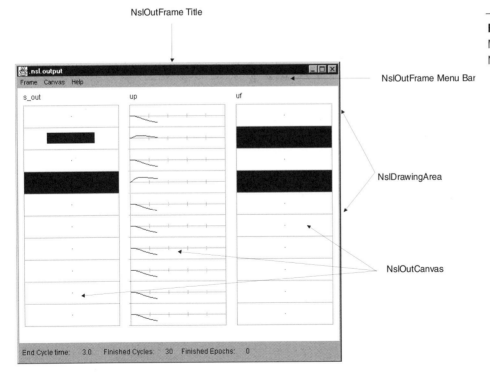

NslOutFrame Title

NslOutFrame Menu Bar

NslDrawingArea

NslOutCanvas

Figure 2.5
MaxSelectorModel
NslOutFrame.

The top part of the window contains the title or frame name and the very bottom of the frame contains the **Status line**. The status line displays the current simulation time, finished cycles, finished epochs, and phase. In the middle, the frame contains the **NslDrawingArea**. In this example, the drawing area contains three **NslOutCanvases**: the first and third corresponds to **Area** graphs while the second corresponds to a **Temporal** graph. (We will describe these graphs in more detail in chapter 5, The User Interface and Graphical Windows.)

2.3 Simulating a Model

If a model is a discrete-event or discrete-time model, the model equations explicitly describe how to go from the state and input of the network at time t to the state and output after the event following t is completed, or at time t+1 on the discrete time scale, respectively. However, if the model is continuous-time, described by differential equations, then simulation of the model requires that we replace the differential equation by some discrete-time, numerical method (e.g., Euler or Runge-Kutta) and choose a simulation time step Δt so that the computer can go from state and input at time t to an *approximation* of the state and output at time t+Δt. In each case, the simulation of the system proceeds in steps, where each *simulation cycle* updates every module within the model once.

In simulating a model, a basic simulation time step must be chosen. Simulation involves the following aspects of model interaction: (1) simulation control, (2) visualization, (3) input assignment and (4) parameter assignment.

Simulation Control Simulation control involves the execution of a model. The Executive window's "Simulation," "Train" and "Run" menus contain options for starting, stopping, continuing and ending a simulation during its training and running phase, respectively.

Visualization Model behavior is visualized via a number of graphics displays. These displays are drawn on canvases, **NslOutCanvas**, each belonging to a **NslOutFrame** output frame. Each **NslOutFrame** represents an independent window on the screen containing any number of **NslOutCanvas** for interactively plotting neural behavior or variables in general. NSL canvases can display many different graph types that display NSL numeric objects—objects containing numeric arrays of varying dimensions. For example the **Area** graph shown in figure 2.5 displays the activity of a one-dimensional object at every simulation cycle. the size of the dark rectangle represents a corresponding activity level. On the other hand, the **Temporal** graph shown displays the activity of a one-dimensional objects as a function of time (in other words, it keeps a history).

Input Assignment Input to a model varies both in terms of the particular model but also in terms of how it is specified. NSL supports input as script commands in the NSLS language using the **Script Window**, by loading script files, as well as by custom-designed input windows.

Parameter Assignment Simulation and model parameters can be interactively assigned by the user. Simulation parameters can be modified via the "Options" menu while model parameters are modified via the **Script Window**. Additionally, some models may have their own custom-designed window interfaces for parameter modification.

The remaining sections of this chapter illustrate model simulation starting with the *Maximum Selector* model then with *Hopfield* and finally with *Backpropagation*.

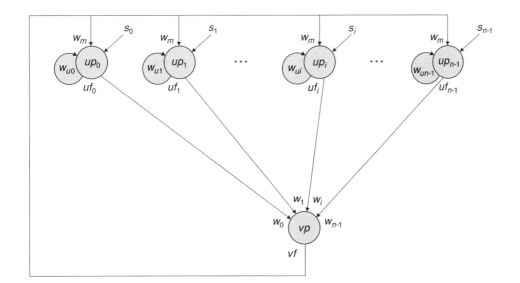

Figure 2.6
The neural network architecture for the Maximum Selector (Didday 1976; Amari and Arbib 1977) where s_i represents input to the network, up_i and vp represent membrane potentials while uf_i and vf represent firing rates. w_m, w_{ui}, and w_i correspond to connection weights.

2.4 Maximum Selector

The *Maximum Selector* neural model (Amari and Arbib 1977) is an example of a biologically inspired neural network. The network is based on the *Didday* model for prey selection (Didday 1976) and is more generally known as a *Winner Take All* (*WTA*) neural network. The model uses competition mechanisms to obtain, in many cases, a single winner in the network where the input signal with the greatest strength is propagated along to the output of the network.

Model Description

The *Maximum Selector* neural network is shown in figure 2.6. External input to the network is represented by s_i (for $0 \leq i \leq n\text{-}1$). The input is fed into neuron u, with up_i representing the membrane potential of neuron u while uf_i represents its output. uf_i is fed into neuron v as well as back into its own neuron. vp represents the membrane potential of neuron v which plays the role of inhibitor in the network. w_m, w_{ui}, and w_i represent connection weights, whose values are not necessarily equal.

The neural network is described by the following set of equations,

$$\tau_u \frac{du_i(t)}{dt} = -u_i + w_u f(u_i) - w_m g(v) - h_1 + s_i \tag{2.1}$$

$$\tau_v \frac{dv}{dt} = -v + w_n \sum_{i=1}^{n} f(u_i) - h_2 \tag{2.2}$$

where w_u is the self-connection weight for each u_i, w_m is the weight for each u_i for feedback from v, and each input s_i acts with unit weight. wn is the weight for input from each u_i to v. The threshold functions involve a *step* for $f(u_i)$

$$f(u_i) = \begin{cases} 1 & u_i > 0 \\ 0 & u_i \leq 0 \end{cases} \tag{2.2}$$

and a *ramp* for $g(v)$

$$g(v) = \begin{cases} v & v > 0 \\ 0 & v \leq 0 \end{cases} \tag{2.3}$$

Again, the range of i is $0 \le i \le n\text{-}1$ where n corresponds to the number of neurons in the neural array u.

Note that the actual simulation will use some numerical method to transform each differential equation of the form $\tau \, dm/dt = f(m,s,t)$ into some approximating difference equation $m(t+\Delta t) = f(m(t), s(t), t)$ which transforms state $m(t)$ and input $s(t)$ at time t into the state $m(t+\Delta t)$ of the neuron one "simulation time step" later.

As the model equations get repeatedly executed, with the right parameter values, u_i values receive positive input from both their corresponding external input and local feedback. At the same time negative feedback is received from v. Since the strength of the negative feedback corresponds to the summation of all neuron output, as execution proceeds only the strongest activity will be preserved, resulting in many cases in a "single winner" in the network.

Simulation Interaction

To execute the simulation, having chosen a differential equation solver (approximation method) and a simulation time step (or having accepted the default values), the user would simply select "Run" from the NSL Executive's Run menu as shown in figure 2.7. We abbreviate this as **Run→Run**.

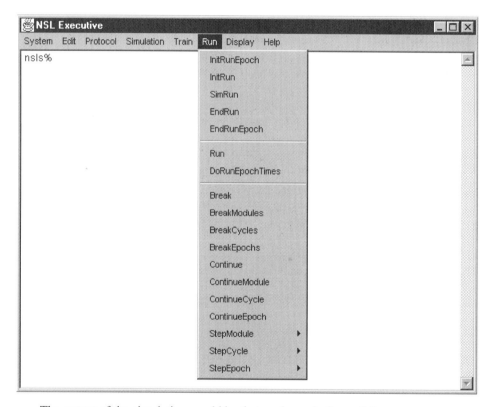

Figure 2.7
The "Run → Run" menu command.

The output of the simulation would be that as shown in figure 2.8.

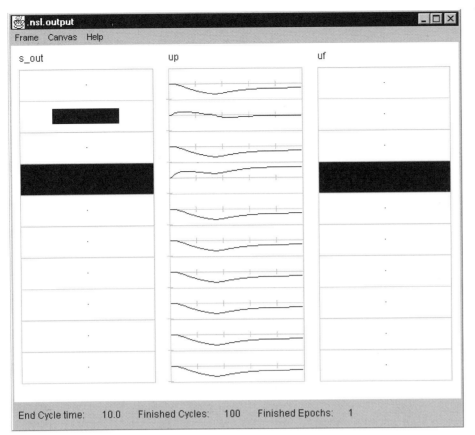

Figure 2.8
Output of the
MaxSelectorModel. Notice
that the second and fourth
elements in the *up*
membrane potential layer are
affected by the input stimuli;
however, the "winner take
all" circuit causes the fourth
element to dominate the
output, as seen in the firing
rate, *uf.*

The resulting written output is displayed in the Executive window's shell, as shown in figure 2.9.

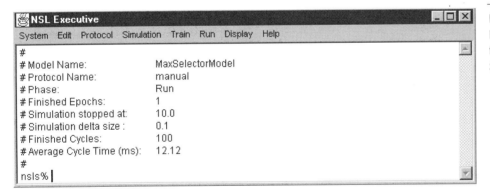

Figure 2.9
Executive window showing
the status from Maximum
Selector execution.

Recall that NSLS is the NSL scripting language in which one may write a script file specifying, e.g., how to run the model and graph the results. The user may thus choose to create a new script, or retrieve an existing one. In the present example, the user gets the system to load the NSLS script file containing preset graphics, parameters, input and simulation time steps by selecting "**System→Nsls file ...**," as shown in figure 2.10.

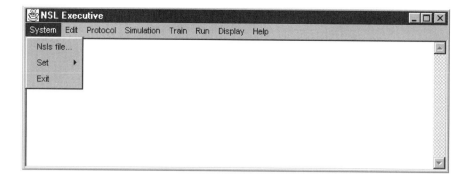

From the file selection pop-up window we first choose the "nsl" directory and then **MaxSelectorModel**, as shown in figure 2.11. Alternatively, the commands found in the file could have been written directly into the **Script Window** but it is more convenient the previous way.

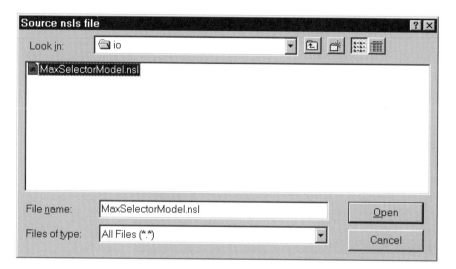

Simulation Control

Simulation control involves setting the duration of the model execution cycle (also known as the delta-t or simulation time step). In all of the models we will present, we will provide default values for the simulation control parameters within the model. However, to override these settings the user can select from **System→Set→RunEndTime** and **System→ Set→RunDelta** as shown in figure 2.12.

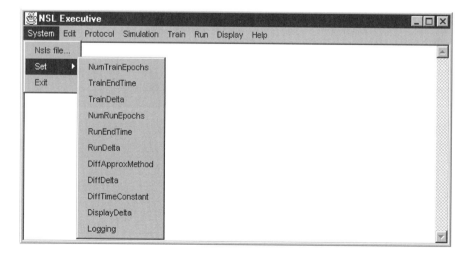

A pop-up window appears showing the current parameter value that may be modified by the user. In this model we have set the *runEndTime* to 10.0, as shown in figure 2.13, and *runDelta* to 0.1 giving a total of 100 execution iterations. These values are long enough for the model to stabilize on a solution.

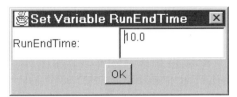

Figure 2.13
RunEndTime parameter setting.

To execute the actual simulation we select "Run" from the "Run" menu, as we did in figure 2.7.

The user may stop the simulation at any time by selecting the "Run" menu and then selecting "Break." We abbreviate this as **Run→Break**. To resume the simulation from the interrupt point select **Run→Continue.**

Visualization

The model output at the end of the simulation is shown in figure 2.8. The display shows input array *sout* with an **Area** type graph, i.e., the area of the black rectangle codes the size of the corresponding input, while array *up*, with a **Temporal** type graph, shows the time course for *up*. The last canvas shows another **Area** type graph for *uf* at the end of the simulation. The largest input in *sout* determines the only element of *sout* whose activity is still positive at the end of the simulation as seen in *uf*—the network indeed acts as a maximum selector.

Input Assignment

The *Maximum Selector* model example is quite simple in that the input *sout* is constant. In the example chosen, is consists of only two different positive values (set to 0.5 and 1.0) while the rest are set to zero (total of 10 elements in the vector). In general, input varies with time. Since input is constant in the present case, it may be set similarly to any model parameter. To assign values to parameters, we use the "nsl set" command followed by the variable and value involved. For example, to specify all ten-element values for *sout* we would do:[1]

```
nsl set maxSelectorModel.stimulus.sout { 0 0 0 1 0 1 0 0 0 0 }
```

Since all variables are stored within modules, being themselves possibly stored in other modules until reaching the top level model, it is necessary to provide a full "path" in order to assign them with new values. (These hierarchies will be made clear in chapter 3. For the moment simply provide the full specified path.) Note that arrays are set by specifying all values within curly brackets. Individual array elements may be set by using parentheses around a specific array index, e.g. to set the value of only array element 3 we would do (array indices starting with 0):

```
nsl set maxSelectorModel.stimulus.sout(3) 1
```

As previously mentioned, this model is atypical in that the input is constant. In general, input varies with time as will be shown in most of the other models in the book. If we are dealing with dynamic input we have different alternatives for setting input. One is to specify a "nsl set" command with appropriate input values every time input changes. Another alternative is to specify the input directly inside the model description or through a custom interface. Both *Hopfield* and *Backpropagation* models give examples on how to dynamically modify input at the script level and through the use of training files described as part of the model definition, respectively. On the other hand, *the Adaptation* model and the *Crowley* model appearing in the second section of the book are examples that set up their input and parameters through custom-designed windows.

Parameter Assignment

Parameters whose values were not originally assigned in the model description, or that we may want to modify, are specified interactively. Two parameters of special interest in the model are the two thresholds, *hu* and *hv*. These two parameters are restricted as follows, $0 \le hu$, and $0 \le hv < 1$. (For the theory behind these restrictions, see Arbib, 1989, Sec.4.4.) Their initial values are set to 0.1 and 0.5 respectively. These parameters have their values specified with the "set" command followed by the variable and value involved

```
nsl set maxSelectorModel.maxselector.u1.hu 0.1
nsl set maxSelectorModel.maxselector.v1.hv 0.5
```

To exercise this model the reader may want to change both the input and parameter values to see different responses from the model. We suggest trying different combinations of input values, such as changing input values as well as specifying different number of array elements receiving these values. In terms of parameters we suggest changing values for *hu* and *hv*, including setting them beyond the mentioned restrictions. Every time parameters or input changes, the model should be reinitialized and executed by selecting the "run" menu option.

2.5 Hopfield

Hopfield networks (Hopfield 1982) are recurrent networks in that their complete output at one time step serves as input during the next processing cycle. These networks rely on locally stable states or *attractors* enabling the association of a particular input pattern to one of its "remembered" patterns. These networks are also known as *associative memories* since they will in many cases transform the input pattern into one of the stored patterns (encoded in the network weights) that it best approximates. Unlike the *Maximum Selector*, a *Hopfield* network involves two processing phases— the training phase where synaptic weights are set to desired values and the running phase where the initial state of each neuron is set to the input pattern being tested.

Hopfield networks have been applied to problems such as optimization as in the famous "Traveling Salesman Problem" (Hopfield and Tank, 1985) where given a number of cities a salesman must choose his travel route in order to minimize distance traveled. In general, it may be quite challenging to go from the specification of an optimization problem to the setting of weight matrices to control memory states of a neural network which will "solve" the problem. This becomes more difficult as the number of inputs, cities in this case, increases. (Due to this difficulty, the "Traveling Salesman Problem" has sometimes been called the "Wandering Salesman Problem"!) What makes the matter worse is that this "solution" may only be *locally* optimal, i.e., it may be better than any similar solution yet not as good as some radically different solution. Attempts to find algorithms that produce better than local optimal solutions (e.g., the introduction of noise) have attracted much effort in the neural networks literature, but lie outside our present concern—to demonstrate NSL simulation of Hopfield networks. Besides optimization, *Hopfield* networks have been used in other practical applications such as error-correcting codes, reconstruction, and pattern recognition. The example presented in this section will be a *Hopfield* network for recognizing letter patterns.

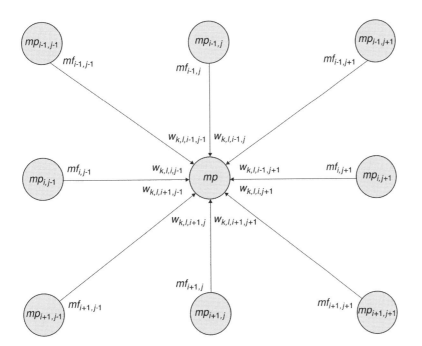

Figure 2.14
The Hopfield network is fully connected with the restriction that no unit may connect to itself.

Model Description

A *Hopfield* network is a discrete-time model consisting of a group of neurons projecting to all other neurons in the network with the restriction that no neuron connects to itself and weights are *symmetric* throughout the network, as shown in figure 2.14. The *Hopfield* model is based on *asynchronous updating* of states: only a single unit, randomly chosen, has its state updated at any given time. As a result the state of the chosen unit may change to reflect prior changes in the states of other units or may remain the same if those changes "cancel out."

The image to be processed does *not*, as might be expected, provide input to the network throughout processing. But rather the input pattern is used to set the initial states of the neurons of the network. To this end, we use double indexing for units m in order to make each unit correspond to a single picture element in a two-dimensional image. The dynamics of the network is then to convert the original pattern into some desired transformation thereof. Each element in the connection matrix w is then specified through four indices. If w_{klij} is the connection between unit m_{ij} and unit m_{kl}, then the activity mp_{kl} of unit m_{kl} is computed directly from the input from all other connections where mf_{ij} is the output from neuron m_{ij}. The computation is given by

$$mp_{kl}(t+1) = \sum_i \sum_j w_{klij} mf_{ij}(t) \tag{2.4}$$

Note that unlike the leaky integrator model, the state of a neuron in this discrete-time model does not depend on its previous state—it is completely determined by the input to the neuron at that time step. For our example, we concentrate on binary *Hopfield* networks using discrete neurons whose values can be either +1 or -1. The state of a neuron is given by

$$mf_{kl} = \begin{cases} 1 & \text{if } mp_{kl} \geq 0 \\ -1 & \text{if } mp_{kl} < 0 \end{cases} \tag{2.5}$$

To analyze the network, Hopfield (1984) suggested viewing the network as minimizing an *energy function E* given by

$$E = -\frac{1}{2} \sum_k \sum_l \sum_i \sum_j w_{klij} mp_{kl} mp_{ij} \qquad (2.6)$$

Each term is composed of the state of the m_{ij} unit, the state of the m_{kl} unit and the strength of the connection w_{klij} between the two units. (Sophisticated readers will note that each neuron has threshold zero.) This energy function may be interpreted as a measure of constraint satisfaction in the network. If we consider that neurons represent hypotheses in a problem, with an assertion of the hypothesis seen as corresponding to the +1 state of a neuron, and connection weights encode constraints between hypotheses, then the energy function is chosen to be a measure of the overall constraint violation in the current hypotheses. A low energy state would correspond to a state of maximum agreement between pairs of coupled assertions, while energy would increase when states become in disagreement. So long as the weights w_{klij} are symmetric, $w_{klij} = w_{lkji}$, some simple algebra (omitted here) shows that changes in state during asynchronous updates always decrease the energy of the system. Of course, if the "update" of a neuron leaves its state unchanged, then the state of the whole system and thus its energy also remain unchanged. Because all terms are finite there is an energy lower bound in the system and the energy function must have at least one minimum, although many minima may exist. As the system evolves with time, its energy decreases to one of the minimum values and stays there since no further decreases are possible. These points are known as *local energy minima*—we say that they are *attractors* because states move as if attracted to them; once at an energy minimum, the state of the network remains there, so we may also speak of these as fixed points. We can arrange the network in such a way that the desired associations occupy low energy points in state space so that the network will seek out these desired associations. In the present section, we look at a network such that we present noisy images and get back the image that most resembles it by comparing corresponding fixed points.

The key to defining a *Hopfield* network is in choosing the weight matrix. In the present image processing example, we initialize the synaptic weights of the network using a given set of input vectors, i.e., n exemplars pat_m for $0 \leq m < n$. We define the weight matrix w as

$$w_{klij} = \begin{cases} 0 & k = i, l = j \\ \sum_m pat_{mkl} \, pat_{mij} & \text{otherwise} \end{cases} \qquad (2.7)$$

for all *n exemplars* or training patterns in the network. If the input vectors are orthogonal (i.e., their scalar product is 0) then *Hopfield* guarantees that each exemplar becomes a fixed point of the network. (The mathematical justification requires some simple linear algebra. See, e.g., Section 8.2 of Arbib 1989.)

Simulation Interaction

We start the simulation interaction by selecting the *Hopfield* model by selecting "HopfieldModel.nsl" as shown in figure 2.15 (after selecting "**system→Nsls file…**" as shown in figure 2.10).

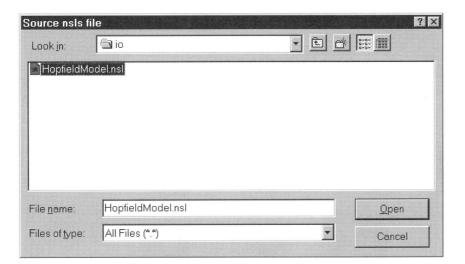

Figure 2.15
The Hopfield model
opened by selecting
HopfieldModel.nsl from
the "io" directory.

The example we have chosen is a pattern recognition problem where we train the network to remember letters A, B, C, D and E, as shown in figure 2.16. During testing we shall use one of these letters or a similar pattern as input. We have designed the particular patterns for each letter trying to keep *orthogonality* between them, that is, they are as distinct as possible. This is an important requisite in *Hopfield* networks for good association.

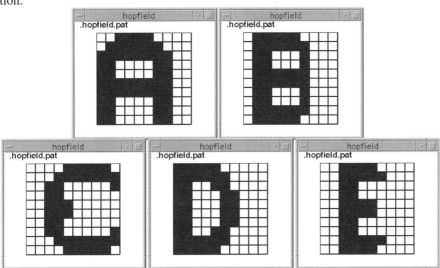

Figure 2.16
Letter A, B, C, D and E,
used for setting the
connection weights of the
Hopfield network. Here we
indicate the connections for
a typical neuron.

Simulation Control

Two simulation phases, for training and running, are involved in the *Hopfield* model as opposed to the single one in the *Maximum Selector* model. The training phase in *Hopfield* is unusual in that connection weights are not learned but adjusted directly from input patterns, as opposed to the training phase in most other training algorithms such as *Backpropagation*. We set *trainEndTime* to 1.0, and also *trainDelta* to 1.0, giving a total of 1 iteration through all the patterns. Additionally, the train cycle is executed for a single *epoch*, a single pass over all training patterns, thus we set *trainEpochSteps* to 1 as well. All the control commands are set in the "hopfield.nsl" file, including specification of the five letters, A, B, C, D and E chosen for the example.

Once all letters have been read we are ready to execute the run phase indefinitely until a stable solution is reached. Depending on the test letter the solution may take a different number of time steps. Thus, the model will stop running only when the solution has stabilized, in other words, when output for a new time step would yield exactly the same output as in the previous time step. To achieve this, we set *runEndTime* to 5000 (corresponding to protracted execution; alternatively, we could specify that detection of a suitable period of constant internal states makes it stop) and *runDelta* is set to 1.0 (this value is arbitrary in discrete-time models). To execute the running phase we select "Run" from the Run menu. To start processing all over again we would execute "Simulation→ initModule" followed by the training phase and then the run phase.

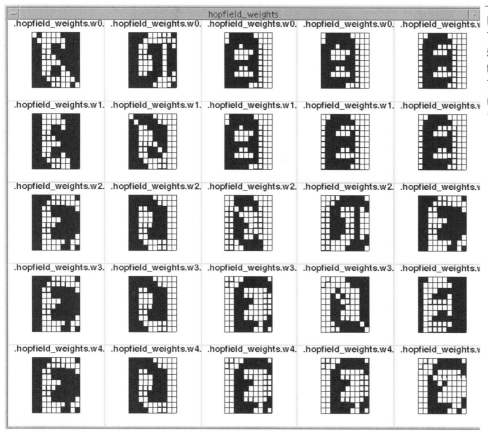

Figure 2.17
The figure presents the 5x5x10x10 weight array after training the Hopfield network. The 5x5 array organization represents the twenty-five 10x10 sub-matrices.

Visualization

The stored script file generates a number of display frames. We show in figure 2.17 the matrix of connection weights that you should obtain after training the model with letters A, B, C, D and E.

Once the network has completed the training cycle we input different letters to recall the memorized letter closer to it. We first try the model by recalling letters from the original ones, as shown in figure 2.18.

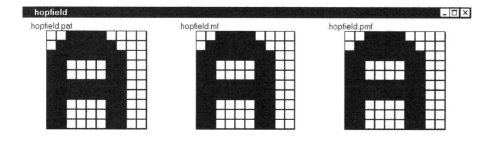

Figure 2.18
The top portion of the figure shows the input letter A, while the lower portion shows the output at the end of the simulation. In this simpler case letter A is recalled exactly as presented.

We show the energy as a function of time in figure 2.19, notice how it goes down as the network settles into a solution.

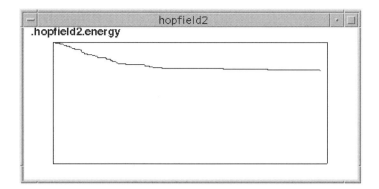

Figure 2.19
Energy as a function of time.

The network is able to recall correct answers from noisy versions of these letters. For example, the input image shown in figure 2.20 would recall letter A. Watch how the isplay reveals the cleaning up of the noisy image.

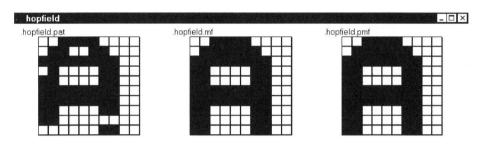

Figure 2.20
Recalling letter A from noisy image.

We can also input a letter such as an F that closely resembles letter E in the training set, as shown in figure 2.21.

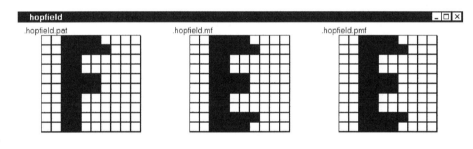

Figure 2.21
Recalling letter E from letter F, the closest to it in the training set.

In some cases the network may "remember" patterns that were not in the original set of examples, as shown in figure 2.22. These are called *spurious* states, unexpected valleys or local minima in the energy function, an unavoidable feature of *Hopfield* networks where processing is "stuck" in intermediate undefined states.

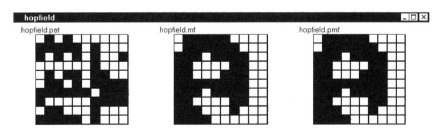

Figure 2.22
Spurious state of the Hopfield network.

This aspect exemplifies one of the shortcomings of *Hopfield* networks in terms of its tendency to stabilize to a local rather that a global minimum of the energy function. Another shortcoming relates to the capacity of *Hopfield* networks is that its capacity goes down as the number of stored patterns increases beyond some critical limit. This results in *crosstalk* from nonorthogonal patterns causing *attractors* to wander away from the desired locations. As more nonorthogonal patterns are stored, the more likely errors become (Abu-Mustafa and St. Jacques 1989). Hopfield (1982) has shown that if more patterns are stored than 15% of the number of units in the network (in our example 15 patterns, compared to 100 units in total), the system randomizes its energy minima. In other words, above this critical value the retrieved pattern has no relation to the stored pattern. (Of course, if there are 100 neurons, then one can store 100 orthogonal patterns. However, "real" patterns such as the letters of the alphabet are very unlikely to form an orthogonal set of vectors. Thus the mathematical results are based on expected performance when vectors are chosen at random. The point here is that if a few vectors are chosen at random, with each "pixel" as likely to be on as off, their pairwise scalar products will be close to zero, but this becomes more and more unlikely as the number of patterns increases. The surprise, to people unacquainted with critical phenomena in statistical mechanics, is that there is a critical number of patterns at which quasi-orthogonality breaks down, rather than a slow degradation of performance as the number of patterns increases.)

Input Assignment

Input plays an important and delicate role in the model. During training, network weights are set according to input matrices representing letters to be remembered. During an execution or simulation run, the network is given an input matrix to be associated with one of its remembered states that best matches the pattern.

In the *Maximum Selector* model we showed how we set constant input, in a manner similar to parameter assignment. In the training phase of the Hopfield model, we need dynamic input to read in a sequence of n input patterns. In the present model, these do not function as neural network inputs (as might happen if we modeled an explicit learning model) but instead serves as input for a process that computes weights according to equation (2.7). Training the *Hopfield* model thus requires dynamic input. We read in the n training patterns by calling the "nsl set" command multiple times. In the example each letter corresponds to a 10x10 matrix. For example, letter "A" is defined as follows:

```
nsl set HopfieldModel.input.out {
{ -1 -1 1 1 1 1 -1 -1 -1 -1 }
{ -1 1 1 1 1 1 1 1 -1 -1 -1 }
{ 1 1 1 1 1 1 1 1 1 -1 -1 }
{ 1 1 -1 -1 -1 -1 1 -1 -1 -1 }
{ 1 1 -1 -1 -1 -1 1 1 -1 -1 }
{ 1 1 1 1 1 1 1 1 1 -1 -1 }
{ 1 1 1 1 1 1 1 1 1 -1 -1 }
{ 1 1 -1 -1 -1 -1 1 1 -1 -1 }
{ 1 1 -1 -1 -1 -1 1 1 -1 -1 }
{ 1 1 -1 -1 -1 -1 1 1 -1 -1 }}
```

Note the curly brackets separating matrix rows. The rest of the letters are defined in a similar way. In order to control the input in a dynamic way we set the input from the script window for each letter being computed by the weight assignment equation followed by the Train command (performs initTrain, simTrain repeated, endTrain) with each epoch incrementing the expressions in Equation (2.7) by adding in the terms corresponding to the current pattern $patt_m$.

```
nsl train
```

We now turn to the "input" for the Running phase. As we have seen, a Hopfield network does not have input in the conventional neural network sense. Instead, the "input" sets the initial state of the network, which then runs to equilibrium, or some other halting condition. The "output" for this particular run is taken from the final state of the network. In each run phase of a simulation, we set the "input" to any arbitrary pattern (i.e., it will probably not belong to the training set) and then run the network as many cycles as necessary. We shall look at the details for defining this model in chapter 3, The Modeling Overview.

Parameter Assignment

There are no parameters that need to be adjusted in the model. Being a discrete-time model, *Hopfield* updates the state directly from its current input and state. Unlike the leaky integrator, there are no time constants. Weights are computed by the training phase and neuron thresholds are set to zero.

You may exercise the model by modifying both the test-input patterns as well as the patterns used for training. They do not even have to be letters.

2.6 Backpropagation

Backpropagation (Werbos 1974; Rumelhart et al. 1986) is an especially widespread neural network architecture embodying *supervised learning* based on gradient descent ("hill climbing" in the downward direction). Supervised learning involves a training set representing both the given problem and the corresponding solution defined as a set of (input, target) training pairs. The goal of successful learning is to acquire general knowledge about the data or training set so the network can use it to resolve similar problems it has not seen before. There are two important factors in building a successful *backpropagation* network: the *training set* and the *network configuration*.

The *training set* consists of a number of training pairs where each pair (input, target) contains a target vector that is deemed the correct response to its corresponding input vector. A "supervisor" compares the resulting network output for a given input vector against the target vector to produce an error. This error is then used to drive the adjustment of weights in the network in such a way that the error is reduced to its minimum. The process of error minimization consists of following a steep path down the input-output error function. Although there is no guarantee of minimizing all errors (*gradient descent* may only find a local minimum, like a valley high in the hills, as for *Hopfield*), a *backpropagation* network is usually able after many training cycles to reduce the errors to a satisfying degree.

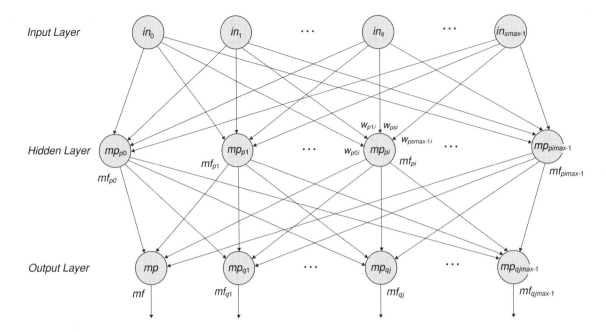

The *network configuration* consists of neurons organized into at least three different layers: an input layer, one or more hidden or middle layers and an output layer (figure 2.23). The network processes information in two distinct modes, a *feedforward* and a *backpropagation* mode. The *feedforward* mode is just the normal mode of operation of a neural network without loops: activity is fed forward from one layer to the next (input to hidden layer, hidden to additional hidden layers if more than one exists, and finally hidden to output layer). There are no loops in strong contrast to the fully recurrent *Hopfield* network. In the *backpropagation* mode, learning propagates backwards by adjusting synaptic weights from output to input layers. The most common configuration is a three-layer network with all possible connections from each layer to the next. Implementing four or more layers is usually discouraged because of the computational burden of the *backpropagation* training process. Both mathematical proof and practical uses of *backpropagation* show that three-layer networks are sufficient for solving most problems (Rumelhart, et al. 1986).

In designing the network configuration, the most important parameter is the network size and the number of units used in the hidden layer to represent features of the problem. There are tradeoffs to consider. With too large a number of hidden units, the network will have the ability to *memorize* each element of the training set separately, and thus will not generalize well. With too small a number of hidden units, there may not be enough memory to store the knowledge (refer to Smith (1993) on how to build appropriate network configurations).

Backpropagation has been applied to a large number of applications in many domain areas, from handwriting recognition and speech synthesis to stock market prediction and on.

Model Description

As we have seen, *Backpropagation* is a typical multi-layer neural network model consisting of an input layer, hidden or middle layer(s), one in this case, and an output layer (figure 2.23). The network is fully connected from one layer to the next, but lacks any connectivity between neurons belonging to the same layer, or back to previous layers.

The *BackPropagation* algorithm works in two phases, as in *Hopfield*. First, a training phase adjusts network weights and then a running phase matches patterns against those

Figure 2.23
The Backpropagation network architecture is made of an input layer connected to a hidden layer that is then connected to an output layer. Units are fully connected between layers without any interconnection to other units in the same layer.

already learned by the network. However, these two phases are not to be confused with a *feedforward* and a *backpropagation* modes introduced above. The training phase is made up of a large number of learning cycles, each comprising a forward pass (*feedforward* mode) and backward pass (*backpropagation* mode). The running phase is made of a single forward pass taking a single cycle although sharing the same forward pass equations (*feedforward* mode) as in the training phase.

Feedforward Mode

During the feedforward mode, the network reads an input vector that is fed into the input layer. The input layer does not do any computation on the input pattern and simply sends it out to the hidden layer. Both the hidden layer and output layer have their neuron activity (corresponding to the membrane potential in more biologically oriented models) defined as a direct summation of all inputs to the neuron multiplied by their respective weights. In the model, *in* represents a unit in the input layer, mp_p represents a neuron in the hidden layer and mp_q a neuron in the output layer.

Hidden Layer

The membrane potential mp_p for a neuron in the hidden layer receives its activation from the input layer multiplied by the respective weights, as described next.

$$mp_p = \sum_s w_{sp} in_s + h_p \qquad (2.8)$$

where h_p is the threshold value.

After mp_p is computed, an activation function is used to produce the output mf_p.

$$mf_p = f\left(mp_p + h_p\right) = \frac{1}{1 + e^{-\left(mp_p + h_p\right)}} \qquad (2.9)$$

where f is a sigmoid function used to compress the range of mp_p so that mf_p lies between zero and one, and e is the mathematical exponential constant. The sigmoid function is used since *Backpropagation* requires the activation function to be everywhere differentiable. The sigmoid function not only satisfies this requirement but also provides a form of automatic gain control. If mp_p is near one or zero, the slope of the input/output curve is shallow and thus provides a low gain. The sigmoid function also has the advantage that large mp_p values will not dominate small mp_p values in influencing the network in going towards the global minimum.

Output Layer

The membrane potential mp_q for a neuron in the output layer receives input from the hidden layer multiplied by the respective weights.

$$mp_q = \sum_p w_{pq} mf_p \qquad (2.10)$$

where h_q is the threshold value.

After mp_q is calculated, an activation function is used to produce the output mf_q.

$$mf_q = f\left(mp_q + h_q\right) = \frac{1}{1 + e^{-\left(mp_q + h_q\right)}} \qquad (2.11)$$

and the activation function f is similar to that defined for neurons in the hidden layer.

Backpropagation Mode

While the feedforward mode is used during both the training and running phases of the network, the backpropagation mode is only used during training. For each cycle of training, the simulator reads a pair of input and target vectors from a training data file. The input vector is fed into the input layer for a feedforward computation, while the target vector is set aside for later error computation. After completion of the forward activation flow, each output neuron will receive an error value—the difference between its actual and desired input—from the training manager module, (the training manager module will be discussed in detail in chapter 3, The Modeling Overview).The backpropagation mode then adjusts the weights according to a modified gradient descent algorithm wherein weight adjustment propagates back from the output layer through the hidden layers of the network.

Output Layer

The error is first calculated for the output layer:

$$error_q = desiredOutput_q - actualOutput_q \qquad (2.12)$$

where *desiredOutput* is obtained from the training file and *actualOutput* is computed by the forward pass output layer firing mf_q.

The accumulated error *tss* is given by the sum of the square of the errors for all neurons of the output layer

$$tss = \sum_t error_q{}^2 \qquad (2.13)$$

To compensate for this error we define δ_q representing the change to be applied to weights and threshold in the output layer given by

$$\delta_q = f'(mp_q) \times error_q \qquad (2.14)$$

where $f'(mp_q)$ is the derivative of squashing function f. With the simple sigmoid function used, the derivative is:

$$f'(mp_q) = mf_q \times (1 - mf_q) \qquad (2.15)$$

The resulting δ_q is then used to modify the thresholds and weights in the output layer as follows

$$\Delta h_q = \eta \delta_q \qquad (2.16)$$
$$h_q(t+1) = h_q(t) + \Delta h_q \qquad (2.17)$$
$$\Delta w_{pq} = \eta \delta_q \times mf_p \qquad (2.18)$$
$$w_{pq}(t+1) = w_{pq}(t) + \Delta w_{pq} \qquad (2.19)$$

where

η represents the learning rate parameter corresponding to how fast learning should be.

$h_q(t)$ represents the threshold value for neuron q in the output layer at step t before adjustment is made.

$h_q(t+1)$ represents the threshold value for neuron q in the output layer at step $t+1$ after adjustment.

$w_{pq}(t)$ represents the weight value from neuron p in the hidden layer to neuron q in the output layer at step t before adjustment is made.

$w_{pq}(t+1)$ represents the value of the weight at step $t+1$ after adjustment.

Hidden Layer

Once the errors are computed and threshold and weight updates have taken place in the output layer, the hidden layer errors need to be computed as well. Since there is no explicit teacher for the hidden units, *Backpropagation* provides a solution by propagating the output error back through the network. To compensate for this error we define δ_p representing the change to be applied to weights and threshold in the hidden layer,

$$\delta_p = f'\!\left(mp_p\right)\!\times\!\sum_q \delta_q w_{pq} \tag{2.20}$$

where $f'(mp_p)$ is the derivative of the sigmoid function in neuron p similar to the $f'(mp_q)$ function in the output layer and w_{pq} is the value of the weight from neuron p in the hidden layer to neuron q in the output layer. As before,

$$f'(mp_p) = mf_p \times (1 - mf_p) \tag{2.21}$$

There is a reason why the hidden layer needs to receive the summation of the products of error δ_q multiplied by weight w_{pq}. Since each neuron contributes differently to the output, its share of the error is also different. By associating the error and the weight, each neuron in the hidden layer will be evaluated by its corresponding contribution to the error and corrected accordingly.

The threshold and weight modification equations are similar in computation to that of the output layer, with delta change δ_p used to modify the thresholds and weights in the output layer,

$$\Delta h_p = \eta \delta_p \tag{2.22}$$
$$h_p(t+1) = h_p(t) + \Delta h_p \tag{2.23}$$
$$\Delta w_{sp} = \eta \delta_p \times in_s \tag{2.24}$$
$$w_{sp}(t+1) = w_{sp}(t) + \Delta w_{sp} \tag{2.25}$$

where

η represents the learning rate parameter corresponding to how fast learning should be.

$h_p(t)$ represents the threshold value for neuron p in the hidden layer at step t before adjustment is made.

$h_p(t+1)$ represents the threshold value for neuron p in the hidden layer at step $t+1$ after adjustment.

$w_{sp}(t)$ represents the weight value from unit s in the input layer to neuron p in the hidden layer at step t before adjustment is made.

$w_{sp}(t+1)$ represents the weight value at step $t+1$ after adjustment.

Simulation Interaction

To illustrate an actual example we will train the network to learn an exclusive or (XOR) function, as shown in the table below. This is a simple although illustrative example in that a simpler Perceptron without the hidden layer would not be able to learn this function. The function is shown in table 2.1.

Input	Output
0 0	0
0 1	1
1 0	1
1 1	0

Table 2.1
Training file format.

We turn now to the NSLS commands stored in "BackPropModel.nsl", where the file is loaded into the NSL Executive in order to simulate the model. We load "BackPropModel.nsl" by selecting the BackPropModel.nsl model as shown in figure 2.24 (after selecting "**system→Nsls file...**" as shown in figure 2.10).

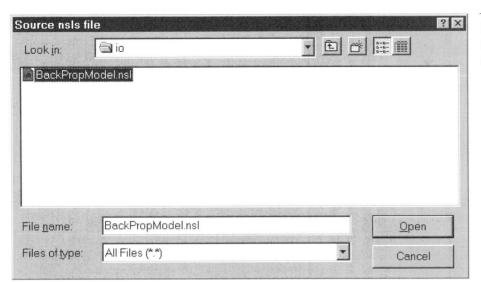

Figure 2.24
Opening the BackPropModel
script file.

Simulation Control

As for *Hopfield*, *Backpropagation* requires both the training and running phases. Simulation control for this model involves setting up the duration for both phases as well. The training phase involves multiple cycles. From the script window we set *trainEndTime* to the number of training patterns specified by *numPats* and *trainDelta* to 1.0 in order to have as many training steps as there are training patterns. (These are also the defaults specified in the model code which we will be discussing in chapter 3, The Modeling Overview.) We then set *runEndTime* to 1.0 and *runDelta* to 1.0.

Additionally, the training cycle will be executed for an unspecified number of *epochs*, where every epoch corresponds to a single pass over all patterns. We set *trainEpochSteps* to 5000 telling the system to train almost indefinitely until some suitable ending makes it stop, in this case, when the error (stopError) is small enough. To make the system learn, we issue the **nsl train** command from the script window. As learning keeps progressing, if the total sum of the square error (*tss*) is not satisfactory, the learning rate η can be adjusted. When the *tss* value reaches a very small *stopError*, the network has been successfully trained. At that point we issue the **"nsl source backproprun"** command from the script window. To reinitialize the system after a complete run, we would issue the "nsl initModule" command.

Visualization

The network training error *tss* can be visualized as the network gets trained, as shown in figure 2.25. As the error gets smaller *tss* approaches 0 meaning the network has learned.

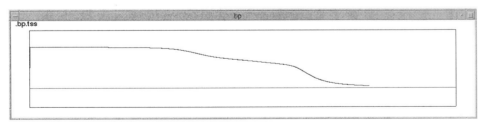

Figure 2.25
The error *tss* is visualized
as a temporal graph as the
network is training with the
XOR example.

Figure 2.26 shows the result of running the trained network with one of the XOR inputs.

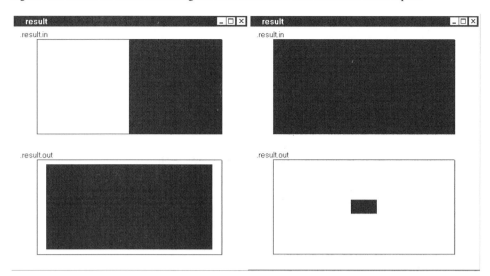

Figure 2.26
The display on the left-hand side shows an input to the network set to "0 1". After the network has been run the output becomes 1, as expected. The display on the right-hand side shows an input to the network set to "1 1" The output this time becomes 0.

Input Assignment

To simplify the training process and to avoid deeper knowledge of NSL, we assign the training set directly to the model as a training array rather than from an external file as is usually the case. (We will show this more "realistic" approach in the NSLM chapter where we go over more extensive details of the modeling language NSLM. Obviously the approach taken will be more involved when dealing with large data sets.) The training set format is shown in table 2.2.

File Format	Example (XOR)
<num_patterns>	4
<input1> <input 2> <output>	0 0 0
<input1> <input 2> <output>	0 1 1
<input1> <input 2> <output>	1 0 1
<input1> <input 2> <output>	1 1 0

Table 2.2
Training file format.

The first row in the file specifies the number of patterns in the file. Training pairs are specified one per row consisting in the XOR example of two inputs `<input1>` and `<input2>` and a single output `<output>`. The training set input is assigned as follows

```
nsl set backPropModel.train.pInput {
{ 0 0 } { 0 1 } { 1 0 } { 1 1 } }
nsl set backPropModel.train.pOutput {
{ 0 } { 1 } { 1 } { 0 } }
```

Note again the curly brackets separating elements in two-dimensional arrays, similar to input in the Hopfield model.

Parameter Assignment

The *Backpropagation* layer sizes are specified within the present implementation of model, i.e., if the number of units in any layer changes, the model has to be modified accordingly and recompiled. The alternative to this example could be to treat layer sizes as model parameters to be set interactively during simulation initialization. While the latter approach is more flexible since layer sizes tend to change a lot between problems, we use the former one to avoid further complexity at this stage. Thus, the user will need to modify and recompile the model when changing layer sizes. In our example we use 2 units for the input layer, 2 for the hidden layer and 1 for the output layer.

Additionally, we set *stopError* to a number that will be small enough for the network to obtain acceptable solutions. For this example, we use 0.1 or 10% of the output value,

```
nsl set backPropModel.layers.be.stopError 0.1
```

The learning parameter η is represented by the *learningRate* parameter determining how big a step the network can take in correcting errors. The learning rate for this problem was set to 0.8 for both the hidden and output layers.

```
nsl set backPropModel.layers.bh.lRate 0.8
nsl set backPropModel.layers.bo.lRate 0.8
```

The training step or delta is typically set between 0.01 to 1.0. The tradeoff is that if the training step is too large—close to 1—the network tends to oscillate and will likely jump over the minimum. On the other hand, if the training step is too small—close to 0—it will require many cycles to complete the training, although it should eventually learn.

This is obviously a very simple model but quite illustrative of *Backpropagation*. As an exercise we encourage you to try different *learningRates (lRate)* and *stopError* values. Additionally, you can modify the training set although keeping the same structure. In section 3.5 you may try changing the layer sizes in designing new problems. Also, if you are not satisfied with the training, there are two ways to keep it going. One is to issue an **initModule** command, adjust *trainEndTime* to a new value, and then train and run again. The other is to save the weights, issue an **initModule**, load the weights again, and then type *simTrain* at the prompt.

2.7 Summary

In this chapter we have given an introduction to NSL simulation as well as an overview of three basic neural models, *Maximum Selector*, *Hopfield* and *Backpropagation* in NSL. These models, although different, take advantage of a consistent simulation interface provided by NSL.

Notes

1. Currently, we are completing the Numerical Editor Input interface/widget which will allow us to set any writable variable within the model from a pop-up window. The widget will eliminate extra typing in the script window.

3 Modeling in NSL

In chapter 2 we introduced model simulation in NSL. The models overviewed were "canned" ready for simulation, having preset parameters as well as visualization specifications. In this chapter we overview how to build neural network models in NSL using the NSLM modeling language. Note that this material is intended for the model builder, as distinct from the model user. We first explain how models are described in terms of *modules* and *neural networks* in NSLM, followed by an introduction to the *Schematic Capture System (SCS)*, our visual tool to create and browse *model architectures*. We then describe the NSL implementation of the *Maximum Selector*, *Hopfield* and *Backpropagation* models introduced in chapter 2.

3.1 Implementing Model Architectures with NSLM

A neural network model is described by a *model architecture* representing its structure and behavior. In NSL, model architectures can be built either top-down or bottom-up. If built top-down, the two step approach to building the model is: first build *modules* to define the overall "black-box" structure of the network and then build the detailed functionality of the *neural networks*. To build bottom-up, we just do the reverse. We illustrate the bottom-up approach with the *Maximum Selector*, *Hopfield*, and *Backpropagation* models.[1]

Modules and Models

At the highest-level model architectures are described in terms of *modules* and *interconnections*. We describe in this section these concepts as well as the *model*, representing the *main* module in the architecture together with a short overview of scheduling and buffering involved with modules.

Modules

The *module*, the basic component in a model architecture, is somewhat analogous to the *object* in object-oriented applications. Additionally, the corresponding module definition is analogous to an object definition, known as the object *class*, used to *instantiate* the actual modules or objects, respectively. A module encapsulates the internal complexity of its implementation by separating the internal details from the external interface. The external portion of the module is the part of the module seen by other modules. The internal portion is not seen by other modules—this makes it easier to create and modify modules independently from each other—and defines the actual module behavior. This behavior need not be reducible to a neural network: (a) it may be an abstraction equivalent to that of a neural network, or (b) it may be a module doing something else, e.g. providing inputs or monitoring behavior.

The most important task of a module's external interface is to permit communication between different modules. As such, a module in NSL includes a set of input and output *data ports* (we shall call them simply *ports*). The port represents an entry or exit point where data may be sent or received to or from other modules, as shown in figure 3.1.

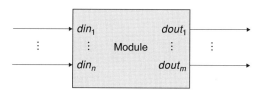

Figure 3.1

The NSL computational model is based on the module concept. Each Module consists of multiple input, din_1, din_n, and output, $dout_1, ..., dout_m$, *data ports* for unidirectional communication. The number of input ports does not have to be the same as the number of output ports.

For example, the *Maximum Selector* model architecture incorporates a module having two input ports *sin* and *vin* together with a single output port *uf*, as shown in figure 3.2.

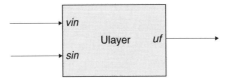

Figure 3.2
The ULayer module of the *Maximum Selector* model has two input ports *sin* and *vin* and a single output port *uf*.

Data sent and received through ports is usually in the form of numerical values. These values may be of different numerical types while varying in dimension. In the simplest form a numerical type may correspond to a single scalar, a one-dimensional array (*vector*), a two-dimensional array (*matrix*), or higher dimensional arrays.[2] For example in the *Ulayer* module shown in figure 3.2, *vin* is made to correspond to a scalar type while *sin* and *uf* both correspond to vector arrays (the reason for this selection will become clear very soon).

In terms of implementation, the NSL *module* specification has been made as similar as possible to a *class* specification in object-oriented languages such as Java and C++ in order to make the learning curve as short as possible for those already having programming background. The general module definition is described in code segment 3.1. The module specification consists of a header and a body. The header comprises the first line of the template, in other words the code outside the curly brackets. The body of the module is specified inside the curly brackets made up of the *structure* and *behavior*, both to be explained later on.

```
nslModule Name (arguments)
{
    structure
    behavior
}
```

Code Segment 3.1
The NslModule definition.

Let us begin with the header (**bold** letters represent NSLM keywords):

- **nslModule** (note the initial lower case "nsl" prefix) specifies the beginning of a module template.
- *Name* (note the initial upper case letter) represents the name of the module to which all module instances will refer.
- *arguments* are an optional variable list useful when passing external information to the module during an instantiation.
- The body of the module consists of two different sections:
- *structure* representing module attributes (data).
- *behavior* representing module methods (operations).

For example, the **Ulayer** module in the *Maximum Selector* model architecture contains the header described in code segment 3.2.

```
nslModule Ulayer (int size)
{
}
```

Code Segment 3.2
MaxSelector Ulayer header.

The header specification consists of:

- nslModule, the always present module definition keyword.
- Ulayer, the name of the module.

- size, an integer type passed as argument to the module.

The module *structure* consists of the module's external interface—its ports, as shown in code segment 3.3.

```
nslModule Ulayer(int size)
{
    public NslDinDouble1 sin(size);
    public NslDinDouble0 vin();
    public NslDoutDouble1 uf(size);
}
```

Code Segment 3.3
MaxSelector's Ulayer external interface.

The **Ulayer** module defines the three ports previously mentioned, *sin*, *vin* and *uf*. Each line ending in a semicolon defines a single port declaration:

- public tells NSLM that the port (or any other specification) is known outside the module—it is part of the module's external interface. (Defining all ports as public is very important if we want to be able to make connections or communication channels with other modules.)
- NslDinDouble1 represents a one-dimensional port array of type "double," where Nsl is the prefix to all NSL defined types. As part of the type description, Din specifies an input data port. Double specifies the primitive data type for the port (other primitive types are Float and Int) while 1 identifies the array dimension, in this case 1, for a vector (other dimensions are 0, 1, 2, 3, or 4).
- sin is the port name used for NSLM referral both from inside the module as well as from its outside.
- The parentheses after sin indicate the instantiation parameter section. In this example the parameter size in the header is passed to the module during its instantiation.
- Ports vin and uf are defined in a similar way. Port vin is of NslDinDouble0 type corresponding to an input port of zero dimensions (i.e., a scalar). uf is of NslDoutDouble1 type corresponding to a one dimensional output port array.

Besides the external interface in the form of ports, the structure of a module may include additional local data. In our example we include three additional "internal" variables *up*, *hu*, and *tau* as shown in code segment 3.4.

```
nslModule Ulayer(int size)
{
    public NslDinDouble1 sin(size);
    public NslDinDouble0 vin();
    public NslDoutDouble1 uf(size);

    private NslDouble1 up(size);
    private NslDouble0 hu();
    private double tau();
}
```

Code Segment 3.4
MaxSelector's Ulayer attribute definition.

up represents an internal module variable of type NslDouble1. Since all attributes, with the exception of ports, should be encapsulated we use the private visibility keyword to specify a local variable not viewed externally to the module. Note how the Din/Dout section of the port types is taken out from a regular variable declaration. The other section, primitive type and dimension are still important, in this case Double and 1, respectively.

- hu and tau represent the offset and approximation method time constant, both of type NslDouble0.

In terms of *behavior*, every module must have methods in order to do something "meaningful." Modules include a number of specific methods called by the simulator during model execution. These methods are used for different purposes, e.g. initialization, execution, termination.

```
nslModule Ulayer(int size)
{
    public NslDinDouble1 sin(size);
    public NslDinDouble0 vin();
    public NslDoutDouble1 uf(size);

    private NslDouble1 up(size);
    private NslDouble0 hu();
    private NslDouble0 tau();
    public void initRun() {
        uf = 0.0
        up = 0.0;
        hu=0.1;
        tau=1.0;
    }
}
```

Code Segment 3.5
MaxSelector's Ulayer attribute and method definition.

For example, the **initRun** method in the **Ulayer** module definition shown in code segment 3.5 is called during the module's run reinitialization. (Additional methods will be defined for this module later in this chapter.) Tasks that we may want to do during reinitialization are for example resetting of all variables to their initial value. (Note that we usually set values for local variables and output ports but not input ports since their values are externally received.) Every method is distinguished by its unique *signature*, consisting of a return type, name and arguments, as well as additional modifiers such as the visibility keyword. In our example the method is defined as follows:

- public is the visibility modifier telling NSLM that the method is to be known outside the module, an important requisite if we want NSL to be able to call this method during module simulation.
- void is the return type from the method, i.e., no value is returned from the method. This is the case with most NSL predefined methods.
- initRun is the name of the method, taken from the set of predefined NSL method names.

Arguments are specified within the parenthesis. In this example no arguments are passed to the method, the case with most NSL predefined methods.

The method body corresponds to the section between curly brackets. Note that the **initRun** defined here sets both the values of arrays **uf** and **up** to 0.0, in other words it assigns zero to every element in the corresponding arrays. On the other hand **hu** and **tau** are initialized to 0.1 and 1.0 respectively.

Interconnections

Interconnections between modules is achieved by interconnecting output ports in one module to input ports in another module. Interconnections free the user from having to specify how data should be sent and received during simulation processing. Communication is unidirectional, flowing from an output port to an input port. Code segment 3.6

shows the **Vlayer** header and structure (we omit its behavior) for the *Maximum Selector* model. It contain s an output **vf**, input port **uin** and three private variables, **vp**, **hv** and **tau**.

```
nslModule Vlayer(int size)
{
    public NslDinDouble1 uin(size);
    public NslDoutDouble0 vf();

    private NslDouble0 vp();
    private NslDouble0 hv();
    private NslDouble0 tau();
}
```

Code Segment 3.6
MaxSelector's Vlayer attribute definition.

The description is very similar to **Ulayer**. The major difference is that **Ulayer**'s output, **uf**, is a vector while **Vlayer**'s output, **vf**, corresponds to a single scalar. figure 3.3 then shows the interconnections between the **Ulayer** module and another, **Vlayer**.

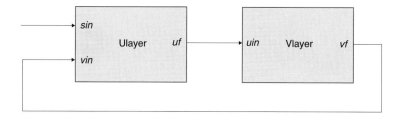

Figure 3.3
Interconnections between modules Ulayer and Vlayer of the *Maximum Selector* model.

In the example, a connection is made from output port **uf** in **Ulayer** to input port **vin** in **Vlayer**; additionally, output port **vf** in **Vlayer** is connected to input port **vin** in **Ulayer**. Note the input port **sin** in **Ulayer** is disconnected at the time. In general, a single output port may be connected to any number of input ports, whereas the opposite is not allowed, i.e., connecting multiple output ports to a single input port. The reason for this restriction is that the input port could receive more than one communication at any given time, resulting in inconsistencies.

This kind of interconnection—output to input port—is considered "same level module connectivity." The alternative to this is known as "different level module connectivity." In this case, an output port from a module at one level is *relabeled* (we use this term instead of *connected* for semantic reasons) to an output port of a module at a different level. Alternatively, an input port at one level module may be *relabeled* to an input port at a different level. For example, in figure 3.4 we introduce the **MaxSelector** module, containing an input port **in** and an output port **out**, encapsulating modules **Ulayer** and **Vlayer**. **MaxSelector** is considered a higher level module to the other two since it contains—and instantiates—them. In general, relabeling lets input and output ports *forward* their data between module levels. (This supports module encapsulation in the sense that a module connected to **MaxSelector** should not connect to ports in either **Ulayer** or **Vlayer** nor be able to get direct access to any of the modules private variables.) Relabelings, similar to connections, are unidirectional, where an input port from one module may be relabeled to a number of input ports at a different level.

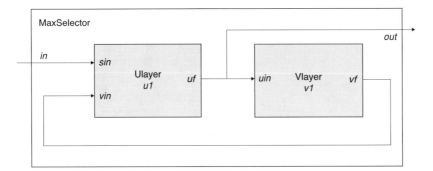

Figure 3.4
Maximum Selector model
architecture contains a
MaxSelector module with
two interconnected modules
Ulayer and Vlayer.

The NSLM specification for figure 3.4 is given in code segment 3.7. the **MaxSelector** module definition incorporates **Ulayer** and **Vlayer** instantiations—**u1** and **v1** are the corresponding instance variables—together with port **in** and **out** instantiations. Note that we have made the instantiations of Ulayer and Vlayer **private** variables. Again this is for encapsulation, or in other words, to protect these module instances from being modified accidentally.

```
nslModule MaxSelector (int size)
{
    public NslDinDouble1 in(size);
    public NslDoutDouble1 out(size);
    private Ulayer u1(size);
    private Vlayer v1(size);

    public void makeConn(){
        nslRelabel(in,u1.sin);
        nslConnect(v1.vf,u1.vin);
        nslConnect(u1.uf,v1.uin);
        nslRelabel(u1.uf,out);
    }
}
```

Code Segment 3.7
MaxSelector top-level
module definition.

In terms of behavior, the **MaxSelector** module includes the predefined **makeConn** method, analogous to the **initRun** method, for specifying port interconnections. (Note that module interconnections are carried out in the *parent*—higher level—**MaxSelector** module, with **Ulayer** and **Vlayer** considered the *children*—lower level—modules.) Connections and relabels between ports are specified as follows:

- nslConnect connects an output port (first argument) to an input port (second argument). In this example we connect output port vf in v1 to input port vin in u1. The second connect statement connects output port uf in u1 to input port uin in v1.

- nslRelabel relabels an input port at a higher module level with an input port at a lower module level, or changing the order, an output port at a lower level with an output port at a higher level. In the example, we relabel input port in in MaxSelector to input port sin belonging to u1 and output port uf belonging to u1 to output port out in MaxSelector.

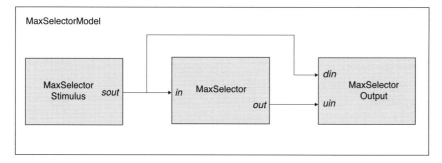

Figure 3.5
MaxSelectorModel
architecture contains the
MaxSelectorStimulus,
MaxSelector, and
MaxSelectorOutput
interconnected module.

Note in the previous examples that specifying connections and relabels is carried out from outside the participating modules—the modules having the actual port to be connected. This way we can design modules independently and without priori knowledge of how they are going to be interconnected promoting module reuse applying them in a number of model architectures.

Models

There is a special module, known as the *model*, which should be present in any model architecture. The *model* is somewhat analogous to a *main* procedure in programming languages in that it is responsible for instantiating the rest of the application. The model contains the complete set of modules defining the particular model architecture. For example, the **MaxSelectorModel** is shown in figure 3.5, which includes two additional modules, **MaxSelectorStimulus** responsible for generating model input, **MaxSelector-Output**, for the processing of module output. These two additional modules may be quite simple, as the case in our example, or may provide sophisticated functionality as probing **MaxSelector** module correctness, or make use of the output as part of further processing. The **MaxSelectorModel** definition is described in code segment 3.8.

```
nslModel MaxSelectorModel ()
{
    private MaxSelector maxselector(10);
    private MaxSelectorStimulus stimulus(10);
    private MaxSelectorOutput output();

    public void makeConn() {
        nslConnect(stimulus.sout,maxselector.in);
        nslConnect(stimulus.sout,output.sin);
        nslConnect(maxselector.out, output.uin);
    }
}
```

Code Segment 3.8
MaxSelectorModel model.

The header specification is similar to the module with the exception that we use the **nslModel** keyword instead of **nslModule**. The model may define both attributes and behavior as part of its body similar to a module. Note how we specify the network sizes and pass them to the two modules. The only restriction is that there may not be more than one model in the application. The *Maximum Selector* model is further described in the *Maximum Selector* section in this chapter. However, before we can describe the complete model, we need to discuss additional issues such as scheduling of modules and buffering of data.

Scheduling and Buffering

Before we get into the detailed implementation of modules we should understand two special aspects in processing models: *scheduling* and *buffering*. Scheduling specifies the order in which modules and their corresponding methods are executed while buffering specifies how often ports read and write data in and out of the module. NSL uses a multi-clock-scheduling algorithm where each module clock may have a different time step although synchronizing between modules during similar time steps. During each cycle, NSL executes the corresponding simulation methods implemented by the user. We will expand upon this later in the chapter and give complete details in the NSLM chapter.

In NSL, buffering relates to the way output ports handle communication. Since models may simulate concurrency, such as with neural network processing, we have provided *immediate* (no buffer) and *buffered* port modes. In the immediate mode (sequential simulation), output ports immediately send their data to the connecting modules. In the buffered mode (pseudo-concurrent simulation), output ports do not send their data to the connecting modules until the following clock cycle. In buffered mode, output ports are double buffered. One buffer contains the data that can be seen by the connecting modules during the current clock cycle, while the other buffer contains the data being currently generated that will only be seen by the connected modules during the next clock cycle. By default NSL uses the non-buffered mode, although the user may change this. Most of the models presented in the book make use of the immediate buffering mode. Full details on scheduling and buffering are given in the NSLM chapter.

Neural Networks

As discussed in the Introduction, NSL favors model architectures where modules are implemented by neural networks. A module defines the structure and behavior of the neural network. The neural network structure consists of a set of neurons and their interconnections, whereas the neural network behavior is defined in terms of non-linear dynamics with connection weights subject to a number of learning rules.

Neurons

Without precluding the importance of other neural models, we focus here on the leaky integrator neuron model. As we described in chapter 1, Neural Networks section, the leaky integrator's internal state is described by its membrane potential or neural activity *mp* and by its output or firing *mf*, specified by some nonlinear function, as shown in figure 3.6 (drawn again from figure 1.6).

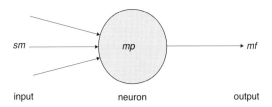

input   neuron   output

Figure 3.6
Single compartment neural model represented by a value *mp* corresponding to its membrane potential, and a value *mf* corresponding to its firing, the only output from the neuron. *sm* represents the set of inputs to the neuron.

In NSL two data structures are required to represent such a neuron in addition to its inputs. One data structure corresponds to the membrane potential and the other one to its firing rate. Different NSLM data types may be used for these structures, for example, **NslFloat0** or **NslDouble0** depending on the numerical type desired.

```
private NslDouble0 mf();
```

Notice the two variables are set to **private** with a scalar type such as **NslDouble0**. (In many cases we may want the value of *mf* to be communicated to other modules. If such is the case, the declaration for *mf* should be modified from a private variable to a public port.)

```
public NslDoutDouble0 mf();
```

In addition to the membrane potential and firing rate we need to define variable *sm* holding a weighted spatial summation of all input to the neuron

```
private NslDouble0 sm();
```

We may also need to declare the "unweighted" input to the neuron. In general, input may be specified as internal to a module or obtained from another module. In the latter case we define input *sin* as a public input port. Note that if *sin* is a vector, then *sm* is a scalar holding the sum of all values in the input vector.

```
public NslDinDouble1 sin(size);
```

The *leaky integrator* model defines the membrane potential *mp* with a first-order differential equation with dependence on its previous history and input *sm* given by equation 3.1 (combining together equations 1.1 and 1.2 and omitting the *t* parameter from both)

$$\tau\frac{dmp}{dt} = -mp + sm \qquad\qquad (3.1)$$

While neural networks are continuous in their nature, their simulated state is approximated by discrete time computations. For this reason we must specify an integration or approximation method to generate as faithfully as possible the corresponding neural state. The dynamics for *mp* are described by the following statement in NSLM

```
mp=nslDiff(mp,tau,-mp+sm);
```

nslDiff defines a first-degree differential equation equal to "*-mp+ sm*" as described by the leaky integrator model. Different approximation methods can be used to approximate the differential equation. The choice of this method may affect both the computation time and its precision. For example, NSL provides Euler and Runge-Kutta II approximation methods. The selection of which method to use is specified during simulation and not as part of the model architecture. We provide further explanation on approximation methods in chapter 6.

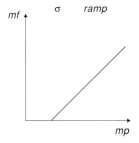
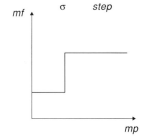
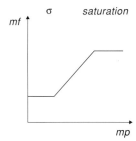
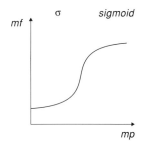

Figure 3.7
Common Threshold Functions.

The *average firing rate* or output of the neuron *mf* is obtained by applying some "threshold function" to the neuron's membrane potential as shown in equation 3.2 (taking out the *t* parameter from previous equation 1.3),

$$mf = \sigma(mp) \tag{3.2}$$

where σ usually is described by a non-linear function. For example, if σ is set to a *step* threshold function, the NSLM equation for the firing rate *mf* would be described by

```
mf = nslStep(mp);
```

where **nslStep** is the corresponding NSLM *step* threshold function. Some of the threshold functions defined in NSL are *step*, *ramp*, *saturation* and *sigmoid*, whose behaviors are plotted in figure 3.7 and described in detail in chapter 6, the NSLM language.

Neural network dynamics are generally specified inside the **simRun** method, as described code segment 3.9.

```
public void simRun()
{
    sm=nslSum(sin);
    mp = nslDiff(mp,tau,-mp+sm);
    mf = nslStep(mp);
}
```

Code Segment 3.9
Leaky Integrator neuron implementation.

While **initRun** is executed once prior to the "run," **simRun** gets executed via multiple iterations during the "run." A "run" is defined as execution over multiple clock cycles (simulation time steps) from time equal zero to the *runEndTime*. Similar to **initRun**, the **simRun** method must also be specified as **public** in order for NSL to be able to process it.

Interconnections

The previous definition specifies a single neuron without any interconnections. An actual neural network is made of a number of interconnected neurons where the output of one neuron serves as input to other neurons. In the leaky integrator neural model, interconnections are very simple structures. On the other hand, *synapses*, the links among neurons, are—in biological systems—complex electrochemical systems and may be modeled in exquisite detail. However, many models have succeeded with a very simple synaptic model: with each synapse carrying a connection weight that describes how neurons affect each other. The most common formula for the input to a neuron is given by equation 3.3 (omitting the *t* parameter from previous equation 1.4),

$$sv_j = \sum_{i=0}^{n-1} w_{ij} uf_i \tag{3.3}$$

where uf_i is the firing of neuron u_i whose output is connected to the *j*th input line of neuron v_j, and w_{ij} is the weight for that link, as shown in figure 3.8 (*up* and *vp* are analogous to *mp*, while *uf* and *vf* are analogous to *mf*).

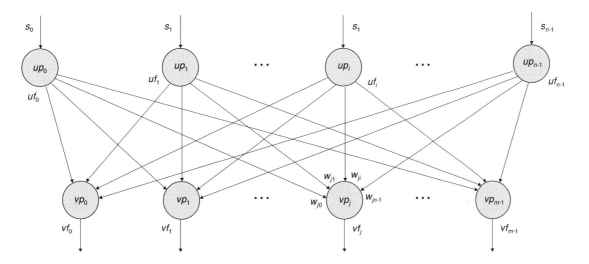

Expanding the summation, input to neuron v_j (identified by its corresponding membrane potential vp_j) is given by sv_j defined by equation 3.4

$$sv_j = w_{0j}uf_0 + w_{1j}uf_1 + w_{2j}uf_2 + ... + w_{n-1,j}uf_{n-1} \qquad (3.4)$$

While module interconnections are specified in NSLM via a **nslConnect** method call, doing this with neurons would in general be prohibitively expensive considering that there may be thousands or millions of neurons in a single neural network. Instead we use mathematical expressions similar to those used for their representation. For example, the input to neuron v_j, represented by svj, would be the sum for all outputs of neuron ufi multiplied (using the '*' operator) by connection weight wij, correspondingly.

```
svj = w0j*uf0 + w1j*uf1 + w2j*uf2 + ...;
```

Note that there exist m such equations in the network shown in figure 3.8. We could describe each neuron's membrane potential and firing rate individually or else we could make all u_i and v_j neuron vector structures. The first approach would be very long, inefficient, and prone to typing errors; thus we present the second approach and describe it in the following section.

Figure 3.8
Neurons vp_j receive input from neuron firings, $uf_0,...,uf_{n-1}$, multiplied by weights $w_{j0},...,w_{jn-1}$, respectively.

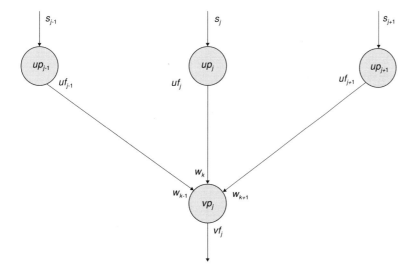

Figure 3.9
Mask connectivity.

Arrays and Masks

Instead of describing neurons and links on a one by one basis, we extend the basic neuron abstraction into *neuron arrays* and *connection masks* describing spatial arrangements among homogeneous neurons and their connections, respectively. We consider uf_j the output from a single neuron in an array of neurons and sv_j the input to a single neuron in another array of neurons. If mask w_k (for $-d \leq k \leq d$) represents the synaptic weights, as shown in figure 3.9, from the uf_{j+k} (for $-d \leq k \leq d$) elements to sv_j, for each j, we then have

$$sv_j = \sum_{k=-d}^{d} w_k uf_{j+k} \tag{3.5}$$

where the same mask w is applied to the output of each neuron uf_{j+k} to obtain input sv_j. In NSLM, the convolution operation is described by a single symbol "@".

```
sv = w@uf;
```

This kind of representation results in great conciseness, an important concern when working with a large number of interconnected neurons. Note that this is possible as long as connections are regular. Otherwise, single neurons would still need to be connected separately on a one by one basis. This also suggests that the operation is best defined when the number of *v* and *u* neurons is the same, although a non-matching number of units can be processed using a more complex notation.

To support arrays and masks, a **NslDouble1** or higher dimensional array structure is used, as was demonstrated in chapter 2, using the Hopfield model. In the Hopfield model neurons are organized as two-dimensional neuron arrays—instead of one dimensional—and weights result in four dimensional arrays—instead of two dimensional. For simplification, both neural arrays and connection masks are represented in NSLM with similar array types. The **simRun** method describing dynamics for neuron *v* would be as shown in code segment 3.10.

```
public void simRun()
{
    sv = w@uf;
    vp = nslDiff(vp,tau,-vp+sv);
    vf = nslStep(vp);
}
```

Code Segment 3.10
Leaky-Integrator **simRun** method implementation.

There are special considerations with convolutions regarding edge effects—a mask centered on an element at the edge of the arrays extends beyond the edge of the array—depending on how out of bound array elements are treated. The most important alternatives are to treat edges as *zero*, *wrap* around array elements such as if the array was continuous at the edges, or *replicate* boundary array elements. We will explain this in more detail in chapter 6, The NSLM Language.

3.2 Visualizing Model Architectures with SCS

There are two ways to develop a model architecture: by direct programming in NSLM as previously explained or by using the *Schematic Capture System* (*SCS*). *SCS* is a visual programming interface to NSLM that serves both as a browser as well as a tool for creating new model architectures as discussed in the Simulation chapter. While *SCS* does not provide the full programming functionality of NSLM, it provides visual support in designing modules and their interconnections. We will show in this section how to visualize already created model architectures with *SCS*. Extended details on how to created new model architectures will be overviewed in chapter 4, the *Schematic Capture System*.

To start executing the *Schematic Capture System* we invoke (see Appendix IV for platform particulars):

```
prompt> scs
```

The system initially presents the *Schematic Editor* (*SE*) window (shown in figure 3.10).

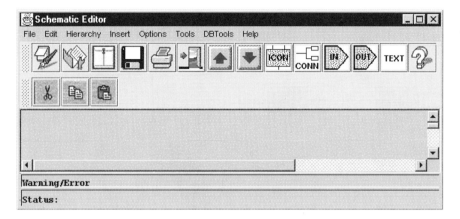

Figure 3.10
Select "Open" from the "File" menu to bring a listing of schematics available in the library of models.

To open the schematic of an existing model from the library of models we select "Open" from the "File" menu, as shown in figure 3.10. *SCS* presents a list of models, where we select for example the *MaxSelectorModel*, as shown in figure 3.11.

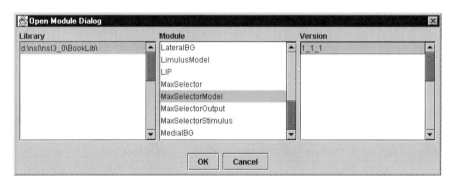

Figure 3.11
Select the MaxSelectorModel Schematic.

Once the model has been selected it is shown in the canvas section of the window, as shown in figure 3.12.

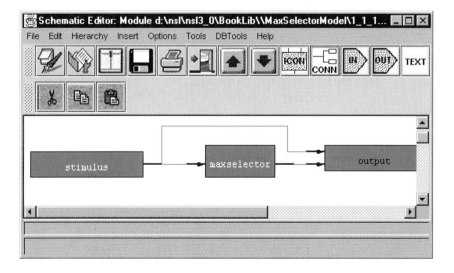

Figure 3.12
MaxSelectorModel Schematic. (The "descend" selection requires us to first select the module that we are to display.)

By "double clicking" on the **MaxSelector** module we will descend one level down the module hierarchy, and the schematics shown in figure 3.13 will be displayed.

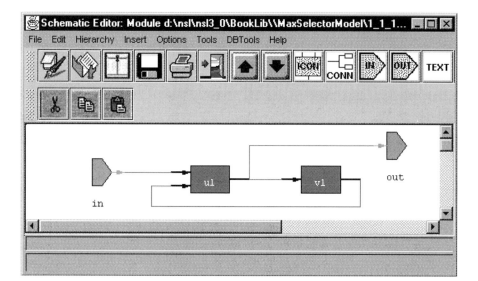

Figure 3.13
MaxSelector module from the MaxSelectorModel.

We can then return one level up by selecting "Ascend" from the "Hierarchy" menu, as shown in figure 3.14. The rest of the SCS interface is described in chapter 4.

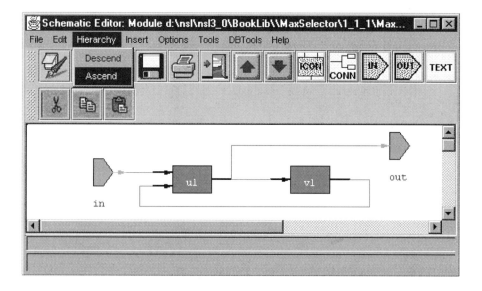

Figure 3.14
Select "ascend" from the "Hierarchy" Menu to go one level up the module hierarchy.

3.3 Maximum Selector

We presented an introduction to *Maximum Selector* model in chapter 2. We now describe its complete model architecture.

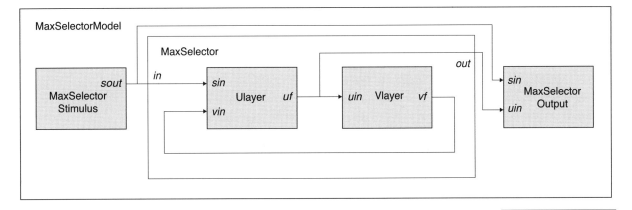

Model Implementation

As we have seen, the **MaxSelectorModel** is composed of five instances of modules: **u1, v1, maxSelector, stimulus, and output** of corresponding module types **Ulayer, Vlayer, MaxSelector, MaxSelectorStimulus**, and **MaxSelectorOutput**, as shown again in figure 3.15. Given an input vector *in* of array size *size*, the **maxSelector** module generates as output a similarly sized vector pattern *out* in which the only active unit (or neuron) corresponds—under suitable conditions—to the largest of the *n* vector inputs. These modules were introduced throughout the chapter so we will quickly recall and extend their description.

Ulayer

For simplicity we have kept only the minimum structure for the model (weights in this module have "1" as their value) described in code segment 3.11.

```
nslModule Ulayer (int size)
{
    public NslDinDouble1 sin(size);
    public NslDinDouble0 vin();
    public NslDoutDouble1 uf(size);
    private NslDouble1 up(size);
    private NslDouble0 hu();
    private NslDouble0 tau();
    public void initRun() {
        up =0;
        uf = 0;
        hu = 0.1;
        tau =1.0;
    }
    public void simRun() {
        up = nslDiff(up, tau, -up + uf - vin - hu + sin);
        uf = nslStep(up,0.1,0.1.0);
    }
}
```

Note that *sin, up,* and *uf* are vector arrays, while *vin, tau* and *hu* are scalar. The module behavior is described by the two equations introduced in chapter 2, with slight modifications for better correspondence with the module structure:

$$tau\frac{dup}{dt} = -up + uf - vin - hu + sin \tag{3.6}$$

Figure 3.15
The MaxSelectorModel contains the MaxSelector module incorporating an input port in used as input to the network and an output port out represents network output, and two module instances of type Ulayer and Vlayer, respectively. Additionally, the MaxSelectorStimulus module generates stimulus for the model and MaxSelectorOutput displays the output results.

Code Segment 3.11
Ulayer module definition.

$$uf = \begin{cases} 1 & \text{if } up > 0 \\ 0 & \text{if } up \leq 0 \end{cases} \tag{3.7}$$

There are two separate initializations: the first, **initModule** gives script access to the *hu* offset variable; the second, **initRun** resets the neuron activity values—the values being computed during the simulation—restarting the network with a new initial state. The **simRun** method contains the above expressions to be repeatedly executed during the simulation process. Note that the two statements for *up* and *uf*, respectively, require vector array return types since both structures are vectors. When adding or subtracting a vector with a scalar, such as "uf—vin" in the **nslDiff** expression, *vin* is subtracted from every element to *uf* as if *vin* were a vector with all elements having the same value.

Vlayer

Again, for simplicity we have kept only the minimum structure for the module without the weight terms, described in code segment 3.12. Note that *uin* is a vector array, while *vp*, *vf*, *tau* and *hv* are scalars.

```
nslModule Vlayer(int size)
{
    public NslDinDouble1 uin(size);
    public NslDoutDouble0 vf();
    private NslDouble0 vp();
    private NslDouble0 hv();
    private NslDouble0 tau();
    public void initRun() {
        vp =0;
        vf = 0;
        hv=0.5;
        tau=1.0;
    }
    public void simRun() {
        vp = nslDiff(vp,tau, -vp + nslSum(uin) - hv);
        vf = nslRamp(vp);
    }
}
```

Code Segment 3.12
MaxSelector's Vlayer module definition.

The module behavior is described by the two equations introduced in chapter 2, with slight modifications for better correspondence with the module structure

$$tau \frac{dvp}{dt} = -vp + \sum_n uin - hv \tag{3.8}$$

$$vf = \begin{cases} vp & \text{if } vp > 0 \\ 0 & \text{if } vp \leq 0 \end{cases} \tag{3.9}$$

These equations are implemented in the **simRun** method above. Note that the two statements for *vp* and *vf*, respectively, require this time a scalar return type since both structures are scalars. For this reason we apply **nslSum()** to all array element values from *uin*, the output received from *uf*, to obtain a single scalar value. **nslRamp** is a *ramp* threshold function.

MaxSelector

The **MaxSelector** module instantiates both **Ulayer** and **Vlayer**, as well as defining two external ports, *in* and *out*, as shown in code segment 3.13. Port interconnections are made inside the **makeConn** method, two connections and two relabels.

```
nslModule MaxSelector (int size)
{
    public Ulayer u1(size);
    public Vlayer v1(size);
    public NslDinDouble1 in(size);
    public NslDoutDouble1 out(size);

    public void makeConn(){
        nslConnect(v1.vf,u1.vin);
        nslConnect(u1.uf,v1.uin);
        nslRelabel(in,u1.sin);
        nslRelabel(u1.uf,out);
    }
}
```

Code Segment 3.13
MaxSelector module.

MaxSelectorStimulus

The **MaxSelectorStimulus** generates the visual stimulus sent to the **MaxSelector** module. The module is described in code segment 3.14. The actual stimulus can be set directly as part of the module definition, or as we discussed in the previous chapter, interactively assigned by the user through the visual interface or through the NSLS shell window. If done directly in the module definition, the **initRun** method would contain for example the corresponding stimulus specification.

```
nslModule MaxSelectorStimulus (int size)
{
    public NslDoutDouble1 sout(size);
    public void initRun(){
        sout=0;
        sout[1]=1.0;
        sout[3]=0.5;
    }
}
```

Code Segment 3.14
MaxSelectorStimulus
module.

MaxSelectorOutput

The **MaxSelectorOutput** receives input from both **MaxSelectorStimulus** and **MaxSelector** modules and generates the canvases/graphs shown in the chapter 2, figure 2.8. For the sake of simplicity we leave the detailed description of this module until chapter 5, The User Interface and Graphical windows.

MaxSelectorModel

The **MaxSelectorModel** instantiates both the **MaxSelectorStimulus, MaxSelector**, and **MaxSelectorOutput** as shown again in code segment 3.15.

```
nslModel MaxSelectorModel()
{
    public MaxSelectorStimulus stimulus(size);
    public MaxSelector maxselector(size);
    public MaxSelectorOutput output(size);
    private int size = 10;

    public void initSys() {
        system.setRunEndTime(10.0);
        system.setRunStepSize(0.1);
    }
    public void makeConn(){
        nslConnect(stimulus.sout,maxselector.in);
        nslConnect(stimulus.sout,output.sin);
        nslConnect(maxselector.out,output.uf);
    }
}
```

As an exercise the user may want to add the different weight parameters specified by the original equations and change their value to see their effect on the model. Additionally, the network could be modeled with different neuron array sizes to see how this affects overall behavior.

3.4 Hopfield

Recall from the Simulation chapter the *Hopfield* model description. We now describe the model architecture.

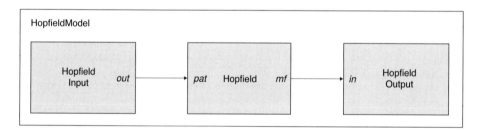

Model Implementation

The *Hopfield* model contains three module instances **hopfield, in, and out** of the corresponding module types **Hopfield**, **HopfieldInput** and **HopfieldOutput** as shown in figure 3.16. Input port *pat* in **Hopfield** receives a number of initial patterns from output port *out* during training to adjust the network's connection weights. During model execution *pat* receives from *out* a single input pattern to be associated to the one that it best approximates.

Hopfield

The **Hopfield** module implements the neural network dynamics. In our example both *pat* and *mf* are set to two- dimensional arrays associating letter images to be tested (although both could have been implemented by vectors). In our example, both input and output ports have the same size for both dimensions. The structure is shown in code segment 3.16.

```
nslModule Hopfield (int size)
{
    public NslDinInt2 pat(size,size);
    public NslDoutInt2 mf(size,size);
    private NslInt2 mp(size,size);
    private NslInt2 pmf(size,size);
    private NslInt4 w(size,size,size,size);
    private NslInt0 energy();
    private NslInt0 change();
}
```

Notice that we are describing a binary *Hopfield* network, thus we implement all types as integers. Two additional two-dimensional arrays are defined, *mp* storing the activity and output of neurons and *pmf* storing previous output. We also define a four-dimensional connection matrix *w*, and two parameters, *energy* and *change*. We define a connection matrix *w* instead of a connection mask due to the varying weight values for all connections. We lose a bit on efficiency due to the higher dimension arrays but we add the ability to better map units to images. The last attribute defined is invisible to the user, but thrown in by the pre-parser. It is a primitive-type integer *size* storing the *size* passed to the module. This variable is later used in the module methods to avoid having to obtain the size each time.

During the training phase, model weights are initialized according to equation 2.7 from chapter 2 and in correspondence to our particular *Hopfield* network application at hand,

$$
w_{klij} = \begin{cases} 0 & k = i, l = j \\ \sum_m pat_{mkl} \, pat_{mij} & \text{otherwise} \end{cases}
\tag{3.10}
$$

Besides the **initRun** and **simRun** methods, the model also requires making use of the **initTrain** and **simTrain** methods for network training. Inside the **initTrain** method, weights are set by going over all *n* input patterns and applying the above equation. Each iteration of the **initTrain** method adds a new pattern to the weight computation. Thus, the **initTrain** method has to be executed for as many times as patterns exist.

```
for (int k=0; k<size; k++)
    for (int l=0; l<size; l++)
        for (int i=0; i<size; i++)
            for (int j=0; j<size; j++)
                if (k==l && l==i && i==j)
                    w[k][l][i][j]=0;
                else

w[k][l][i][j]=w[k][l][i][j]+pat[k][l]*pat[i][j];
```

Notice that NSLM enables the user to write his/her own matrix manipulation functions when necessary, such as in the above example.

After weights have been set, the network executes according to equations 2.4 and 2.5 from chapter 2

$$
mp_{kl} = \sum_i \sum_j w_{klij} mf_{ij}
\tag{3.11}
$$

$$mf_{kl} = \begin{cases} 1 & \text{if } mp_{kl} \geq 0 \\ -1 & \text{if } mp_{kl} < 0 \end{cases} \qquad (3.12)$$

The **initRun** method initializes neuron activity to the input pattern. One important aspect previously mentioned in the Simulation chapter is that the network gets updated asynchronously, with neurons randomly chosen for update. Thus, we compute the output for each neuron immediately after computing its activity, so it can be used as input by the next neuron chosen for update. The neuron activity *mp* and the neuron output *mf* are computed according to the above equations. The simulation proceeds as described in the **simRun** method. Since it contains a number of interesting expressions, we explain each one separately.

We first obtain two random integer values, *k* and *l*, used as indices in selecting the next neuron to be updated. Recall that all neurons are stored in a two-dimensional array and thus the need for the two indices.

```
int k = nslRandom(0,(size-1));
int l = nslRandom(0,(size-1));
```

The method **nslRandom** is one of a number of NSL library methods (described in more detail in the NSLM chapter) for numerical computations, in this case to obtain an integer random number between 0 and "size-1." Since array indices start at 0 we do not want numbers that are equal to or larger than the size of the arrays. We then apply a summation over all inputs to the randomly selected neuron multiplied by the respective connection weights—we use the "^" operator for *pointwise* array multiplication, i.e., multiplication between corresponding array elements.

```
mp[k][l] = nslSum(w[k][l]^mf);
```

Note that "w[k][l]" generates a matrix array, resulting in a valid operation. Once we get the activity for the neuron we compute its firing with a *step* function with outputs set to either -1 or 1, as specified by the last two parameters of the following **nslStep** expression. (The zero term specifies the threshold.)

```
mf[k][l] = nslStep(mp[k][l],0,-1,1);
```

We then check if the error is zero, corresponding to the output of all neurons generating exactly the same values as in the previous computation—previous values are stored in *pmf*. This is done by first subtracting *mf* from *pmf*, and then transforming the result to its absolute value to make sure all differences are positive. Finally, we add the resulting absolute values together to generate the *change*, as shown next,

```
change = nslSum(nslAbs(pmf-mf));
```

If *change* is zero, convergence has occurred, we print out a "Convergence" message—we use the **nslPrintln** printing method—and we break the simulation cycle effectively stopping execution by using the **system.breakCycles** method as follows

```
if (change == 0)
    nslPrintln("Convergence");
    system.breakCycles();
}
```

The module conditional ending is very common in many neural networks, especially those involving training, as will also be seen in the *Backpropagation* model.

The last expression in the **simRun** method sets the new *mf* value to the previous *pmf* value for the next simulation iteration.

```
pmf[k][l] = mf[k][l];
```

Additionally, we compute the energy in the network, described by equation 2.6 from chapter 2,

$$E = -\frac{1}{2}\sum_k \sum_l \sum_i \sum_j w_{klij} mp_{kl} mp_{ij} \qquad (3.13)$$

This equation is implemented as follows

```
energy = 0;
for (int k=0; k<size; k++)
    for (int l=0; l<size; l++)
        for (int i=0; i<size; i++)
            for (int j=0; j<size; j++)
                energy=energy+w[k][l][i][j]*mp[k][l]*mp[i][j];
energy = -0.5*energy;
```

Again we need to do our own element by element multiplication.

HopfieldModel

The **HopfieldModel** instantiates the **Hopfield**, **HopfieldInput** and **HopfieldOutput** modules. Both the **HopfieldInput** and **HopfieldOutput** modules are quite simple, analogous to the MaxSelectorModel, and we leave their description until chapter 5, The User Interface and Graphical Windows. Model input can be set directly as part of the module definition or, as we discussed in the previous chapter, interactively assigned by the user via the script or menu interface. We pass the network size to the two modules, in this case "10." Module connections are made inside the **makeConn** method as described in code segment 3.17.

As an exercise the user may want to change network size as well as extend the model to make use of two different sizes for array rows and columns, respectively, instead of a single one. If you have a different problem at hand, such as the "Traveling Salesman," you may want to modify the equation for weights as well as the energy function. The rest of the computation should be the same.

```
nslModel HopfieldModel ()
{
    private int size = 10;
    public Hopfield hopfield(size);
    public HopfieldInput in(size);
    public HopfieldOutput out(size);

    public void makeConn(){
            nslConnect(in.out,hopfield.pat);
            nslConnect(hopfield.mf,out.in);
    }
}
```

Code Segment 3.17
HopefieldModel model definition.

3.5 Backpropagation

Recall from Section 2.6 the *Backpropagation* model description. We now describe the model architecture.

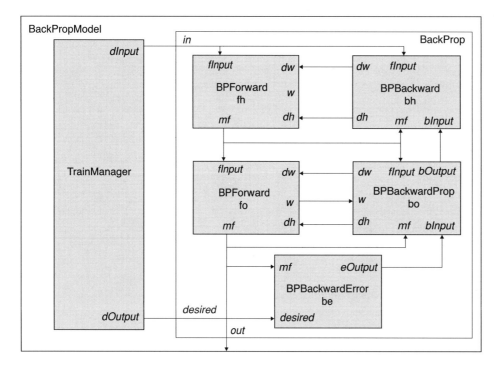

Model Implementation

The model architecture is shown in figure 3.17. The **BackPropModel** is decomposed into a **TrainManager** module and a **BackPropLayers** module. The **TrainManager** module reads training data and sends it one cycle at a time to the **BackPropLayers** module. The **BackPropLayers** module communicates with to **BPForward**, **BPBackward**, **BPBackwardProp** and **BPBackwardProp** modules to implement neural behavior. Note that there could be more modules if there were additional hidden layers in the network. Also note that we do not model the input layer as a separate module since this layer simply reads training or simulation data without any additional processing. Thus, the input layer can be directly mapped to the input port of the **BackPropLayers** module. All ports in the network are set to a one-dimensional array or vector of similar size.

The network is processed in two modes, training and simulation. Training proceeds itself in two modes:

- A feedforward mode where an input is selected and processed by the network in order to generate an output vector.

- A backpropagation mode where the error is computed as the difference between the current output vector and the desired or target output vector. The backward pass then adjusts the synaptic weights of the output layer neurons and then the hidden layer neurons, in that particular order.

As a result of this continual "wearing away" of the synaptic weights, the network will, in general, come to provide outputs that better and better approximate the target values.

Once the network has been completely trained, a process that finishes depending on the error produced simulation, the simulation run proceeds in a single mode:

A **feedforward mode** where an input vector is processed by the network to generate an output vector. The forward pass is executed a single time with the desired input pattern.

It is the job of the **BackPropLayers** module (and **BPForward**, **BPBackward**, **BPBackwardProp** and **BPBackwardProp** submodules) to conduct the forward pass and backward pass after being supplied by the **TrainManager** module with the training pair. It is the job of the **TrainManager** to take a whole training set and cycle through calling **BackPropLayers** for each pair.

We next describe the different modules top-down: **TrainManager**, **BackPropLayers**, **BPForward**, **BPBackward**, **BPBackwardProp**, **BPBackwardProp** and finally **BackPropModel**.

```
nslModule TrainManager (int nPats, int inSize, int outSize)
{
    public NslDoutFloat1 dInput(inSize);
    public NslDoutFloat1 dOutput(outSize);
    private NslFloat2 pInput(nPats, inSize);
    private NslFloat2 pOutput(nPats, outSize);
    private int counter = 0;
    private int numPats = nPats;
}
```

Code Segment 3.18
TrainManager attribute definition.

TrainManager

The **TrainManager** module reads training data from a training file and sends them one cycle at a time to the **BackPropLayers** module. The module structure is described in code segment 3.18.

The model structure includes two output ports sending both input and desired output data, *dInput* and *dOutput*, respectively. To simplify the example, we directly assign the training data into two-dimensional variables *pInput* and *pOuput*. This is quite efficient when having small training sets such as in this case. With very large data sets this would not be possible since data files may be too large to store in memory and it will be more efficient to load them from a file as needed. We include two additional parameters, *counter* and *numPats*. Variable *counter* is used to control the particular data being sent during the training cycle as will be explained next. Variable *numPats* stores the number of patterns being used for training. The actual layer sizes are passed into the module during module instantiation.

The module's main responsibility is to provide with training data to the rest of the model. Recall the training set format from table 3.1.

<num_patterns>
<input1> ... <inputN> <output1> ... <outputM>
<input1> ... <inputN> <output1> ... <outputM>
:
<input1> ... <inputN> <output1> ... <outputM>

Table 3.1
TrainManager input file format.

During model training, the **simTrain** method sends out the data. This is achieved by grabbing the next (input, desired output) pair in the given order, as shown in code segment 3.19.

```
public void simTrain()
{
    counter++;
    int pat = counter%numPats;
    dInput = pInput[pat];
    dOutput = pOutput[pat];
}
```

Code Segment 3.19
TrainManager simTrain
method.

Note how we control this by doing a "mod"—operator %—of the current cycle
counter over the number of total patterns in *numPats*. Although the training procedure is
in the given order or *sequential*, where the total number of training steps is set equal to
the total number of patterns, it does not have to be always that way. There are many other
approaches, e.g., having the training given as a random choice of next (input, desired
output) pair.

BackPropLayers

The **BackPropLayers** module is responsible for controlling the detailed training cycle. It
defines data structures and simulation methods for the network necessary to execute the
feedforward (activation) mode and backpropagation (adaptation) mode. The module
instantiates five modules, two **BPForward** modules and single **BPBackward**,
BPBackwardProp, and **BPBackwardError** modules. The module also defines two
input ports and two output ports to receive and send information from and to the
TrainManager module, respectively. The module definition is described in code
segment 3.20.

```
nslModule BackPropLayers (int inSize, int hidSize, int outSize)
{
    public BPForward fh(inSize,hidSize);
    public BPForward fo(hidSize,outSize);
    public BPBackwardError be(outSize);
    public BPBackwardProp bo(hidSize,outSize);
    public BPBackward bh(inSize,hidSize);

    public NslDinFloat1 in(inSize);
    public NslDinFloat1 desired(outSize);
    public NslDoutFloat1 out(outSize);
}
```

Code Segment 3.20
BackPropLayers module
attributes.

Two input ports *in* and *desired* receive their data from the **TrainManager** and are
relabeled to *fInput* and *desired* in the respective submodules. *fInput* represents the input
layer feeding data into the hidden layer corresponding to both the first **BPForward** and
the **BPBackward** modules. On the other hand *desired* is used to compute the backward
error in the **BPBackwardError** module. In terms of **BackPropLayers** output ports, *out*
is relabeled from the output *mf* of the second **BPForward** module representing the
feedforward mode output. Note the specific order in specifying the five submodules.
Since we are using immediate mode buffering this order is significant and results in the
following:

1. **Process** fh BPForward **module.**
2. **Process** fo BPForward **module.**
3. **Process** be **BPBackwardError module.**
4. **Process** bo BPBackwardProp **module.**
5. **Process** bh BPBackward **module.**

Remember that two processing modes are involved in the model. It is crucial that the feedforward mode for both hidden and output layer be completed before the backpropagation mode on both layers. After each training *epoch*—a complete pass through all the training patterns—the network should have learned something and can use the new weights to estimate better and fine-tune itself. The network requires many epochs for training. While **BPForward** modules are processed in both modes, the last three modules are only involved in the backpropagation mode as will be seen in the rest of the section.

BPForward

The **BPForward** module implements both the hidden and output layers in the "forward" computations. The module attributes, three input ports, *fInput*, *dw* and *dh*, two output ports *mf* and *w*, and two internal variables *mp* and *h*, as shown in code segment 3.21.

```
nslModule BPForward (int inSize, int hidSize)
{
    public NslDinFloat1 fInput(inSize);
    public NslDinFloat1 dh(hidSize);
    public NslDinFloat2 dw(inSize, hidSize);
    public NslDoutFloat1 mf(hidSize);
    public NslDoutFloat2 w(inSize, hidSize);

    private NslFloat1 mp(hidSize);
    private NslFloat1 h(hidSize);
}
```

Code Segment 3.21
BPForward module attributes.

This module is involved in both feedforward and backpropagation modes. Since backpropagation mode is processed before the feedforward mode let us start describing first the module's behavior during the backpropagation mode.

Backpropagation mode

The module first initializes network thresholds and weights to random values inside the **initSys** method that gets executed every time the complete model gets reinitialized, as shown in code segment 3.22.

```
public void initSys()
{
    nslRandom(h,-1.0, 1.0);
    nslRandom(w,- 1.0, 1.0);

    dw = 0.0;
    dh = 0.0;
}
```

Code Segment 3.22
BPForward initSys method.

The **nslRandom** function sets the variables, *h* and *w*, to random values between the two limits, -0.5 and 0.5, in this case. The model also sets the two "deltas," *dw* and *dh* to 0.

We then define a "forward" computation (used in both the backpropagation and feedforward modes) calculating the activity *mp* by doing a weight matrix multiplication with over input vector *fInput*. This input is received from the previous stage, i.e. hidden layer receives input from the input layer and the output layer receives input from the hidden layer output. The output *mf* is computed by applying a *sigmoid* threshold function over the activity. This output will then be fed into the next **BPForward** module in the case of the hidden layer, or to the **BPBackwardError** module in the case of the output layer.

The two equations (for every *i*) are as follows,

$$mp_i(t) = \sum_j w_{ji}(t) fInput_i(t) \tag{3.14}$$

$$mf_i(t) = f(mp_i(t) + h_i(t)) = \frac{1}{1 + e^{-(mp_i(t) + h_i(t))}} \tag{3.15}$$

Since we define a single **BPForward** module to define both the hidden layer and output layer "forward" dynamics, we use a single set of equations for the two, using the indices *i* and *j* instead of *s, p,* and *q* as originally used in Section 2.6 for the two layers. These two statements are stored in the **forward** method shown in code segment 3.23.

```
public void forward()
{
    mp = w*fInput;
    mf = nslSigmoid(mp + h);
}
```

Code Segment 3.23
BPForward forward method.

Notice that *fInput_i* corresponds to *in_s* (we use *fInput* instead of the original *in* to be consistent with the rest of the modules here to distinguish between forward and backward input), while **nslSigmoid** is a NSL library function computing the *sigmoid* transfer function in the above equation.

In the backpropagation mode the thresholds and weights get updated by adding in new "deltas," *dh* and *dw* (for every *i*) computed from the previous backpropagation cycle.

$$h_i(t+1) = h_i(t) + \Delta h_i(t) \tag{3.16}$$

$$w_{ji}(t+1) = w_{ji}(t) + \Delta w_{ji}(t) \tag{3.17}$$

The backpropagation mode is stored in the **simTrain** method as described in code segment 3.24. It consists of the two updates with the "deltas" and the "forward" computation.

```
public void simTrain()
{
    w = w + dw;
    h = h + dh;
    forward();
}
```

Code Segment 3.24
BPForward simTrain method.

Feedforward mode

During the feedforward mode the **simRun** method is executed as described in code segment 3.25. It simply calls the "forward" computation.

```
public void simRun()
{
    forward();
}
```

Code Segment 3.25
BPForward simRun method.

BPBackwardError

The **BPBackwardError** module does only backpropagation mode computation. The module includes two input ports *mf* and *desired*, an output port *eOutput* and three local parameters *change*, *tss* and *pss*, as shown in code segment 3.26.

```
nslModule BPBackwardError (int outSize)
{
    public NslDinFloat1 mf(outSize);
    public NslDinFloat1 desired(outSize);
    public NslDoutFloat1 eOutput(outSize);

    private NslFloat1 stopError();
    private NslFloat0 pss();
    private NslFloat0 tss();
    public void initModule() {
            stopError.nslSetAccess('W');
    }
}
```

Code Segment 3.26
BPBackwardError module attributes.

The module receives the output *mf* from the **fo BPForward** output layer and compares its value against the desired value being forwarded from the **TrainManager** as follows

$$eOutput(t) = desired(t) - mf(t) \tag{3.18}$$

The network stops its training when a small enough error *tss* has been reached. The error calculation is as follows,

$$tss = \sum_t eOutput^2(t) \tag{3.19}$$

The computation is implemented in the **simTrain** method as shown in code segment 3.27. In order to compute the epoch error *tss* we compute first a train cycle error *pss* being accumulated through the epoch.

```
public void simTrain()
{
    eOutput = desired - mf;
    pss = pss + nslSum(eOutput ^ eOutput);
}
```

Code Segment 3.27
BPBackwardError simTrain method.

To stop training we compare the tss value against a previously set *change* value—telling the model when to stop learning—as given in the **endTrain** method, a method called at the end of every epoch completion, shown in code segment 3.28.

```
public void endTrain()
{
    tss = pss;
    if (tss < change) {
            nslPrintln("Convergence");
            system.breakEpochs();
            return;
    }
}
```

Code Segment 3.28
BPBackwardError endTrain method.

We first print a message ("Convergence") telling the user that we have completed the training cycle. This completion is actually achieved through the **system.breakEpochs** method specifying that epoch processing should be interrupted (as opposed to a **system.breakCycles** method for breaking a single training cycle). The interruption is only processed internally by NSL after the return statement.

BPBackwardProp

The **BPBackwardProp** module is only involved in the backpropagation mode. The module is defined in code segment 3.29 and it contains four input ports, *fInput*, *bInput*, *mf* and *w*, three output ports, *bOutput*, *dw* and *dh*, and two variables, *delta* and *lrate*.

```
nslModule BPBackwardProp (int hidSize, int outSize)
{
    public NslDinFloat1 bInput(outSize);
    public NslDinFloat1 fInput(hidSize);
    public NslDinFloat1 mf(outSize);
    public NslDinFloat2 w(hidSize, outSize);
    public NslDoutFloat1 dh(outSize);
    public NslDoutFloat2 dw(hidSize, outSize);
    public NslDoutFloat1 bOutput(hidSize);


    private NslFloat1 delta(outSize);
    private NslFloat0 lrate();
}
```

Code Segment 3.29
BPBackwardProp module attributes.

The module receives the **BPBackwardError** output layer error *eOuput* in *bInput* using it to compute output layer "deltas." The computation is as follows (η represents the learning rate *lrate*),

$$\delta_q(t) = mf_q(t) \times (1 - mf_q(t)) \times bInput_e(t) \tag{3.20}$$

$$\Delta h_q(t) = \eta \delta_q(t) \tag{3.21}$$

$$\Delta w_{pq}(t) = \eta \delta_q(t) \times fInput_p(t) \tag{3.22}$$

$$bOutput_p(t) = \sum_q w_{qp}(t) \delta_q(t) \tag{3.23}$$

The **simTrain** method computes output the deltas, δ, *dh* and *dw*, and the output *bOutput* sent to the hidden layer as shown in code segment 3.30.

```
public void simTrain()
{
    delta = (mf * (1.0 - mf)) * bInput;
    dw = lrate * delta * fInput;
    dh = lrate * delta;
    bOutput = w*delta; //this is the product of a matrix
        times a vector
}
```

Code Segment 3.30
BPBackwardProp simTrain method.

BPBackward

The **BPBackward** module is similar to **BPBackwardProp** module except that it does not compute the additional *bOutput* (unless additional hidden layers are present). The module is defined in code segment 3.31 and it contains three input ports, *fInput*, *bInput*, and *mf*, two output ports, *dw* and *dh*, and two variables, *delta* and *lrate*.

```
nslModule BPBackward (int inSize, int hidSize)
{
    public NslDinFloat1 bInput(hidSize);
    public NslDinFloat1 fInput(inSize);
    public NslDinFloat1 mf(hidSize);
    public NslDoutFloat1 dh(hidSize);
    public NslDoutFloat2 dw(inSize, hidSize);

    private NslFloat1 delta(hidSize);
    private NslFloat0 lrate();
}
```

Code Segment 3.31
BPBackward module attributes.

The computation is as follows,

$$\delta_p(t) = mf(t) \times (1 - mf_p) \times bInput_q \qquad (3.24)$$

$$\Delta h_p(t) = \eta \delta_p(t) \qquad (3.25)$$

$$\Delta w_{sp}(t) = \eta \delta_p(t) \times fInput_p(t) \qquad (3.26)$$

The **simTrain** method computes output the deltas, δ, dh and dw, as shown in code segment 3.32.

```
public void backwardPass()
{
    delta = mf * (1.0-mf) * bInput;
    dw = lrate * delta * fInput;
    dh = lrate * delta;
}
```

Code Segment 3.32
BPBackward simTrain
method.

BackPropModel

The **BackPropModel** is responsible for instantiating its two submodules, **BackPropLayers** and **TrainManager**, as well as initializing the appropriate layer sizes and the number of patterns to be stored. The code is shown in code segment 3.33.

```
nslModel BackPropModel ()
{
    int inSize = 2;
    int hidSize = 2;
    int outSize = 1;
    int nPats = 4;
    public TrainManager train(nPats,inSize,outSize);
    public BackPropAllLayers layers(inSize,hidSize,outSize);
}
```

Code Segment 3.33
BackPropModel model
attributes.

There are a number of exercises that can be done on this model. In particular, since *Backpropagation* is a gradient descent algorithm, there are concerns that the slope of the error surface could contain local minima that the network could become stuck in. An additional training parameter known as *momentum* (identified by α) could be defined in the BPBackwardProp module. The momentum variable is quite useful in order to keep the network from becoming stuck in local minima. In such a way, the error computation equations would be modified to contain both the training rate and momentum terms as follows, for the hidden layer

$$\Delta h_p(t+1) = \eta \delta_p + \alpha \Delta h_p(t) \tag{3.27}$$

$$\Delta w_{sp}(t+1) = \eta \delta_p \times fInput_p + \alpha \Delta w_{sp}(t) \tag{3.28}$$

and for the output layer

$$\Delta h_q(t+1) = \eta \delta_q + \alpha \Delta h_q(t) \tag{3.29}$$

$$\Delta w_{pq}(t+1) = \eta \delta_q \times fInput_q + \alpha \Delta w_{pq}(t) \tag{3.30}$$

Parameter α, the momentum constant, is commonly set to around 0.9.

An additional common modification to the algorithm is to update thresholds and weights at the end of each epoch instead of every training cycle. You can modify this and see the effect on model training as well.

On a different perspective, most of the modifications on the *Backpropagation* model are usually in terms of layer sizes and input file structure. We invite the user to make the layer sizes parameters of the model instead of constant. The actual values could then be interactively assigned or read from a NSLS script file. The model would require the use of dynamic memory allocation (the **nslMemAlloc** method handling dynamic memory allocation described in the NSLM chapter).

Another possible modification is to take advantage of NSL object-oriented programming, in particular *inheritance*. Inheritance is quite useful in avoiding class definition duplication. For example, **BPBackward** and **BPBackwardProp** are quite similar. We could make **BPBackwardProp** definition inherit from **BPBackward** where we would only need to add the backward output port *bOutput* to the **BPBackwardProp** definition while the rest gets inherited. Again, we invite the user to exercise this but only after having read the NSLM chapter.

3.6 Summary

We have shown how modeling of neural architectures is done following the module approach in NSL. The three models described in this chapter, *Maximum Selector*, *Hopfield* and *Backpropagation*, use different features of NSL although keeping a very consistent organization based on the NSL module architecture.

Notes

1. The complete syntax for NSLM as well as further descriptions is found in chapter 6.

2. At the moment NSL supports up to 4-dimensional array ports and in general numerical type arrays.

4 Schematic Capture System

The Schematic Capture System (SCS) provides graphical tools to build hierarchical neural models either by a top-down or bottom-up approach. SCS consists of the Schematic Editor, Icon Editor, NSLM Editor, Library Path Editor, Consistency Checker, Library Manager, NSLM Code Generator, and NSLM Viewer. SCS allows one to build a model graphically by connecting icons together into what we call a schematic. Each icon can then be decomposed further into a schematic of its own. In addition, SCS also provides an interface to the USC Brain Project, Brain Models on the Web database (BMW)

The Schematic Capture System (SCS) is an important component of the NSL system. SCS is primarily used to generate NSL models as shown in figure 4.1.[1] (This chapter covers the latest version of the software found in NSL3_0_n., database version 4.)

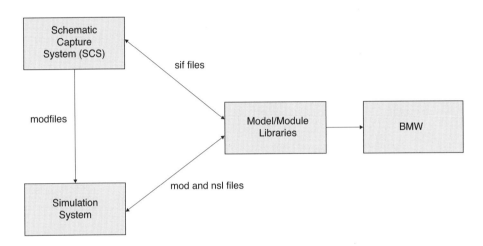

Figure 4.1
NSL System Diagram.

4.1 SCS Tools
The Schematic Capture System consists of many subsystems—the Schematic Editor, the Icon Editor, the NSLM Editor, the Library Path Editor, the Library Manager, the Consistency Checker, the NSLM Generator, and the NSLM Viewer.

Schematic Editor (SE)
The Schematic Editor is responsible for building the structure of the model. It is also serves as the control window for the Schematic Capture System. From the Schematic Editor window we can start any of the other SCS tools, load a model or module into the Schematic Editor, or descend/ascend into a schematic. When selecting icons to use in the schematic, SE allows the user to pick which version of a module to use: the user can choose a floating version that can change at any time or a fixed version, which cannot change.

When opening other tools from the Schematic Editor it is import to note that each new tool pops up in its own window and we can have as many open as we would like. However, there is always one and only one Schematic Editor Window open at any time.

Icon Editor (IE)
The Icon Editor allows the user to build the graphical appearance of the individual icons (modules).

NSLM Editor (NE)

The NSLM Editor allows the user to add NSLM code to the code that SCS has generated. This is particularly important for "leaf" level modules since they contain most of the functionality of the module.

Library Path Editor (LPE)

The Library Path Editor allows the user to modify the list of libraries in use.

Library Manager (LM)

The Library Manager allows the user to access and create new libraries of models and modules within the file system, move module from one library to another, and edit module attributes.

Consistency Checker (CC)

The Consistency Checker is responsible for keeping track of the versions of the modules that the model contains and checking that the ports from one level match those of the next level. The Consistency Checker is called automatically when a model is generated (NSLM Generator) or when a module is saved using Schematic, Icon, or NSLM editors.

NSLM Generator (NG)

The NSLM Generator generates the code from the schematic structure of the model. It also calls the Consistency Checker

NSLM Viewer (NV)

The NSLM Viewer displays the code generated by the NSLM Generator.

4.2 An Example Using SCS

We start by invoking the *Schematic Capture System* with scs.

The *Schematic Editor* window is shown in figure 4.2.

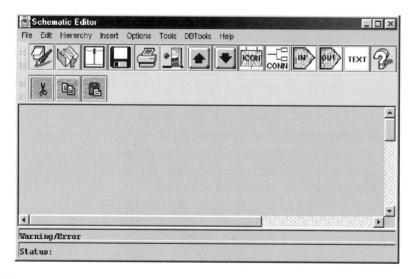

Figure 4.2
The Schematic Editor Window.

There are a number of steps to follow in creating a new schematic: (1) Create a library to save your work in; (2) Create the icons or borrow existing ones; (3) Place the icons in the schematics(4) Connect the icons together; (5) Save the schematic back to one of the libraries; and (6) Generate the NSLM file.

Create a Library

From the Schematic Editor window choose the Tools menu and then select the Library Manager option. (We will abbreviate this to: "**Tools→Library Manager**" in the future.) The system opens the window shown in figure 4.3.

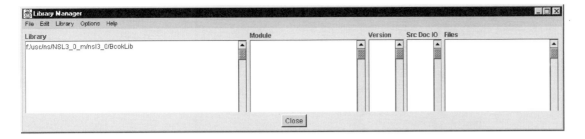

Verify that the first library is "<somepath>/nsl3_0/BookLib" (the "/" directory symbol in UNIX corresponds to a "\" symbol in a PC) where *somepath* is where your administrator installed the basic SCS library. Create another library in which to save your schematics by selecting **Library→New Library**. A popup will appear as shown in figure 4.4.

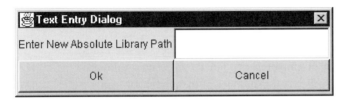

Enter the path where you wish to create your library, **in our case it is f:/usc/ns/NSL3_0_m/nsl3_0/FirstLib**. Then select **OK.** When you are finished, select **Close** from the Library Management Window.

Create Icons

To create a schematic, we first need to verify that the icons we want exist. In this example, we will start from scratch and create icons for the **Ulayer** and **Vlayer** modules we wrote earlier. First open the *Icon Editor* where individual icons/modules are edited. This is achieved by **Tools→IconEditor** from the Schematic Editor Window. A pop-up window will appear as shown in figure 4.5.

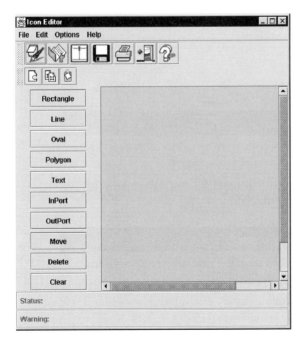

Since we want to create a new icon we select **File→New** from the top menu bar. In response to this option we get the window shown in figure 4.6.

Figure 4.3
The SCS Library Manager Window

Figure 4.4
New Library Path Prompy

Figure 4.5
The picture shows the layout of the Icon Editor Window. The top row of menu options allows us to create new icons, edit old ones, and change the graphical options. The left tool bar is in charge of the graphical editing commands.

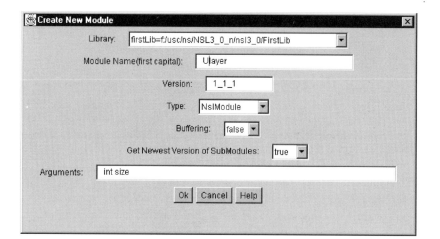

Figure 4.6
New Icon Prompt

In figure 4.6 we note that the first thing in the Icon Prompt Window is the library name. By default the last library we enter is the first library on the list. Next, we type in the name **Ulayer as the icon or module name (the icon is just one view of the module).** We also note here that the first letter of **Ulayer** is capitalized since it is a module and not an instance of one. Next we specify the version number of the module or icon we are creating. We will take the default 1_1_1. Next we specify the icon type corresponding to the type of template that we want to specify. At this point we choose **NslModule** since we are about to specify a module (see table 4.1), and we would like the buffering to be "false" for non-double buffering (see table 4.2). Next we select the option of "float all submodules" which allows specify the default option to apply to submodule of this module (see table 4.3). This will be explained in more detail later. Finally, we specify the arguments for this module/icon, and there is only one "int size".

Module Types	Description
NslModule	leaf and middle level modules
NslModel	top level module
NslClass	user defined class
NslInModule	stimuli
NslOutModule	output displays

Table 4.1
Module Types

Buffering Choices	Description
true	double buffering of output ports—this option is for simulated parallel processing
false	no buffering—this option is for sequential processing (default)

Table 4.2
Buffering Choices

Get Newest Version of Submodules	Description
true	Specify a default that submodule versions may change
false	Specify a default that submodule versions may not change.

Table 4.3
"Get Newest Version of Submodules" Choices

When we are finished we select "OK". You should see a figure similar to that shown in figure 4.7.

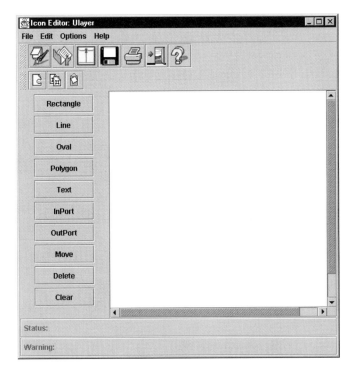

Figure 4.7
Icon Editor Window after
Ulayer Module just created.

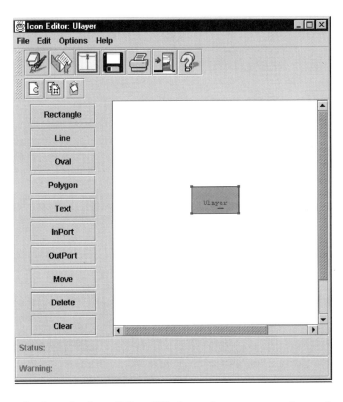

Figure 4.8
The Ulayer's Icon without
Ports.

We then go back to the Icon Editor Window where we press the **rectangle** button. To get the rectangle icon in the canvas we first move the mouse to the canvas window and then drag the mouse across the screen until the rectangle is the desired size. The output of this is shown in figure 4.8.

Specifying the Ports on the Icon

Now we want to add two input ports, *v_in and s_in,* and one output port, *uf,* to the icon. This is done by selecting "InPort" and then selecting "OutPort". A popup window will appear similar to the one in figure 4.9.

In this window we first type the name, *s_in*. Then a window which looks like that in figure 4.10 will appear. We specify what kind of data structure the port will hold, mainly **NslDinInt, NslDinFloat** or **NslDinDouble**. In this case we choose NslDinDouble. Next we specify the Dimension X where *X* represents the dimension: 0, 1, 2, 3, 4, or higher-Dim. Nsl currently only handles dimension of 4 or less but you can create your own user defined type with more than 4 dimensions. In this example, we choose "1" as the dimension. Direction indicates the direction the user would like the port to point "left→right", "right→left", "up→down", or "down→up". We choose "left→right". The "Signal Type" indicates whether the port has an excitatory or inhibitory affect on the module. We choose the signal type to be "excitatory", and the parameters to be just the "size" of the array used. The parameters correspond to the same parameters we would provide in the NSLM language. (*s_in* has 10 elements which will be defined through the "size" parameter.) When done entering, select "**OK**" from the bottom of the window. See figure 4.10.

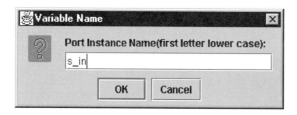

Figure 4.9
Input Port Name s_in on the Ulayer module.

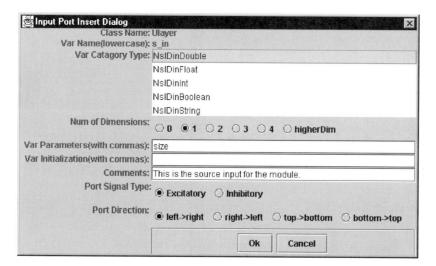

Figure 4.10
Input Port information for s_in on the Ulayer module

Once entered, you will need to specify the position of the pin or port. For convenience, select any spot on the Icon Canvas where you would like the end point of the pin to go. We have selected a location such that it looks like the input is going into the rectangle. See figure 4.11.

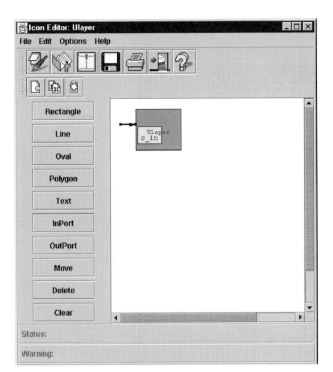

Figure 4.11
Input Port s_in on the Ulayer module

For input port *v_in*, we choose type NslDinDouble0, and we choose "left→right" as the direction. We choose the "excitatory" signal type, and there are no parameters. When done entering, select "**OK**" from the bottom. See figure 4.12.

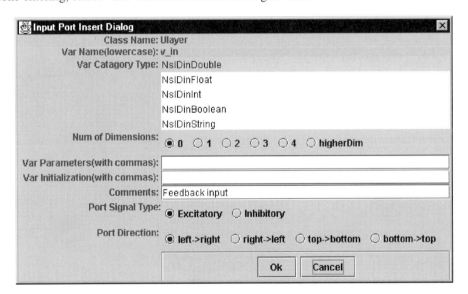

Figure 4.12
Input Port Information for *v_in*

The resulting port is shown in figure 4.13.

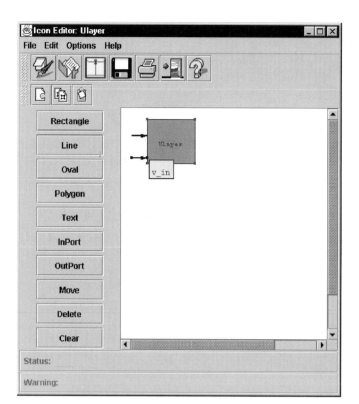

Figure 4.13
Input Port picture for *v_in*.

For port *uf*, we select the "OutPort" button, and type the name *uf*, choose the option "NslDoutDouble1", with direction "left→right", and parameter "size". When done entering select "OK" from the bottom as shown in figure 4.14.

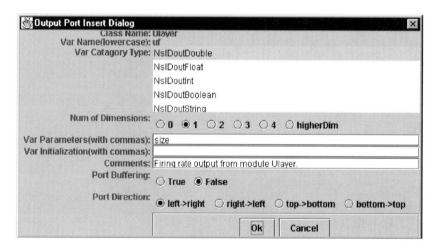

Figure 4.14
Output Port Information for *uf*.

We next save the icon by selecting the **File→Save** menu option from the Icon Editor window. We have now completed the icon creation process and should have an icon with port entries as shown in figure 4.15.

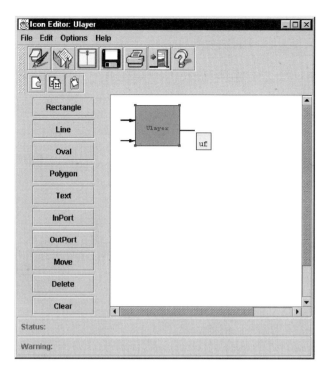

Figure 4.15
Output Port picture for uf.

Now it is time to create the second icon, **Vlayer**. **Vlayer** is created in exactly the same manner as **Ulayer**, except that its input port is *u_in* (with dimension 1 and parameter *"size" without the quotes*) and its output port is *vf* (with no dimension). After completing it, we are ready to move on to creating the schematic of the **MaxSelector** module itself.

Creating the Schematic

To create a schematic from the Schematic Editor Window select the **Module→New Module** menu option. A window should appear similar to the one below. Type in the name "MaxSelector" and version number "1_1_1". Specify the library as the **c:\users\me\nsl3_0\FirstLib** or whatever library you are using. Since this module is going to be a middle level module, we will declare it to be of type "NslModule". When you are finished select "OK" as shown in figure 4.16.

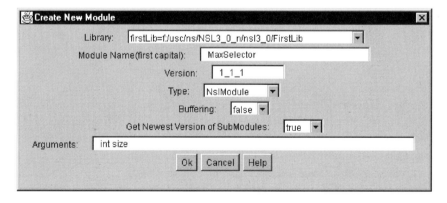

Figure 4.16
New Module Creation Window for MaxSelector.

Now we are going to add the two icons we just created and then connect them. First select the **Insert→Icon** menu option. A popup window will appear, similar to figure 4.17. We type in the instance name of u1.

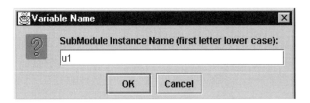

Figure 4.17
Submodule instance name
popup dialog.

Next, a popup window similar to the one in figure 4.18 appears. We fill in the instance information: which is the instance name and the instance parameters. In this case, u1 and size. Instead of typing in the name of the library, module, and version, we simple select the "Or Choose File" option and select the **Ulayer** icon from the library as shown in figure 4.19.

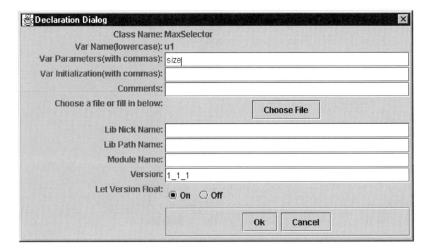

Figure 4.18
Choose submodule or icon
popup window.

In figure 4.19 if we click on the library name we want (in this case the first line), then we will see a list of modules to choose from. If we click on the **Ulayer** module, we will see the different versions of this module as shown. For this exercise, we will version "1_1_1".

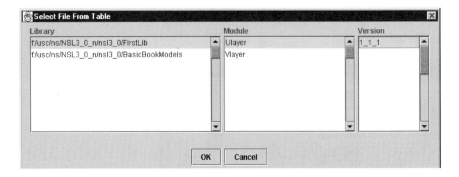

Figure 4.19
Selection of the Ulayer module
from the Declaration Dialog
"Choose File" popup.

Finally, we return to the Declaration Dialog box, and the fields for library, module and version are filled in for us as show in figure 4.20. The "Let Version Float" option allows us to specify that we want to take the most recent version of the module or icon— always. This means that even if someone else changes a submodule, we want the latest updates. If we do not want the changes to the submodule, say **Ulayer,** to affect our schematic, then we should set the option to "Let Version Float" to false. Finally, we select "OK" as shown in figure 4.20.

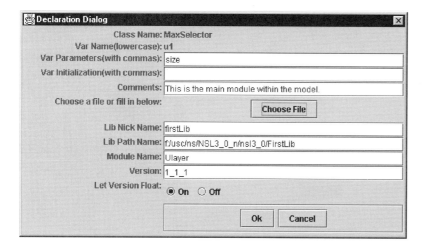

Figure 4.20
Filled in Open Module Dialog
Box.

The **Ulayer** icon with an instance name of **u1** will appear on the Schematic Canvas. You will need to take your mouse and select the icon and move it to where you would like it to be located. See where we put it in figure 4.21.

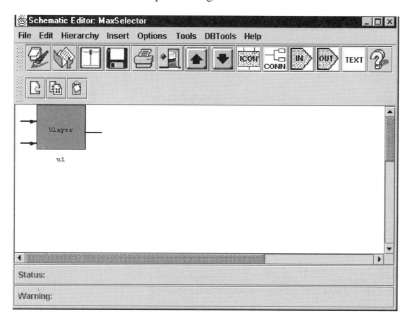

Figure 4.21
Icon placed on schematic.

Next select the "Insert→Icon" command, and use the **Choose File** button to find the **Vlayer** icon template name we just created. Give it an instance name of **v1**. And again, you will need to move *v1* to where you would like it to be located. See figure 4.22.

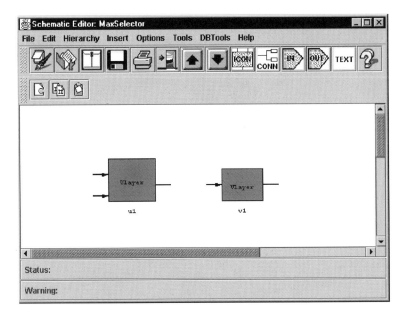

Figure 4.22
The u1 instance and v1 instance placed in a schematic.

Next we must add input and output ports to the MaxSelector schematic. We select the "Insert→Inport" menu option and a pop-up window appears. The name is "in", the type is "NslDinDouble1", the direction is "left→right", the signal type is excitatory, and the parameter is *size*. See figure 4.23.

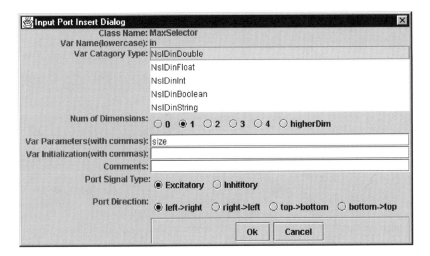

Figure 4.23
MaxSelector input port specification.

Again, move the input port icon into position as shown in figure 4.24. (We sometimes call these ports "inports".)

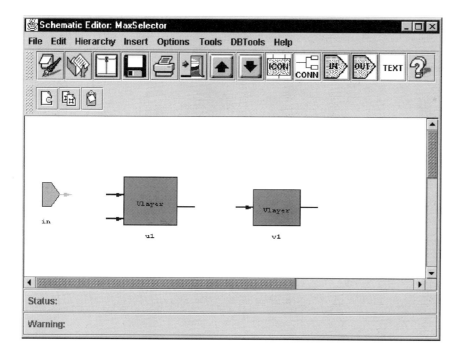

Figure 4.24
MaxSelector input port
specification.

We also must add an output port to this schematic. Add an output port by selecting "Insert→Outport" from the menu. The name of this port should be "out", the type is "NslDoutDouble0", the direction is "left-→right", the buffering is set to true, and the parameter is "size". See figure 4.25.

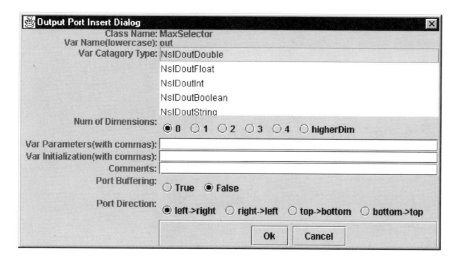

Figure 4.25
MaxSelector output port
specification.

You should now see the picture in figure 4.26.

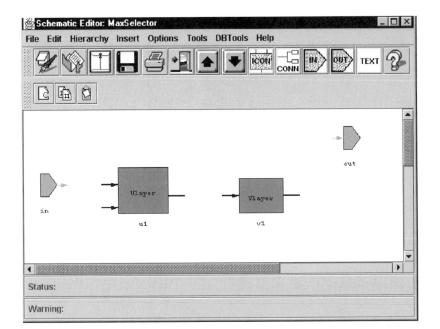

Figure 4.26
All icons placed in the
MaxSelector module.

Finally, with all of the icons in place we are ready to add the "interconnect". Select **insert→connection** from the Schematic Editor menu. (But before doing so make sure you do not have anything else selected. You can unselect an object by click on the right mouse button.) You can tell that you are in "connection" mode by the status window at the bottom. It should say "Insert Connection". Let us connect the icons moving from left to right. First, place your mouse over the output pin of the input port "in". Push the mouse button down. Next, drag the mouse to the upper input pin on the "u1" icon. Release the mouse about in the middle of the pin. You should see a picture similar to figure 4.27.

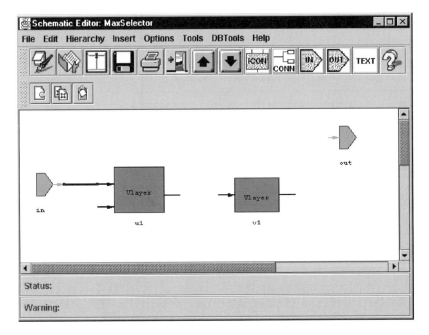

Figure 4.27
First line of interconnect
between "in" and "u1".

Next, place your mouse over the output port of the "u1" instance. (First, a little flag with the name of the pin should appear.) Push the mouse down and drag the mouse to the inport of the v1 instance and release the mouse button. Next, place your mouse over the outport of the v1 instance, push the mouse down, and drag the mouse to the right by about one half inch, release the mouse. With the mouse in the same place, press the mouse down and drag it downward one inch. Release the mouse. With the mouse in the same place, press the mouse down and drag it to the left until it is just past the "u1" input pins. Release the mouse. With the mouse in the same place, press the mouse down and drag it to the lower input pin of the "u1" icon. You should then see the picture in figure 4.28.

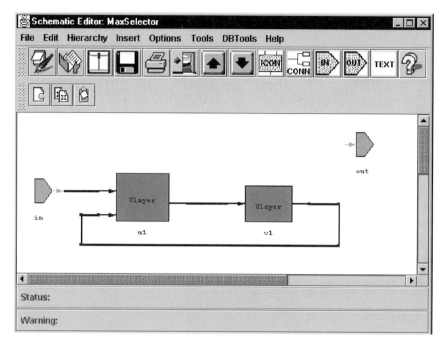

Figure 4.28
Connection between the output port of v1 and the input port of u1.

The last connection we need to make is from the "u1" output port to the output port of the MaxSelector schematic itself. Move the mouse over the output pin of the icon "u1" and push down. Next drag the mouse up about three-quarters of an inch, and release the mouse. With the mouse in the same position, drag it to the input side of the "out" output port icon, and release the mouse.

At this point, we have just completed our first schematic. The result is shown in figure 4.29.

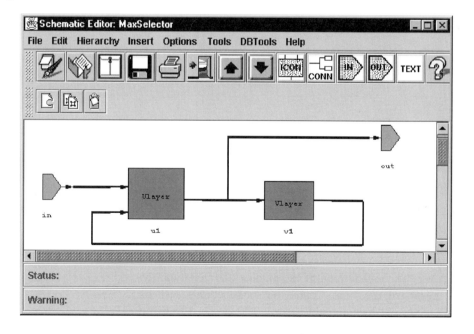

Figure 4.29
Finished Schematic of MaxSelector module.

Mouse Action Commands

Before we move on, we would also like to describe some of the mouse action commands that SCS provides. We have already mentioned the "unselect" option, and here are three more.

- Select one object—The user clicks on any object in the schematic canvas and that object will be highlighted, indicating that it is selected. If the user keeps pressing the Shift key down, then the selected objects will be this newly selected one plus previous selected ones.

- Unselect object—When an object is in a selected mode, then clicking with the right mouse button again will make it unselected.

- Move object—The user can move any object (individual or group object) in the canvas by first clicking on it and then dragging the mouse.

- Descend—In current schematic page, if the user double clicks on a module, then the detailed layer corresponding to that module will be shown in the canvas.

Automatic Generation of Code

After completing the schematic we can see the NSLM code that it generates by selecting **Tools→View NSLM** from the Schematic Editor window. Next, select **File→Open** from the **NSLM Viewer** window and open the MaxSelector module we just created, as shown in figure 4.30.

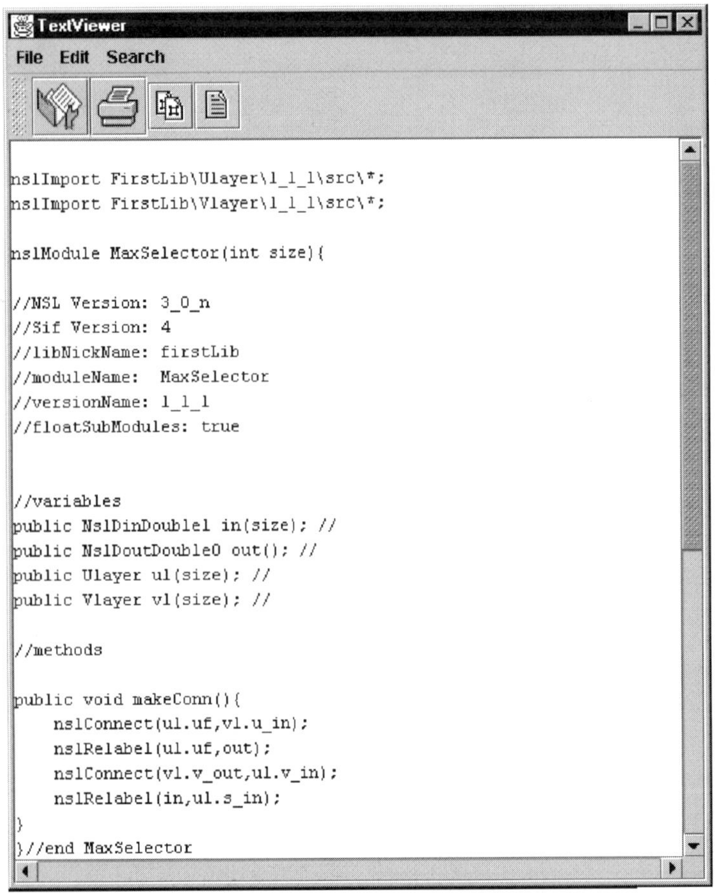

Figure 4.30
NSLM Viewer with MaxSelector module.

```
nslImport FirstLib\Ulayer\1_1_1\src\*;
nslImport FirstLib\Vlayer\1_1_1\src\*;

nslModule MaxSelector(int size){

//NSL Version: 3_0_n
//Sif Version: 4
//libNickName: firstLib
//moduleName:  MaxSelector
//versionName: 1_1_1
//floatSubModules: true


//variables
public NslDinDouble1 in(size); //
public NslDoutDouble0 out(); //
public Ulayer ul(size); //
public Vlayer vl(size); //

//methods

public void makeConn(){
    nslConnect(ul.uf,vl.u_in);
    nslRelabel(ul.uf,out);
    nslConnect(vl.v_out,ul.v_in);
    nslRelabel(in,ul.s_in);
}
}//end MaxSelector
```

We notice that SCS has generated the definition of the module, the ports and the variables for us. It has also generated the "makeConn", but not methods such as "initModule", "initTrain", and "initRun" which are still needed. The we need to fill in these other methods using the NSLM editor. We will examine how to use the NSLM Editor next.

Manual Generation of Leaf Level Code

Although a lot of the code has been automatically generated, we still need to fill in the code for both the **Ulayer** and **Vlayer** modules. We do this with the NSLM editor. Select **Tools→NSLM Editor** from the Schematic Editor window. Next select **File→Open**, from the NSLM Editor window and then select **Ulayer** version "1_1_1" from the list. An editor similar to the following should appear. Notice how **template oriented** this editor is, as shown in figure 4.31.

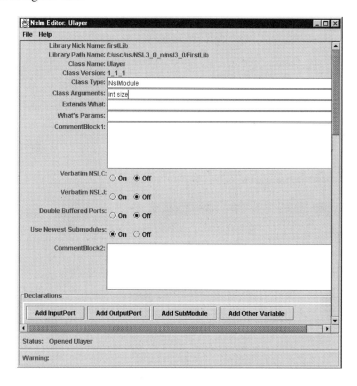

Figure 4.31
The First Half of the NSLM Editor Window showing the Name, Arguments, and Flags.

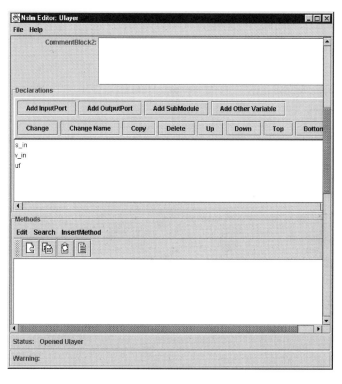

Figure 4.32
Second half of the NSLM Editor Window showing the variables and the Methods Editor.

Now we just need to add the internal variables *up,* and *h1.* Add these variables and give them the same data types and parameters as in the figure 4.33 and figure 4.34

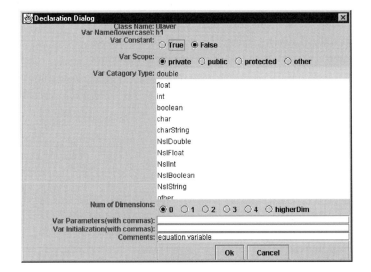

Figure 4.33
Adding the Equation Variable h1 to the Ulayer.

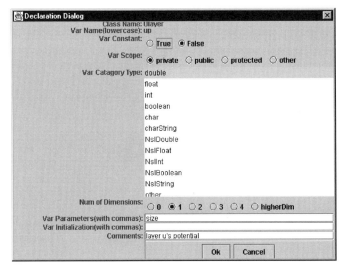

Figure 4.34
Adding Ulayer's potential layer *up*

We note that the output port variables are already declared but not initialized; thus we will initialize them in the initModule and initRun methods within the Methods Window. See figure 4.35.

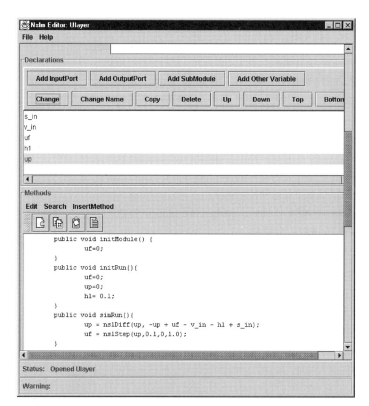

Figure 4.35
The Ulayer NSLM code.

```
public void initModule() {
        uf=0;
}
public void initRun(){
        uf=0;
        up=0;
        h1= 0.1;
}
public void simRun(){
        up = nslDiff(up, -up + uf - v_in - h1 + s_in);
        uf = nslStep(up,0.1,0,1.0);
}
```

Next, add the **initRun** method and the **simRun** method as shown in the figure 4.34. And then select **File→Save**. Now do the same for **Vlayer** using the code in figure 4.36.

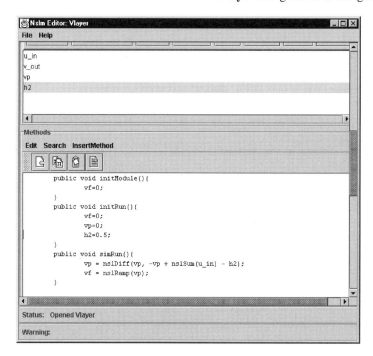

Figure 4.36
The Vlayer NSLM code.

```
public void initModule(){
        vf=0;
}
public void initRun(){
        vf=0;
        vp=0;
        h2=0.5;
}
public void simRun(){
        vp = nslDiff(vp, -vp + nslSum(u_in) - h2);
        vf = nslRamp(vp);
}
```

Generating NSLM Code

We can generate the NSLM code for our modules at any point in the development. For the MaxSelectorModel we need to generate the top level module called the model—MaxSelectorModel (A popup window will appear similar to figure 4.16). We also need to create the modules "MaxSelectorStimulus" and "MaxSelectorOutput", see figure (3.12) and code segments 3.13, 3.14, and 3.15.

To generate the NSLM (mod or module) files for both the NSLJ System and the NSLC System, the Schematic Editor menu select "Tools-→Generate NSLM". The program performs automatic checks to make sure that the icons used in the schematic match what is contained in the NSLM View, it then generates the NSLM code. Once the icons, schematics, and leaf level modules have been created we are ready to make a *Makefile* and executable code.

Compiling and Generating the Executable File

To generate the *Makefile* and executable code, select "Tools→Build Java Version" or select "Tools→Build C++ Version". (When building the executable code, the system checks to see that all of the "mod" files are created and the proper time stamps are on the files. Thus, we can actually skip the "Generate NSLM Code" step if we plan to make an executable file anyway.) We provide both generate options so that we can execute both systems if we desire. Both commands will prompt for the name of the model executable to be built. (This window is the same as that in figure 4.19) The *Makefile* and the executable file will be generated for your particular platform that you are running on and the particular operating system that you are using. These files can be found in the subdirectory "exe" directory below the version directory. Additionally, models can be compiled from a system shell writing 'nsljc model' for Java and 'nslcc model' for C++. For additional compilation and execution details see Appendix V where web site links are specified".

Reusing Modules and Models

To re-use an existing module, simply select it from one of the libraries and include it the schematic for your new module. To reuse a model, you must rename it. If you add ports to an existing model, it them becomes a module, and you must specify the type as such when you go to save your new module.

Copying Existing Modules and Models

As mentioned above we can copy modules, modify them, and give them new names. To copy a module, simply open the existing module in any editor and save it under a new name (you can also save it under the same name but a different version number).

4.3 Summary

We have introduced the different tools available in the Schematic Capture System in helping the user with model creation. In particular, we have shown how to visually build modules and automatically generate code. Some of the tools we covered where the Schematic Editor, the Icon Editor, the NSLM Editor, the Library Path Editor, and the Library Manager. We also showed how to create a library, an icon, and a schematic.[2]

Notes

1. The NSL Schematic Capture System version is based on Sun Microsystem's Java 1.2 programming language and virtual machine. SCS can only be executed as an application and not as an applet since applets put security restrictions on generating output files. We assume that the user has a two-button mouse attached to the computer.

2. Since SCS is one of our newer applications, we encourage the reader to review the latest documentation and technical reports on the NSL web site. See Appendix V for details.

5 User Interface and Graphical Windows

The NSL graphical user interface provides interactive simulation control by means of the NSL Executive Window and different types of input and output displays customized for every model. Each model may include a number of *protocols* corresponding to different experiments involving different sets of input, parameters and graphics displays. In a well-written model, every model experiment should correspond to one of these protocols. Sometimes, however, models only come with scripts that must be read via the Script Window and sometimes they only come with "README" files that describe the proper script command sequences that should be issued to get the different results. (The script language is described in chapter 7.) The NSL graphical user interface is designed to provide an environment that protects as much as possible the novice model user from having to type too many commands. At the same time, the graphical interface provides flexibility for the advanced model builder to experiment with multiple simulation options in analyzing model results.

Ideally every model executes with just selecting one of the protocols from the Protocol menu, and then selecting the Simulation, TrainAndRunAll menu item.

5.1 NSL Executive User Interface
When NSL is first invoked, the NSL Executive Window is displayed as shown in figure 5.1. From the Executive window the user controls the simulation and brings up other display windows or frames.

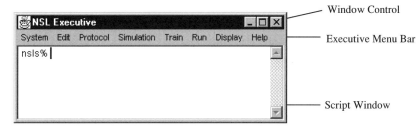

Window Control

Executive Menu Bar

Script Window

Figure 5.1
The NSL Executive Window controls model simulation. It includes menu options as well as a script window for written commands.

The top portion of the NSL executive window corresponds to the "Window Control" section containing a title and three buttons for window control. Underneath the "Window Control" the "Executive Menu Bar" contains five menu buttons: **System, Edit, Protocol, Simulation, Train, Run, Display,** and **Help**, discussed in the following sections. The bottom portion of the window corresponds to the "Script Window" allowing the user to interactively type commands. Any command that can be selected from one of the menu pull-downs can also be typed in the Script Window as well as stored in files for later retrieval. Script commands are discussed more thoroughly in chapter 7.

System Menu
The **System** menu contains commands related to general system aspects. In particular, the menu contains the following items:

- **Source**—to read NSLS model scripts.
- **Set**—to read or modify system parameter values.
- **Exit**—to stop the simulation, close all windows, and exit.

Edit Menu
The **Edit** menu allows the user to select text from the script window, copy text from the script window into the clipboard or paste text into the script window from the clipboard. These commands are quite handy when importing commands to the script window or saving script commands into another file. The menu contains the following items:

- **Select**—select text from the script window.
- **Copy**—copy text from the script window into the clipboard.
- **Paste**—paste text from clipboard into the script window.

Protocol Menu

The **Protocol** menu specifies the *protocols* or experiments included with each model. Protocols are model driven, i.e. the modeler decides which protocols should be placed in the menu. The default "manual" protocol is always provided allowing the user to write script commands to set up stimuli and parameters for the simulation. Protocols are an easy way for the model builder to setup customized input and output windows to handle model input and output respectively. This customization takes place directly in NSLM. The protocol menu contains the following items:

- **Manual**—default user specified input by means of scripts.
- *Additional Protocols*—Modeler define additional protocols (none by default).

Simulation Menu

The **Simulation** menu contains different options to control the general aspects of the simulation, such as setting up system variables and global initialization of the modules (see chapter 6, The NSLM Language). The following menu options exist:

- The **InitSys** menu item executes the *initSys* method for every module.
- The **InitModule** menu item executes the *initModule* method for every module.
- The **TrainAndRunAll** menu item executes the initialization of the training epochs, all of the epochs for the training phase of simulation as well as the initialization of the run epochs and all of the epochs for the run phase of simulation.
- The **EndModule** menu item executes the *EndModule* method of every module.
- The **EndSys** menu item executes the *EndSys* method of every module.

Train Menu

The **Train** menu item executes all the methods necessary to train the model. The menu contains the following options:

- The **InitTrainEpochs** menu item executes all of the "initTrainEpochs" methods for all modules.
- The **InitTrain** menu item executes all of the "initTrain" methods for all modules.
- The **SimTrain** menu item executes all of the "simTrain" methods over and over again until "system.trainEndTime" is reached. The system.trainEndTime is the system variable that specifies how long the training process should last. Based on the training delta used, the system.trainEndTime is used to calculate the number of cycles for each epoch.
- The **EndTrain** menu item executes all of the "endTrain" methods.
- The **EndTrainEpochs** menu item executes all of the "endTrainEpochs" methods.
- The **Train** menu item executes one epoch that includes the execution of initTrain, simTrain for the number of cycles or steps specified, and finally endTrain.
- The **DoTrainEpochTimes** menu item executes the initTrainEpochs method for all modules, then executes the initTrain, simTrain (repeated for n cycles), and endTrain methods for however many training epochs have been specified with system.numTrainEpochs. And finally, it executes the endTrainEpochs method for all modules.
- We can execute the **Break** command to stop the simulation between cycles. We can then use the "continue" menu option to continue the simulation.
- We can execute the **BreakModules** command to stop the simulation between modules.
- We can execute the **BreakCycles** command to stop the simulation between cycles.
- We can execute the **BreakEpochs** command to stop the simulation between epochs.

- The **Continue** menu item continues the simulation from the last break point. It then executes all of the "simTrain" methods over and over again until "system.trainEndTime" is reached.
- The **ContinueModule** menu item continues the simulation from the last break point. If the last break was with BreakModules, then it continues with the next module in the scheduler. It then executes all of the "simTrain" methods over and over again until the last module in the scheduler is executed.
- The **ContinueCycle** menu item continues the simulation from the last break point. If the last break was with BreakCycles, then it continues with the next cycle. It then executes all of the "simTrain" methods over and over again until "system.trainEndTime" is reached.
- The **ContinueEpoch** menu item continues the simulation from the last break point. If the last break was with BreakEpochs, then it continues with the next epoch. It then executes all of the epochs over and over again until **numTrainEpochs** is reached.
- The **StepModule** menu item executes the "simTrain" method of the next module in the scheduler.
- The **StepCycle** menu item executes all of the "simTrain" method once for each module in the scheduler.
- The **StepEpoch** menu item executes one epoch that includes the initTrain method, the simTrain methods for however many cycles are specified, and the endTrain method.

Run Menu

The **Run** menu item executes all the methods necessary to run the model. The menu contains the following options:

- The **InitRunEpochs** menu item executes all of the "initRunEpochs" methods for all of the modules
- The **InitRun** menu item executes all of the "initRun" methods for all of the modules
- The **SimRun** menu item executes all of the "simRun" methods over and over again until "system.runEndTime" is reached. The system.runEndTime is the system variable that specifies how long the Running process should last. Based on the Run delta used, the system.runEndTime is used to calculate the number of cycles for each epoch.
- The **EndRun** menu item executes all of the "endRun" methods.
- The **EndRunEpochs** menu item executes all of the "endRunEpochs" methods.
- The **Run** menu item executes one epoch that includes the execution of initRun, simRun for the number of cycles or steps specified, and finally endRun.
- The **DoRunEpochTimes** menu item executes the initRunEpochs method for all modules, then executes the initRun, simRun (repeated for n cycles), and endRun methods for however many training epochs have been specified with system.numRunEpochs. And finally, it executes the endRunEpochs method for all modules.
- We can execute the **Break** command to stop the simulation between cycles. We can then use the "continue" menu option to continue the simulation.
- We can execute the **BreakModules** command to stop the simulation between modules.
- We can execute the **BreakCycles** command to stop the simulation between cycles.
- We can execute the **BreakEpochs** command to stop the simulation between epochs.
- The **Continue** menu item continues the simulation from the last break point. It then executes all of the "simRun" methods over and over again until "system.RunEndTime" is reached.
- The **ContinueModule** menu item continues the simulation from the last break point. If the last break was with BreakModules, then it continues with the next module in

the scheduler. It then executes all of the "simRun" methods over and over again until the last module in the scheduler is executed.

- The **ContinueCycle** menu item continues the simulation from the last break point. If the last break was with BreakCycles, then it continues with the next cycle. It then executes all of the "simRun" methods over and over again until "system.RunEndTime" is reached.

- The **ContinueEpoch** menu item continues the simulation from the last break point. If the last break was with BreakEpochs, then it continues with the next epoch. It then executes all of the epochs over and over again until **numRunEpochs** is reached.

- The **StepModule** menu item executes the "simRun" method of the next module in the scheduler.

- The **StepCycle** menu item executes all of the "simRun" method once for each module in the scheduler.

- The **StepEpoch** menu item executes one epoch that includes the initRun method, the simRun methods for however many cycles are specified, and the endRun method.

Display Menu

The **Display** menu contains commands to control output and input display window creation. The display options in the menu are,

- **NslOutFrame** used to create a frame to display results of model variables,
- **NslInFrame** used to create a frame to control input stimulus and model parameters.

The two frame types are described in the following sections.

Help menu

The **Help** menu retrieves help on any command. It contains three types of help: "How To", "Command Help", and "Setup".

5.2 NslOutFrames

Upon selection of a new **NslOutFrame** from the executive window, a **NslOutFrame** will appear with a long name in the form of ".nsl.*frameNameX*" where the ".nsl" comes from the fact that all windows are actually subwindows of the **NslExecutiveWindow** associated with ".nsl" prefix. The *frameName* is set to "OutModule" when selecting an output frame ("InModule" when selecting an input frame). The *X* is assigned to an incremental integer number resulting in names such as ".nsl.OutModule2". A popup window will appear first requesting a protocol name to be associated with the new **NslOutFrame**, as seen in figure 5.2. Note that if no protocols exist for the model then only the "manual" option on the right hand side will appear.

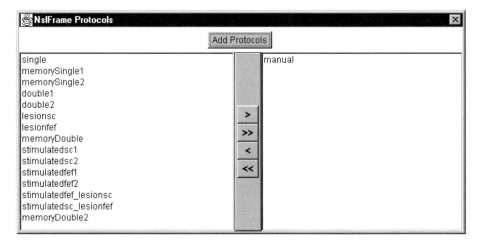

Figure 5.2
Popup Window for Adding a New NslOutFrame

Once the OutputFrame or more appropriately, the OutputModule has registered for certain protocols, a new window is instantiated as shown in figure 5.3. At the top is the **title** or frame name. Underneath the frame's title is the **frame's menu bar**. In this menu bar we have the **Frame**, **Canvas**, and **Help** menus, as follows,

- **Frame**—The **Frame** menu items are responsible for changing the items and attributes of the frame.
- **Canvas**—The **Canvas** menu items are responsible for changing the items and attributes of a selected canvas.
- **Help**—The **Help** menu displays information on any command.

In the middle of the frame is the **drawing area** or the place where canvases can be placed. And at the bottom of the frame is the **status bar**.

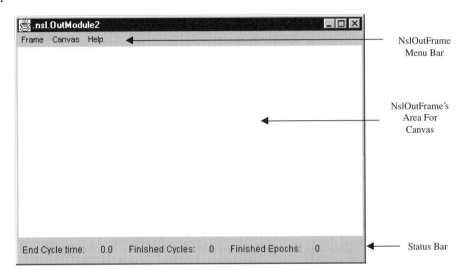

Figure 5.3
The NslOutFrame without any canvases

The NslOutFrame's Frame Menu

A **NslOutFrame** is basically a container for **NslOutCanvases** displays of NSL variables. All NSL variables that have been declared to have either "Read" or "Write" visibility can be displayed in a **NslOutFrame**. The **NslOutFrame** contains a menu bar for adding new canvases/variables and for manipulating the canvases, as shown in figure 5.4.

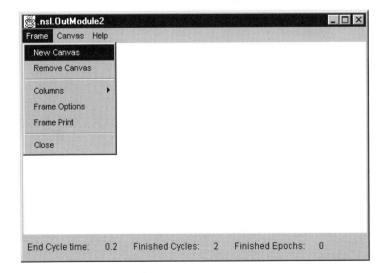

Figure 5.4
NslOutFrame's Menu

The **Frame** menu contains commands necessary to change the contents and attributes of the frame. These commands are **New Canvas, Remove Canvas, Columns, Frame Options, Frame Print,** and **Close.** The following describes these commands.

Create a New Canvas Containing a Plot of a NSL Variable

To add a variable display to an existing **NslOutFrame**, you go to the **NslOutFrame**'s menu bar and select "Frame→New Canvas" as shown in figure 5.4. A popup window as shown in figure 5.5 will appear.

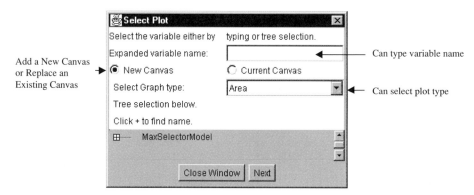

Figure 5.5
Add New or Change Current Canvas-Popup Window

At the top of the window, we have the choice of typing a full path variable name, or we can select the variable by tracing down the hierarchy tree in the lower gray area of the window. In this example, we will select the variable from the hierarchy tree. To do this, we first click on the little "plus sign" icon next to the word "**MaxSelectorModel**". Next we click on the "**plus sign**" icon next to the word "**stimulus**", and then the plus of **s_out**. At this point the tree should look like that in figure 5.6.

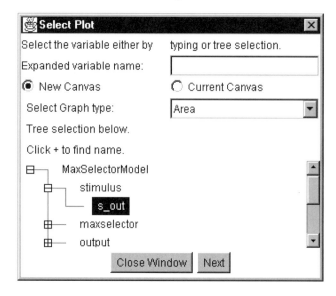

Figure 5.6
New Canvas or Change Current Canvas Popup Window with selection of **s_out**

To add the selection to the **NslOutFrame**, we select the **Next** button at the bottom of the window. We repeat the process again this time selecting a different type of plot. In the "Graph Type Selector" we change the graph or plot type to "**Temporal**". (The plot types are **Area, Bar, Dot, Spatial, String, Temporal, AreaColor, MultiTemporal** and **XY** being described in the section titled "Output Graph Types".) This time we expand the plus sign next to the **maxselector** module, then **u1**, then **up**. The window should look like that in figure 5.7.

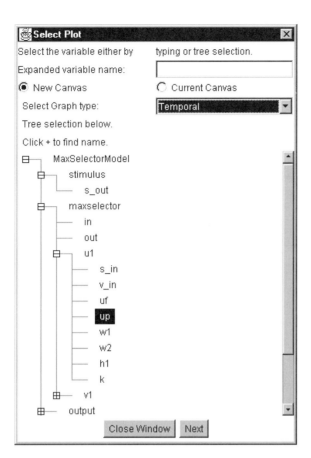

Figure 5.7
New Canvas or Change Current
Canvas Popup Window with
selection of **up**.

We select the **Next** button to add **up** to the NslOutFrame, and then we add **uf.** To add **uf,** we change the graph type back to **Area** and select the NSL variable "maxselector.u1.uf". After we have done this, we select the "**Next**" button at the bottom of the window. The resulting canvases are shown in figure 5.8.

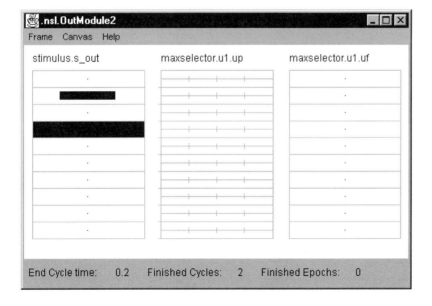

Figure 5.8
An example of a NslOutFrame
that contains a menu bar,
drawing area, and three
NslOutCanvases corresponding
to the variables stimulus.s_out,
maxselector.u1.up, and
maxselector.u1.uf.

Selecting and Deselecting a Canvas from a Frame

We can select a specific canvas in a frame by moving the mouse to the desired canvas and then clicking the left mouse button on it. The canvas will become highlighted in the default highlighting color. Once selected there are a number of operations that can be applied to the canvas as will be seen later on such as changing the type of graph or variable being displayed. To deselect the canvas either click the mouse's right button or select another canvas.

Deleting a Canvas from a Frame

To delete a canvas from a frame, first select the canvas and then choose "Frame→Delete Canvas" from the Frame's menu.

Modifying the Number of Rows and Columns in a NslOutFrame

To modify the number of rows or columns **NslOutFrame** displays, select "Frame→Columns" and then the number of columns desired. This will also affect the number of rows displayed since if we display 8 canvases, we can display them in 1 row with 8 columns, or 2 rows with 4 columns, or 4 rows and 2 columns, etc.

Positioning and Resizing a Canvas

To change the position of a canvas, you need to delete it first and then re-add it in the desired location. To resize a canvas we can only make the frame larger or smaller. Currently all canvas sizes are the same in every frame as seen in figure 5.8.

Changing Options that Effect All Canvases

To change the update time, the starting graph time, ending graph time, the vertical minimum, vertical maximum, the default colors (background, grid color, drawing color) in every canvas currently displayed or later instantiated in this frame, select the "Frame→Frame Options" menu item. This will cause the popup window shown in figure 5.9. to appear. The "Apply to Future" button causes the canvases that are created in the future to have these default properties. The "Apply to All" button causes all of the current and future canvas to have these properties. And the "Cancel" button takes no action.

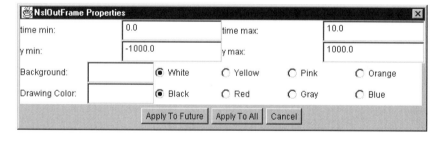

Figure 5.9
The NslOutFrame's Options for Properties Popup Menu

Printing a Frame

To print a **NslOutFrame** or to save an image of a **NslOutFrame** in any of the supported formats[1] select the **NslOutFrame**'s "Frame→Frame Print" menu item. To print one of the **NslOutCanvases**, first select that canvas and then select the "Frame→Print option". A print popup window will appear. The look of this window varies depending on the environment.

Closing a NslOutFrame

To close a **NslOutFrame**, simply select the "Frame→Close" option. This will close the frame, but will leave the simulation still executing. To exit the NSL System, select "System→Exit" from the Executive window.

The NslOutFrame's Canvas Menu

All of the Frame's Canvas Menu items pertain to changing the properties of a particular canvas. A canvas must first be selected with the mouse. Once selected the canvas will become highlighted in the default highlighting color, as shown in figure 5.10 where the "**maxselector.u1.up**" graph has been selected.

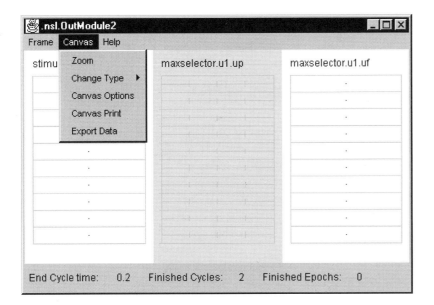

Change Type of Graph in Canvas

To change the type of graph displayed within the canvas, select "Canvas→Change Type". A submenu will appear with the following graph type options: Area, Bar, Dot, Spatial, String, **Temporal**, **AreaColor**, **ImageColor**, **MultiTemporal** and **XY**. All of these graph types are described in the section titled "**Output Graph Types**".

Zoom Canvas

To see the labels on the axis and tick marks, first select the canvas, and then select "Canvas→Zoom". A separate Zoom window will appear, as shown in figure 5.11. Once the window appears, drag the mouse over the area of interest starting in one corner and holding down the mouse button, drag mouse to the opposite corner. Then select "ZoomIn", and the window should now magnify the area selected. (In figure 5.11, we have actually executed the model before selecting the graph, and then we selected zoom.)

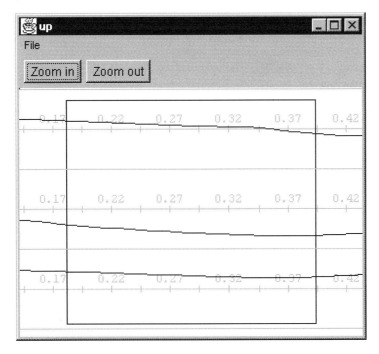

Options for a Canvas

To change the property options of a selected canvas, choose "Canvas→Canvas Options" from the NslOutFrame menu bar. A Properties popup window based on the graph type displayed will appear. figure 5.12 displays the options for the "Area Level Graph".

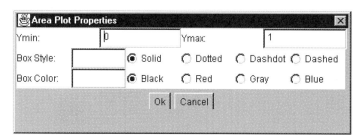

Figure 5.12
Canvas Options—Change Area
Level Graph Plot Properties

The Canvas or Plot Properties that can be changed are the *y* minimum, *y* maximum values, the style of the box, and the color of the box.

Print a Canvas

To print a canvas in any of the predetermined formats, first select the canvas and then the "Canvas→Canvas Print" menu item. A popup window should appear that looks exactly like that of the "Frame→Frame Print" menu.

Exporting the Data from a Canvas Window to a File

To export the data from a Canvas Window in one of the specified binary formats first select the canvas and then select "Canvas→Export Data". A pop-up window will appear as explained in more detail in Appendix II.

NSL Output Graph Types

NSL canvases can display different graph types, as either a basic intensity plot (shows variable's values at the current time) or a temporal plot (shows a variable's values over a certain time period). This list of graph types will grow as more and more modelers add their custom output widgets or graph types to the standard set of Nsl Output Widgets or Graphs. Thus it is recommended that you consult the NSL web site for new widgets and graphs that have been added (see Appendix II). The graph types are the following:

- **Area**—The window is divided into small rectangular boxes each representing the activity of an element of the variable during one cycle. Negative values are drawn with an open box while positive values are shaded. The shaded boxes are centered in the middle of the element and the stronger the element value, the larger the box. The graph is updated every Display Delta increment. figure 5.13 shows two such canvases, the one on the left (s_out) and the one on the right (uf).

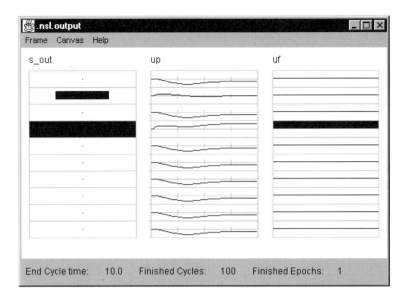

Figure 5.13
Examples of **Area** Level and
Temporal Graph Types

- **Bar**—The bar graph is similar to the area plot. Instead of drawing a box representing the value of the element, a bar is drawn instead. The bottom of the box represents the y minimum value and the top of the box the y maximum value. Positive values display a filled in bar while negative values display an open bar. The graph is updated every Display Delta increment.

- **Dot**—The dot plot is most similar to the area plot, however, instead of plotting each element as a box, a small "dot" is drawn instead and no grid is displayed. Typically, the dot plot is only applied to two-dimensional matrices and the location of the dot represents x and y coordinates. If a value is zero or negative, it is not drawn. The graph is updated every Display Delta increment. The graph on the right-hand side of figure 5.14 contains a dot plot.

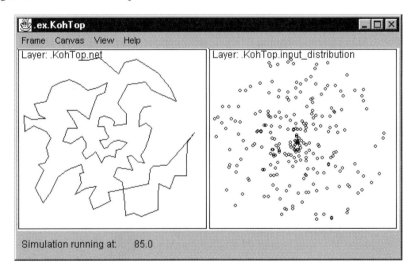

Figure 5.14
Example of **String** and **Dot**
Plots

- **Spatial**—The Spatial plot is similar to the Area plot, however, instead of shading the boxes, a point is drawn on the y-axis representing the activity of the variable. Negative values are drawn below the zero line. Positive values are drawn above the zero line. Once all elements are plotted, a line is drawn connecting the points. For two-dimensional data, the plot is draw in three dimensions. The graph is updated every Display Delta increment. figure 5.15 shows a canvas containing a three dimension spatial plot.

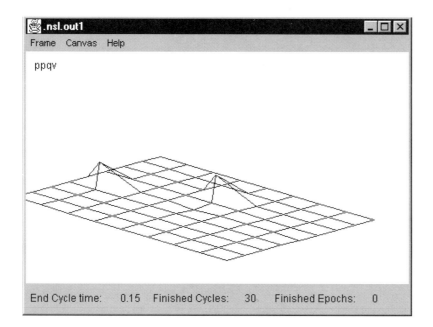

Figure 5.15
Example of Spatial Graph or Three Dimensional graph.

- **String**—The String plot is similar to the Dot plot, however, the dots are much smaller and a line is draw between consecutive dots (time wise). The graph is updated every Display Delta increment. The graph on the left-hand side of figure 5.14 contains a String plot.

- **Temporal**—The Temporal graph represents Time along the horizontal axis and the value of the element of the variable along the vertical axis. In the current version, only 1000 cycles can be viewed at any given time. If a variable has several elements, as in one and two-dimensional arrays, each element will be displayed in its own temporal plot. The middle graph shown in figure 5.13 contains a temporal plot

- **AreaColor**—For the area-level graph in color is just like the area level graph except that it uses both size denote the value of the element represented by the box and color to represent the data type of the element within the box. Each different color can represent a different type of data, such as a special type of neuron. The graph is updated every Display Delta increment.

- **ImageColor**—The color scale map represents each element of a color array as a pixel. The greater the value of the element the warmer the color.

- **MultiTemporal**—The Multi-variable Temporal graph is just like the regular temporal plot, only instead of plotting one variable it can plot up to ten variables each in its own color and line style.

- **XY**—The x axis represents one variable and the y axis represents another variable.

5.3 NslInFrames

NslInFrame is a container for one or more **NslInCanvases** that contain widgets that control the input to NSL variables. Just like the **NslOutFrames**, **NslInFrames** have a standard menu system.

The NslInFrame's Menu

The Frame menu contains all of the commands necessary to change the contents and attributes of the frame. These commands are **New Canvas, Remove Canvas, Columns, Frame Options, Frame Print,** and **Close**. These commands have already been described in section 5.2 except for the types of input widgets that can be placed on the frame when a "New Canvas" command is selected, as shown in figure 5.16.

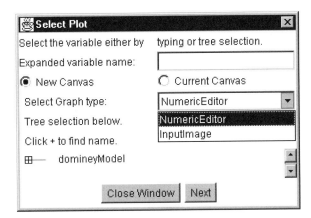

Figure 5.16

Input Widget Types that can be selected at Run-time and placed on a NslInFrame.

The NslInFrame's Canvas Menu

All of the Frame's Canvas Menu items pertain to changing the properties of a particular canvas. The canvas menu options are the same as they are in section 5.3 for the NslOutFrame.

NSL Input Graph Types

The input graph type options currently supported are:

- **NumericEditor**—The NumericEditor graph displays a one-dimensional or a two-dimensional grid containing the values of the elements. It is unique in that the values shown can also be modified for input to the simulation. figure 5.17 shows three canvases containing a numeric editor each.

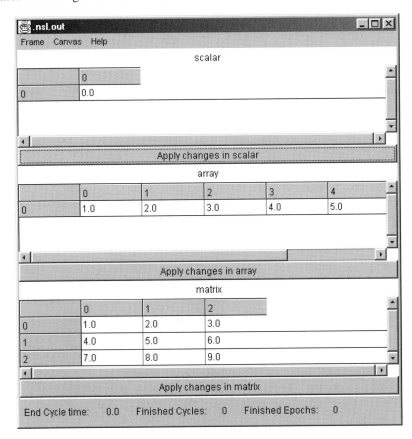

Figure 5.17

Example of the Three **NumericEditor** Canvases. The first canvas shows the variable **scalar**, and the single value it contains as well as an Apply button. The second canvas shows the variable **array**, and the four values it contains as well as an Apply button. The third canvas shows the variable **matrix**, and the nine values it contains as well as an Apply button. The values are updated every Display Delta increment.

- **InputImage**—InputImage graphs divides a canvas into small boxes; each box represents the absolute value of an element of the variable during one cycle. If the box is not selected the variable will take *wymin* value, otherwise it will be *wymax*. figure 5.18 shows two canvases containing the second one an image editor.

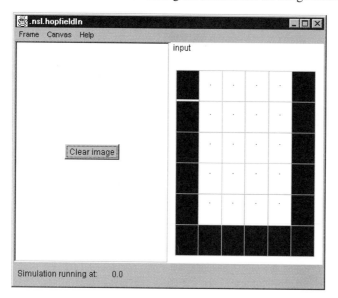

Figure 5.18
The Hopfield Example (chapter 3) of an input image editor.

5.4 Summary

In this chapter we have demonstrated the NSL user interface. We showed how the NSL Executive window is used to control the complete simulation as well as to display new windows via pull-down menus. (Users more comfortable with scripts can use the scripting language within the NSL Script window to accomplish the same tasks as explained in chapter 7.) We have also demonstrated how users can use the built-in graph types to display the results of their simulation, or as input to the simulation.

Notes

1. Different formats depending on the particular environment are PostScript (PS), Graphics Interchange Format (GIF), or Joint Picture Extraction Group (JPEG).

6 The Modeling Language NSLM

In this chapter we describe the NSLM modeling language. NSLM is a high-level programming language designed to support the construction of model architectures in NSL. For efficiency and extensibility reasons, the NSLM language is translated into either C++ or Java, depending on the chosen environment. While NSLM is a *self-contained* programming language supporting a complete set of types and expressions—the user may take advantage of the full power of C++ and Java when necessary. Yet, we strongly recommend avoiding as much as possible writing "direct" Java or C++ code but try to follow NSLM modeling philosophy and expressions as much as possible. This will result in more consistent and extensible code. In general terms, NSLM is actually a superset of either language in that it provides a set of types and expressions common to both languages together with a library of classes useful in constructing and simulating models in NSL. NSLM syntax has been kept as close as possible to Java with slight variations to simplify the task of building model architecture while at the same time supporting C++ translation as well. Once translated into either Java or C++, an appropriate compiler should process the resulting code (refer to Appendix II for supported compilers). If you are already familiar with either C++ or Java you will find much of the material discussed in this chapter quite familiar, with some aspects such as modules and ports going beyond the semantics provided by either C++ or Java. If you are not familiar with either of the two languages, we recommend getting acquainted with the basic concepts found in object-oriented programming. We recommend reading one of the introductory texts such as The C++ Programming Language by Stroustrup (1997) or Core Java by Cay Horstmann and Gary Cornell (1999), among others.

This chapter is given more as a reference for the NSLM Language than a tutorial. It and the *NSLM Methods Appendix I* reviews more structures and expressions found in the language. We start by giving an overview of general aspects followed by a description of the different language components.

6.1 Overview

There are a number of general aspects in NSLM that we will overview in this section.

General Conventions

We shall be using throughout this chapter a number of general conventions used in NSLM:

- Comments are denoted by "/*" at the beginning and "*/" at the end. Single line comments are denoted with "//" at the beginning of the comment.

- All statements end with a semicolon ";".

- We consider *object types*, *object classes* or simply *classes* as equivalent terms (some programming languages distinguish between the concept of *class* and *type*). In general, *objects* represent instances of *classes*.

- We consider *module objects* as instances of *module classes*. Similarly, *model objects* represent instances of *model classes*. We treat module classes and model classes as special kinds of object classes in the programming language sense, where module objects and model objects become special kinds of objects.

- Classes—model classes, module classes and any other object classes—begin their names with an uppercase alphabetic character, e.g. *MaxSelectorModel* or *MaxSelectorStimulus*.

- Objects—model objects, module objects and objects in general—together with variables and function begin their names with a lowercase alphabetic character, e.g. *maxSelectorModel*, *maxSelectorStimulus* or *var*.

- File names storing NSLM model definitions should have a ".mod" suffix (analogous to ".C" and ".java" suffixes generated by the NSLM compiler translation).

Types

NSLM is a *typed-language*, similar to C++ and Java, supporting different types of structures. In particular, NSLM supports the following general types:

- The *primitive* or *native* data type corresponds to the basic types available in most languages, such as C and Pascal, as well as in object-oriented languages such as C++ and Java. These types always start with a lowercase letter and consist of the ubiquitous: **int**, **float**, **double**, **char** and **void** (the null type). NSLM adds two more types to this short list: **charString** and **boolean**. The **charString** type translates into "String" in Java and "char*" in C++. The **boolean** type translates into "boolean" in Java and into an enumerated type in C++ containing 1 (true) and 0 (false).

- The general *object class* data type corresponds to the basic types available only in object-oriented languages, such as C++ and Java. As opposed to the limited set of predefined *native* or *primitive* types, *object* types represent an extensible family of *classes*, either specified by the user or provided by the language in the form of libraries. The classes included in the NSLM class library are an essential component of the system and includes types, such as the scalar **NslFloat0** or the input port vector **NslDinDouble1**, used in describing neural elements, data ports or any other structure.

- The *module class* and *model class* data types corresponds to the unique family of NSLM types, distinguishing it from other object-oriented languages, such as C++ and Java. While *module classes* and *model classes* are object-oriented structures in their nature, they go beyond the basic semantics of an *object class*. *Module classes* and *model classes* incorporate semantics for input and output port based communication, something not found in "regular" object classes.

Variables, Attributes and Methods

Variables are the most basic entity in a programming language. Variables provide dual function-ality, they are used to hold either *values* (e.g. 0.5) or *references* (i.e., a virtual memory address indirectly specifying where to find the actual *values* in memory). As in most object-oriented languages, NSLM variables may not exist as independent global entities but only within an object, module or model class—being called class *attributes*. This is also the case with *functions* that may only be defined within an object, module or model class as well—being called class *methods*. Since NSLM is a typed language, every variable or attribute must first be declared according to an existing type.

- When a variable refers to a *native primitive* type, the variable will store a *value*. These types will be defined in section 6.2, *Primitives Types*.

- When a variable refers to a *module*, *model* or *class* type, the variable will store a *reference* to the particular object instead of holding a simple value. This is quite common, since objects are more complex than primitive types and thus require more sophisticated handling. (As a general comment to those users familiar with the concept of *pointers*—pointers exist in C++ but not in Java—NSLM does not include any pointer computation, only *references*.) Note that variables never refer to a class but to an object instantiated from that class. These types will be defined in sections 6.4 and 6.6, Creation of Module Types and Creation of Class Types respectively.

Attribute Reference Hierarchies

Since attributes belong to classes and attributes may provide references to other objects, we end up with attribute reference hierarchies or simply *Attribute Trees*. By providing the starting point of a tree—the root—we can access any attribute by knowing all references in its path. When NSL is running, there are two different trees present in the system:

- The *system* tree for storing NSL specific attributes, and
- The *model* tree for storing user defined attributes.

Actually, every model and module has its own attribute reference tree. If we examine one of these attribute reference trees we see that attributes of a primitive type (to be discussed below)—can only be *leaves* in the tree while attributes holding references are considered *nodes* of the tree. For example, the model attribute reference tree for the *Maximum Selector* model (as we saw in chapter 3), is shown in figure 6.1. The instance **maxSelectorModel** is the root.

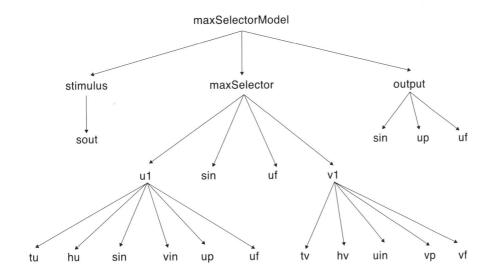

Figure 6.1
Reference tree of the *Maximum Selector* model. Note all instances of objects, or references to objects, are in lowercase, where **maxSelectorModel** is the root of the hierarchy. The model object is implicitly instantiated by NSL when simulating it (see chapter 3).

Note that every entry in the tree corresponds to a variable referencing an object and not the name of a class.

To refer to any variable we use the "dot" notation, i.e. *var1.var2*. There exist two ways of referencing a variable in the tree: *absolute* and *relative* referencing format.

- The *absolute* reference notation starts from the root of the tree specifying the complete path from there. For example, in the *Maximum Selector* model to refer to variable *vp* we must use

    maxSelectorModel.maxSelector.v1.vp

    All references for the model tree start with the name of the model.

- The *relative* reference notation starts from a particular node in the tree and continues on from there. For the previous example, if we currently reference *maxSelectorModel.maxSelector*, we would then refer to *vp* by

    v1.vp

Note that referencing a variable requires specifying its visibility as *public* (described in section 6.2) effectively breaking up the module encapsulation (where variables are defined as *private* instead). (We will also describe a similar concept called *accessibility* in section 6.3.) These concepts are analogous to how directories are made readable or not in a file system.

Class Reference Hierarchies

A different reference hierarchy also exists in all object-oriented languages. This hierarchy or tree defines references between classes as opposed to objects and it is known as the *Class Tree*. Since classes primarily exist to help define object instances, class trees are used to organize the different class definitions. The goal behind this hierarchical organization is to avoid duplicate attributes and methods by specifying common ones in the *base class* or *super class* (the class where common attributes and functions are first defined) while having other classes, known as *subclasses*, *inherit* these common attributes and methods from the *super class*. Class Inheritance Specification is quite useful in building systems and NSL takes advantage of this mechanism both internally and in letting the user build classes in general. We introduce in this section the main class hierarchy in NSL while describing how to build user-defined class trees in section 6.4 and 6.6. (Please see the NSL web site for the complete NSL Class Hierarchy details.)

Predefined Reference Variables

NSLM includes a number of pre-defined reference variables:

- **nslName** represents a **charString** type variable referencing the name of a particular object. For example, **nslName** within the *maxSelector* module object would refer to "**maxSelector**".

- **nslParent** provides a reference from any object back to where it was instantiated. For example, any reference within the **Vlayer** module instance would refer back to the **maxSelector** module instance where **Vlayer** was instantiated.

- **this** provides a reference to the current object. **this** is particularly important as a *return* reference inside functions as well as passing it as argument to another function.

- **super** provides a reference from any class back to its base class, in other words, the class from which it inherits. The **super** reference is used to retrieve attributes or methods defined in the base class, used in conjunction with inheritance. For example, a reference such as **super**.*method*()would call the function *method*() defined in its base class. In general, unless specified otherwise **super** refers to the **NslModule** base module class since all modules by default inherit from it. (We will discuss this in more detail in section 6.3.).

- **null** represents the *null* or invalid reference. It is primarily used within expressions that check the validity of a reference variable.

Importing Libraries

NSLM lets the user call external libraries within a model description by using the **nslImport** statement. As in most programming languages, NSLM requires all definitions to be present during compilation. Since the user may call externally defined classes, it is necessary to include an import statement specifying what additional definitions are needed and where they should be found. For example a class defined in a file called *moreobjects.class* in Java or *moreobjects.h* in C++ would be imported using the following format,

```
nslImport moreobjects;
```

Since Java and C++ use different syntax for defining a path to an imported file, the *NSL verbatim* statement allows us to block off a section of and make it a purely Java code or C++ code. We will discuss verbatim in more detail in section 6.2.

Verbatim

NSLM includes a *verbatim* keyword telling the compiler that part of the code contains C++ or Java specific statements, as opposed to NSLM general statements, that should not be parsed by the NSLM compiler but left intact for direct C++ or Java compiler processing. For example, if the user needs more complex import statements than the ones offered in the previous section, then the *verbatim* keyword could be used. We mark *verbatim* sections in the following way:

C++-only sections of code use the notation:

```
verbatim_NSLC;
```

and Java-only sections of code use the notation:

```
verbatim_NSLJ;
```

To end the C++ or Java section of code use:

```
verbatim_off;
```

While the use of *verbatim* should be avoided, we do offer such an option when there is no appropriate NSLM construct. Note that if you use a verbatim section, the NSL preparser will not preprocess that section of code and many of the NSL constructs will need to be manually expanded to their Java or C++ correct forms. For instance all NSL library module and object instantiations actually take two extra parameters, a *charString name* and *NslModule parent*,

```
NslDouble2 someobj("someobj",this,4,5);
SomeModule somemod("somemod",this,..otherparams..);
```

We thus recommend being extremely careful when adding verbatim sections.[1]

6.2 Primitive Types

As previously mentioned, *native* or *primitive* data types store values.[2]

Defined Types

The primitive types in NSLM are shown in table 6.1. They include *numeric, string, boolean* and *void* types.

Type	Description	Initial Value
int	integer type	0
float	single precision floating point number	0
double	double precision floating point number	0
boolean	**true** or **false**	false
char	single character	null
charString	string of characters	null
void	non type	

Table 6.1

Native or *Primitive* types in NSLM with their initial default value.

It is a good practice to always set the initial value of a variable in one of the initialization methods, as will be discussed in section 6.3. It should also be noted that **void** is not actually a type but a *non-type*. It represents the lack of a type and it is used, for example, when a method returns nothing.

Declarations

Specifying the type of a variable is known as a *declaration*. In NSLM variables are declared and defined (assigning automatic space for storing values) as follows:

```
VisibilitySpec PrimitiveType varName;
```

The *VisibilitySpec* is discussed in the next section. *PrimitiveType* is the corresponding type, such as **int**; *varName* is the name of the variable storing values according to the associated type.

An example of a primitive type variable declaration with the optional initialization is as:

```
private double x = 1.0;
```

Note that we also include a *private* visibility specification in front of the declaration of *x* (described in the next section). The variable initialization is given by "=" followed by a numerical value in this case "1.0".

Visibility

Visibility specifies attributes (variables) and methods can be seen from outside a class or module. This is a very important aspect in object-oriented programming since it is the basis for *encapsulation*. Three levels of visibility are supported by NSLM, *private*, *protected* and *public*. (This is similar to visibility levels available in both C++ and Java.) The three levels are defined as follows,

- **private**—attributes and methods are local to every object instantiated from the particular class,
- **protected**—attributes and methods are local to every object instantiated from the particular class or from any of its subclasses,
- **publi**—attributes and methods are both local and external to every object instantiated from any class.

In general all attributes should be defined as *private* for encapsulation reasons. The exception to this rule is the declaration of the *ports* (to be described below) and external methods. Ports need to be available for external referencing, as do some external methods. Methods that are only used within the class should be defined as *private*. (You should be careful if omitting visibility specifications since the defaults are inconsistent between C++ and Java: C++ considers the default to be *private,* while Java considers the default to be *public* to classes defined in the same directory.) Also, the above rules only apply to attributes and methods; the visibility specification is not need if variables are declared within a method. The same visibility rules apply to object and modules types.

Arrays

NSLM supports multiple dimension arrays on all primitive types with the exception of **void**. For example a single dimension *array* of integers is defined as

```
private int alpha[10];
```

where the array *alpha* consists of 10 integers accessed each by its *index*,

```
alpha[index];
```

an integer going from 0 to the array size minus one, in this case 9.

For example, a two-dimension array or matrix is defined as

```
private float beta[10][5];
```

where the array *beta* consists of 10 by 5 float number accessed each by its *row* and *col*,

```
private beta[row][col];
```

an integer going from 0 to the array size minus one, in this case up to 9 for the *row* number and an integer going from 0, in this case up to 4, for the *col* number.[3]

Constants

The *nslConstant* keyword can be used to specify certain variables of primitive types to be constants, in other words variables that will not change over the course of the execution of the program. The syntax to do this is:

```
nslConstant VisibilitySpec type var = value;
```

For example a *public* constant would be specified as follows,

```
nslConstant public float pi = 3.14;
```

Expressions

NSLM supports primitive type expressions mainly in the form of operators similar to those common to Java and C++. Primitive expressions may be part of independent statements, passed as parameters to a method, or even as part of a return statement.

Numeric

Arithmetic operators can only be applied to numerical types—**int**, **float** or **double**—as shown in table 6.2. (Note that "unary" operators take a single argument, e.g. "-*alpha*," while "binary" operators take two arguments, e.g. "*beta-alpha*.")

Table 6.2
Operators that may be applied to numerical type variables, i.e., int, **float**, and **double**.

Operator	Usage	Description
++	++*a* or *a*++	pre-or-post increment (unary)
--	--*b* or *b*--	pre-or-post decrement (unary)
+	+*b* or *a*+*b*	positive (unary) or addition (binary)
-	-*b* or *a*-*b*	negative (unary) or subtraction (binary)
*	*a**b	multiplication
/	*a*/*b*	division for doubles and floats, or modulus for integer values
%	*a*%*b*	remainder
=	*a*=*b*	assignment
*=	*a**=*b*	*a*=*a**b
/=	*a*/=*b*	*a*=*a*/*b*
+=	*a*+=*b*	*a*=*a*+*b*
-=	*a*-=*b*	*a*=*a*-*b*

For example, the assignment operator "=" assigns one number to a variable:

```
int x;
x = 5;
```

The first line defines the variable x to be of integer type, while the second line assigns a value of 5 to the variable. The two can be combined into a single statement as follows (this is known as *initialization*),

```
int x = 5;
```

Other operators are used in a similar fashion.

Logical operators compare numerical—**int**, **float** or **double**—values to obtain a boolean type value—either **true** or **false**—as shown in the table 6.3.

Operator	Usage	Description
<	a < b	less than
>	a > b	greater than
<=	$a <= b$	less than or equal
>=	$a >= b$	greater than or equal
==	$a == b$	equal
!=	$a != b$	not equal

Table 6.3
Logical operators that may be applied to numerical type variables, i.e., **int**, **float**, and **double**. Returns **true** or **false**.

Boolean

Boolean operators are usually seen in control statements (described in the next section): *if, while, for,* and *switch.* Operators that can be applied to boolean types are shown in table 6.4.

Operator	Usage	Description
=	$a=b$	Assignment among boolean values
==	$a == b$	Return true if the two boolean values are equal
!=	$a != b$	Return true if the two boolean values are not equal
&&	a && b	Logical AND
||	a || b	Logical OR
!	!a	Logical NOT

Table 6.4.
Assignment and logical operators that may be applied on boolean types.

String

Operators that can be applied to charString types are shown in table 6.5.

Operator	Usage	Description
=	$a=b$	Copy one string to the other one
+	$a+b$	String concatenation
==	$a == b$	Return true if the two string values are equal
!=	$a != b$	Return true if the two string values are not equal

Table 6.5.
Assignment, concatenation and logical operators that may be applied on string types.

Control Statements

Control statements control the flow of execution by incorporating conditions on statements. The *while, do* and *for* statements allows the execution flow to loop over one section of code several times until a particular condition is met. The *if* and *switch* statements execute a certain section of code once if a certain condition is met. NSLM includes the standard control statements shown in table 6.6. (square brackets represent optional control expressions).

Statement	Usage Example	Description
if (*condition*) { *statements* } [**else if** (*condition*) { *statements* }] [**else** { *statements* }]	**if** (*a>b*) { *a* = 2; } **else if** (*a>c*) { *a* = 1; } **else** { *a* = 0; }	*if*-else statement with optional intermediate *else-if* expressions and a final optional *else* expression. When *condition* is **true** the corresponding *statements* are processed.
while (*condition*) { *statements* }	**while** (*a<b*) { *a* ++; *c*= *a* *2; }	*while* statement. While *condition* is **true** process *statements*.
do { *statements* } **while** (*condition*);	**do** { *a* ++; *c* = *a* *2; } **while** (*a<b*);	*do-while* statement. Process *statements* until *condition* becomes **false**.
for (*initial-expression; continuation-condition; continuation-expression*) { *statements* }	**for** (*a* =0; *a< b*; *a* ++) { *c* = *a* *2; }	*for* statement. Execute *initial-expression*; then execute *statements* while *continuation-condition* is **true**. After each successful continuation execute *continuation-expression*.

switch (*variable*) {
 case *value: statements* **break**;
 [**case** *value: statements* **break**;]
 [**default**: *statements*]
 }
	switch (a) {
	 case 0: *c* = 0; **break**;
	 case 1: *c* = 2; **break**;
	 default: *c* = *a*;
	 }
		switch statement. Choose from the appropriate *variable* value the equivalent *value* **case** statement (as many as cases as necessary); then execute the corresponding *statements*, with an optional **default** when no matching value is found. This is equivalent to an *if-else* statement with multiple sections. At the end of each switch section a **break** statement is added.

*condition***?***statement-true***:***statement-false*	*c>d?a:b*	if *condition*, then *statement-true* else *statement-false*

In general, all control statements can include both a **break** and **continue** statement used to either *break* or stop processing the control statement or *continue* with the next cycle in the control statement without completing the current one. Both the break and continue statements search for the closest loop (*while, do, for*) to escape from when many nested control statements exist.

Table 6.6
Control statements: *if, while, do, for* and *switch*.

Conversions, Casting, and Promotions

As in most languages, expression return a type that can be deduced from the structure of the expression and the types of the *literals* or *operands* involved (numbers, characters, etc.). Variables may not be used in expressions where their type does not match the expected one. However, in some cases such restrictions are loosened. For example, in a method requiring an argument of type **double**, it would not be appropriate to supply a parameter of **int** type. However, languages such as C++ and Java, perform an implicit *conversion* from the deduced expression type to a type acceptable for its surrounding context, such as implicitly converting an **int** type to a **double**. In general, NSLM supports all conversions permitted by both C++ and Java on primitives, such as assignment conversion, method parameter conversion, and numeric promotion (or casting).

An assignment conversion between an integer and a float would involve an implicit *cast or conversion*:

```
private int x = 5;
private float y;
y = x;
```

where *y* stores the **float** version of *x*, in other words, 5.0.

A method invocation conversion between an integer and a float for a method defined as

```
private void func(float x) { ... }
```

would involve an *implicit cast*:

```
private int x = 5;
func(x);
```

converting *x* into a **float** when passed as an argument to the function.

Numeric promotion between an integer and a float would involve an *explicit cast or conversion*:

```
private int x = 5;
private float y;
y = (float) x;
```

where *x* gets promoted to a **float** before doing the assignment.

6.3 Object Types

NSLM *object types* or *classes* are analogous to those found in object-oriented languages, having both *attributes* (data) with corresponding *methods* (functions) to manipulate them. NSLM lets the user define new object classes as well as instantiate from a number of predefined ones, organized as *numeric*, *string*, and *boolean* classes.

Defined Types

We describe these structures followed by operators and expressions that can be applied to them.

Numeric

NSLM defines set of numeric object types varying in their dimension particularly useful for arithmetic computations. These classes vary according to the underlying numeric attribute type, **int**, **float** or **double**, and its corresponding dimension (0-4), as shown in table 6.7.

Dimension Type	0	1	2	3	4
float	NslFloat0	NslFloat1	NslFloat2	NslFloat3	NslFloat4
double	NslDouble0	NslDouble1	NslDouble2	NslDouble3	NslDouble4
int	NslInt0	NslInt1	NslInt2	NslInt3	NslInt4

The reason for providing these special types is that by encapsulating the dimension within the object, NSLM is able to *overload* a number of operators that the user would otherwise have to explicitly define. For example, additions may be specified in a single "+" statement avoiding the use of multiple "for" loops going through one primitive numeric element addition one at a time. Additionally, NSL protects the user from accessing undefined index elements (overflows), a major headache when doing direct array manipulations at the primitive level.

Boolean

NSL defines several **boolean** object types with varying dimensions as shown in table 6.8.

Dimension Type	0	1	2	3	4
boolean	NslBoolean0	NslBoolean1	NslBoolean2	NslBoolean3	NslBoolean4

As with the primitive **boolean** types the values any element of a **NslBoolean** array can hold is either **true** or **false**. **NslBoolean** object methods are discussed in more detail in the Appendix.[4]

String

NSL defines a **charString** object type useful in storing single strings of characters[5] as shown in table 6.9.

Dimension Type	0	1	2	3	4
charString	NslString0				

The **NslString0** type, together with **charString**, are introduced in NSLM to overcome the different handling of strings in C++ and Java as well as enable the user to use strings as parameters. The methods that apply to **NslString0** types are discussed in Appendix I, *NSLM Methods*.

Ports

Ports are special object types that by linking them together enable data communication between modules—as opposed to simply storing private data within objects or modules. Ports have all the functionality defined of analogous "non-port" object types, and as such they can be used in any expression having been previously defined. Port specific expressions are described in the following sections. Ports are organized in two categories according to their semantics, *output ports* (**Dout**) and *input ports* (**Din**). We describe them according to their underlying object type.

Numeric

The numeric output and input port types are shown in table 6.10.

Dimension Type	0	1	2	3	4
float	NslDoutFloat0	NslDoutFloat1	NslDoutFloat2	NslDoutFloat3	NslDoutFloat4
	NslDinFloat0	NslDinFloat1	NslDinFloat2	NslDinFloat3	NslDinFloat4
double	NslDoutDouble0	NslDoutDouble1	NslDoutDouble2	NslDoutDouble3	NslDoutDouble4
	NslDinDouble0	NslDinDouble1	NslDinDouble2	NslDinDouble3	NslDinDouble4
int	NslDoutInt0	NslDoutInt1	NslDoutInt2	NslDoutInt3	NslDoutInt4
	NslDinInt0	NslDinInt1	NslDinInt2	NslDinInt3	NslDinInt4

Boolean

The boolean output and input port types are shown in table 6.11.

Dimension Type	0	1	2	3	4
boolean	NslDoutBoolean0	NslDoutBoolean1	NslDoutBoolean2	NslDoutBoolean3	NslDoutBoolean4
	NslDinBoolean0	NslDinBoolean1	NslDinBoolean2	NslDinBoolean3	NslDinBoolean4

String

The string output and input port types are shown in table 6.12.

Dimension Type	0	1	2	3	4
charString	NslDoutString0				
	NslDinString0				

Declarations and Instantiations

While classes define types, actual objects are required to exist for a program to do anything meaningful. In NSLM as in typed languages such as C++ or Java, objects are identified through variables referencing them. Specifying the type of a variable is known as a *declaration*, while actually defining the objects to which the variable refers is known as *instantiation*—creating the object for the first time. In NSLM variables are declared and have their referred object instantiated together in a single expression as follows:

```
VisibilitySpec ObjectType varName(paramList);
```

The *VisibilitySpec* is similar to that of primitive types as discussed in the next section. *ObjectType* is the corresponding object type, such as **NslInt0**, *varName* is the name of the variable storing the reference to the new instantiated object, and *paramList* is a list of instantiation parameters that vary depending on the associated type.

Instantiation Parameters

While declarations and instantiations are similar for any NSLM or user defined types, instantiation parameters (*paramList*) vary depending on the specific type. In particular, NSLM defines certain types with a corresponding dimension suffix as shown in table 6.13.

Table 6.10
Numeric output and input port types.

Table 6.11
Boolean output and input port types.

Table 6.12
String output and input port types. (Only "0" dimension string ports are currently defined.)

ObjectType	paramList
Nsl*Type*0	
Nsl*Type*1	*size*
Nsl*Type*2	*row* , *col*
Nsl*Type*3	*dim*, *row* , *col*
Nsl*Type*4	*dim1* , *dim2* , *row* , *col*

For example:

```
private NslInt0 x();
```

declares and instantiates an object of type **NslInt0** referenced by variable *x*. Note that NSLM automatically creates the C++ or Java code needed to allocate memory space for the new variable *x*.[6] Examples of object instantiations for different dimensions and types are,

```
private NslDouble1 y(10);
private NslFloat2 z(10,5);
```

where 10 is the *size* of object *y* and 10 by 5 is the size (*row,col*) of object *z*.

In the case of ports, the syntax to declare and instantiate a port type is similar to that used for normal NSL numeric types, namely:

```
public NslDinInt0 xp();
```

declares and instantiates an object of type **NslDinInt0** referenced by variable *xp*. Examples of object instantiations for different dimensions and types are,

```
public NslDinDouble1 yp(10);
public NslDoutFloat2 zp(10,5);
```

where 10 is the *size* of object *yp* and 10 by 5 is the size (*row,col*) of object *zp*. Also note that we always include the visibility declaration of "public" since other modules need to be able to connect to these ports. Ports should only be defined as attributes and not within methods.

There is an alternative option for defining objects without fully assigning its internal size during instantiation. This is particularly useful when providing array sizes in a dynamic way. The format is as follows:

```
private NslDouble1 r();
private NslFloat2 s();
```

where no specific values are given for the *r* or *s* corresponding dimensions. The dimensions are set at a later time using the *var*.**nslMemAlloc**(*sizeList*) method (see Appendix I for further details) where *sizeList* represents the corresponding sizes from the original *paramList* in one of the constructor or initialization methods discussed in section 6.3. Defining objects this way provides great flexibility since models may have their internal sizes dynamically assigned during model execution avoiding recompilation such as in the extensions mentioned for the *Backpropagation* model described at the end of chapter 3.

Arrays

Array usage with object types varies from that of primitive types. In the current NSLM version the user may define arrays of primitive types but they may not define object type arrays. This is because of the differences of array handling in Java and C++. Yet, the NSL C++ version does support C++ arrays of NSL types as described in Appendix III (NSLC extensions). On the other hand, since NSL predefined object types already include up to four dimensions, NSL includes array-style data accessing in those types.

In general, accessing data from an object is done through method invocations or in the case of NSL dimensional objects, it varies depending on the particular dimension objects may have. To access an element within an object, NSLM provides array indexing using the conventional bracket pair "[ ]" according to the following considerations (note that all array indices start at zero).

- **Zero:** A zero-dimensional type stores a single primitive type value or scalar. For example **NslFloat0** type stores a **float** type.

- **One:** A one-dimensional type stores a one-dimensional primitive type array (considered a row vector). For example **NslFloat1** type stores a **float** type array. In a one-dimensional object m, $m[j]$ returns the $j+1$-th element in m, where j must be a positive integer value (or an expression returning a positive integer value).

- **Two:** A two-dimensional type stores a two-dimensional primitive type array (considered a matrix). For example **NslFloat2** type stores a **float** type two-dimensional array. The first dimension of the array represents the rows while the second dimension represents the column. In a two-dimensional object m, $m[i]$ returns the $i+1$-th row of the array, which is a one-dimensional array. $m[i][j]$ returns the element at the $i+1$-th row and $j+1$-th column of the array.

- **Three:** A three-dimensional type stores a three-dimensional primitive type array (considered a vector of matrices). For example **NslFloat3** type stores a **float** type vector containing two-dimensional arrays. The left-most dimension identifies the vector while the other two represent the rows and columns of the matrix, respectively. In a three-dimensional object m, $m[h]$ returns the $h+1$-th two-dimensional array. $m[h][i][j]$ returns the element at the $h+1$-th array, $i+1$-th row and $j+1$-th column of the two-dimensional array.

- **Four:** A four-dimensional type stores a four-dimensional primitive type array (considered a vector of three-dimensional matrices). For example **NslFloat4** type stores a **float** type array of a **float** type array that stores a two-dimensional arrays. In a four-dimensional object m, $m[g]$ returns the $g+1$-th three-dimensional array, $m[g][h]$ returns the $g+1$-th and $h+1$-th two-dimensional array. $m[g][h][i]$ returns the $g+1$-th, $h+1$-th, $i+1$-th vector. $m[g][h][i][j]$ returns the $g+1$-th, $h+1$-th, $i+1$-th , $j+1$-th element of the array.

(A number of methods manipulation objects with different dimensions are described in Appendix I.) table 6.14 summarizes array indexing and partial indexing.

ObjectType	Indexing	ResultType
Ns*lType*1	var[index]	type
NslType2	var[row]	Ns*lType*1
	var[row] [col]	type
NslType3	var[index1]	Ns*lType*2
	var[index1] [row]	Ns*lType*1
	var[index1] [row] [col]	type
NslType4	var[index1]	Ns*lType*3
	var[index1] [index2]	Ns*lType*2
	var[index1] [index2] [row]	Ns*lType*1
	var[index1] [index2] [row] [col]	type

Table 6.14
Indexing for dimensional object types. *Type* corresponds to either Int, Float, Double, Boolean or String for their correspondingly defined dimensions (similarly with port types). Again, *index*, *row*, *col*, *index1* and *index2* are integer values specifying the corresponding index number. *type* would correspond to a primitve type either int, float, double, boolean or charString respectively.

Constants

Similar to primitive types, the *nslConstant* keyword can be used in conjunction with object types in order to for them to be constants, in other words variables that will not change over the course of the execution of the program. The syntax to do this is:

```
nslConstant visibilitySpec objectType varName(paramList) =
value;
```

For example a public constant would be specified as follows,

```
nslConstant public NslFloat0 pi = 3.14;
```

Expressions

NSLM supports a number of expressions on the different defined types. We will described them according to *numeric*, *boolean*, *string* and *port* types.

Numeric

NSLM supports most numeric operators to those defined for primitive numeric types (this applies to both numeric and numeric port types). The supported arithmetic expressions are shown in the table 6.15.

Operator	Usage	Description
=	a=b	Assignment
+	+b or a+b	Unary Positive or Two Parameter Addition
-	-b or a-b	Unary Negative or Two Parameter Subtraction
/	a/b	Pointwise Division
^	a^b	Pointwise Multiplication
*	a*b	Scalar Multiplication or Vector/Matrix Product
@	a@ b	Vector/Matrix Convolution (see Appendix II)

Table 6.15
Arithmetic operators for object numeric types. Typically, operands required on each side of the operator (except in the case of the unary operators) must be of a similar type and dimension although in some cases parameter may be of different dimension. More details on valid operands are described in Appendix II.

For instance, a NSL **NslFloat0** object would have its value assigned as follows:

```
private NslFloat0 x();
x = 5.0;
```

If the assignment takes place on the same line as the declaration and instantiation then it is known as *initialization*:

```
private NslFloat0 x() = 5.0;
```

A NSL **NslFloat2** object would have one of its elements assigned a value as follows:

```
private NslFloat2 y(2,3);
y[0][1] = 5.0;
```

or all its elements as follows,

```
y = 5.0;
```

where 5.0 is assigned to every element in *y*.

Note that assignment copies values from one object to another one. This is not a copy of references (as opposed to Java handling of object to object assignment). For example

```
private NslFloat2 z(2,3);
z = y;
```

assigns every element value in *y* to every element value in *z*, where *y* and *z* must be equally sized.

Also note that numeric objects on the left-hand side of an assignment statement may be assigned with primitive types returned on the right-hand side. For example, the following code works without having to add an explicit cast. (Explicit cast is covered in this section on *Conversions, Casting, and Promotions*.)

```
private NslFloat1 phi(5);
private NslFloat0 force();
private float mu;
phi=22;
mu=phi[0];
force=phi[0];
```

The previous to last equation copies the content of *phi*[0] into *mu*, while the last statement copies *phi*[0] to *force*.

NSLM also provides logical operators for numeric port types. The logical operators are shown in table 6.16.

Operator	Usage	Description
<	a < b	less than
>	a > b	greater than
<=	$a <= b$	less than or equal
>=	$a >= b$	greater than or equal
==	$a == b$	equal
!=	a != b	not equal

Table 6.16
Logical operators for object numeric types.

All logical operators are applied as pointwise to arrays and return an array of similar size. If the arrays are of different dimension or size, an error will occur.

Boolean

Boolean types are mainly used as resulting values from statement conditions. For example all expressions in table 6.15 return a boolean value. Since boolean values can only be true or false, the only expression that can be applied to this values are the ones shown in table 6.17.

Operator	Usage	Description
=	$a=b$	Assignment among boolean values
==	$a == b$	Return true if the two boolean values are equal
!=	a!= b	Return true if the two boolean values are not equal
&&	a && b	Logical AND
||	$a \| \| b$	Logical OR
!	! a	Logical NOT

String

String type expressions are shown in table 6.18.

Operator	Usage	Description
=	$a=b$	Copy one string to the other one
+	$a + b$	String concatenation
==	$a == b$	Return true if the two string values are equal
!=	$a!= b$	Return true if the two string values are not equal

For example, to declare as well as initialize a variable of type NslString0 we type:

```
private NslString0 protocol()= "Protocol";
```

Ports

In general all "non-port" expressions apply to port types, i.e., numeric type expressions apply to numeric port types, similarly with booleans and strings. There a number of additional expressions, in the form of methods particular to port types defined for specifying *connections* and *relabels* between them. When connecting or relabeling ports the type and dimension of the ports must match or a compilation error will occur, the only exception is connecting among different numeric port types. In order to illustrate these expressions in more detail we present in figure 6.2 a comprehensive diagram of the *Maximum Selector* model previously described in chapter 3.

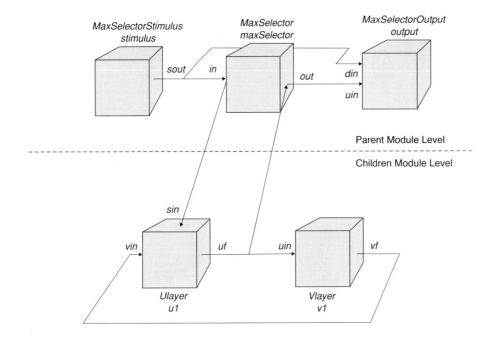

Figure 6.2
Complete diagram
representation for the
Maximum Selector presented
in chapter 3. The model
contains a top-level (*Parent
Module Level*) consisting of
the the **MaxSelector** module
and both the
MaxSelectorStimulus and
MaxSelectorOutput
modules. The **MaxSelector**
module is decomposed at the
bottom-level (*Children
Module Level*) into the
Ulayer and **Vlayer** modules.
Connections are made
between modules at the top-
level or bottom-level,
respectively. Relabels are
made across modules in the
top-level and bottom-level.

Connections

NSL provides the user with a special function nslConnect to make connections between ports. Connections are always specified from output ports to input ports as follows,

```
nslConnect (m1.dout,m2.din);
```

where output port *dout* in module *m1* is connected to input port *din* in module *m2*. This statement, specified within the **makeConn** method, shows how to specify port connections between modules and should be specified at the parent module level, that is inside the module that actually instantiated both *m1* and *m2*. For example, at the *parent module level* the following three connections are made in figure 6.2,

```
nslConnect(stimulus.sout,maxselector.in);
nslConnect(stimulus.sout,output.sin);
nslConnect(maxselector.out, output.uin);
```

At the *children module level* the following two connections are made in figure 6.2,

```
nslConnect(v1.vf,u1.vin);
nslConnect(u1.uf,v1.uin);
```

As an additional consideration, in order to refer to a port it must have been defined with visibility public, otherwise the above connection statement would cause a compilation error.

Relabels

Besides connections NSL provides a special connectivity function **nslRelabel** to forward data between ports belonging to modules at different levels in the module tree hierarchy. Recall that connections are done between an output port and an input port belonging to different modules at the same decomposition level. On the other hand, relabeling is specified between a *parent module* input port and a *child module* input port or between a *child module* output port and a *parent module* output port, respectively. Relabeling plays an important role when building module *compositions* or *assemblages*. For example, the following statements would relabel an input port *din* at the parent module level to *din* in *m1* and an output port *dout* in *m1* to *din* at the parent module level,

nslRelabel*(din,m1.din);*
nslRelabel*(m1.dout,dout);*

For example, the following two relabels are made in figure 6.2,

```
nslRelabel(in,u1.sin);
nslRelabel(u1.uf,out);
```

Note that we do not need a module reference in the first argument since the reference is the actual module where the relabel is taking place—the "**this**" module.

Control Statements

Previously defined control statements (see "Primitive Types" section) support the use of object types as long as the corresponding expressions allow it. For example, boolean conditions permit the use of object type expressions returning boolean types. More generally, statement accept any object type defined expressions.

Conversions, Casting, and Promotions

Analogous to primitive types, object type variables may not be used in expressions where their type does not match the expected one. However, in some cases such restrictions are also loosened. For example, in a method requiring an argument of type **NslDouble0** a **NslInt0** type would be accepted as well. This applies between all numeric types as long as their dimension corresponds. In particular port types can be used whenever "non-port" types correspond. (The opposite is not true since "non-port" types cannot be connected among themselves.) No conversions, castings or promotions may be applied between primitive and object types.

6.4 Creation of New Object Types

NSLM allows for the creation of new object-oriented style classes (creation of new module and model types is described in section 6.5 and 6.6 respectively). As will be seen later, the major differences between modules and classes is their lack of ports and any control from the NSL scheduler. Defining a new class involves defining attributes and methods common to all its objects. New objects may be instantiated only if there exists a previously defined corresponding class as in most object-oriented languages. The class definition format is somewhat similar to that in C++ or Java. (The user can also define native C++ or Java classes with the use of the verbatim modifiers.)

Template

To define a new class we use the special **nslClass** keyword in the class definition header, as shown in code segment 6.1.

```
nslClass class-name ( class-instantiation-spec ) class-
inheritance-spec
{
    class-attribute-spec
    class-method-spec
}
```

Code Segment 6.1
nslClass definition template.

The code section outside the curly brackets corresponds to the class *header*, consisting of the following:

- *class-name* represents the name identifying the class.
- *class-instantiation-spec* defines instantiation arguments (type-name pairs separated by commas) that must be passed when instantiating a new object. (This corresponds to the header of the object constructor in either C++ or Java.)
- *class-template-inheritance-spec* defines the inheritance specification for the class.
- The code section that appears inside the curly brackets defines the actual structure and functionality of the class:
- *class-attribute-spec* defines the structure of the class in terms of its attributes, primitive and object type variables.
- *class-method-spec* defines the behavior of the class in terms of local function or method definitions.

Header

The basic class header includes the **nslClass** keyword, the *class-name*, and the *class-instantiation-spec*. For example, code segment 6.2 describes the main header section for a **MemoryCalc** class.

```
nslClass MemoryCalc (int size) class-inheritance-spec
{
    class-attribute-spec
    class-method-spec
}
```

The *class-instantiation-spec* defines a single instantiation parameter *size* passed to class **MemoryCalc**.

Inheritance

Every class definition in NSLM requires a *class-inheritance-spec*. Inheritance is an important feature present in all truly object-oriented languages permitting the definition of new classes as extensions to already existing ones. The inheritance scheme provides the new class with all the attributes and methods (except for the *private* ones) of the *superclass* or *baseclass*, where the new class is known as the *subclass*. Inheritance is also the basis for code reuse in an application. As an aside for those users familiar with the concept, NSL supports only single inheritance—as opposed to multiple inheritance. In order to show how the *class-inheritance-spec* is used, we will create another class called *MovementCalc* that inherits from *MemoryCalc* as shown in code segment 6.3.

```
nslClass MovementCalc (int size) extends MemoryCalc (size)
{
    class-attribute-spec
    class-method-spec
}
```

We define **MovementCalc** as a subclass of **MemoryCalc**. Recall that **MemoryCalc** requires an instantiation argument. Thus, we must pass *size* to **MemoryCalc** as shown in the inheritance specification to avoid an error. Note the difference between the instantiation argument specification containing the type of the argument—int for *size*—and the parameter passed to the base class containing only the parameter name and not its type.

Also note that **MovementCalc** can use all of the *public* and *protected* attributes and methods from **MemoryCalc** class.

NSLM provides a default empty inheritance specification on the previous **MemoryCalc** class definition as shown in code segment 6.4. In this case, the NSLM compiler generates the default inheritance specification "**extends NslClass(charString** nslName, **NslModule nslParent)**" when none is provided. **NslClass** is directly or indirectly the highest superclass for all class objects.

```
nslClass MemoryCalc (int size)
{
    class-attribute-spec
    class-method-spec
}
```

Attributes

Attributes define the structure of the class. Attributes may be either primitive or object types. For example, in code segment 6.5 we add a private object to the **MovementCalc** class.

```
nslClass MovementCalc (int size) extends MemoryCalc (size)
{
    private NslInt1 vector1(size);
    class-method-spec
}
```

The attribute section consists of a **private NslInt1** type object referenced by variable named *vector1*, with instantiation argument *size* corresponding to the vector size. Variable *size* is part of the instantiation arguments. Note that we should not name attributes the same as instantiation arguments since that will cause a compilation error. Furthermore, since we also have a base class containing its own attributes and methods, we must avoid conflicts with attributes with similar names in base classes.

Methods

Methods or functions define the behavior of the class. Methods correspond to functions in structured languages such as C and directly correspond to those defined in object-oriented languages. Methods must always be defined within a class corresponding to the *class-method-spec* section. The body of a method—its implementation—supports expres-sions and statements similar to those used in C++ or Java, involving both primitive and object types. Methods can take any number of parameters and may or may not have a return type. Both arguments and the return type may be either objects or primitive types. As an example, we add a *print* method to the **MemoryCalc** example as shown in code segment 6.6.

```
nslClass MovementCalc (int size) extends MemoryCalc (size)
{
    private NslInt1 vector1(size);
    public int print() {
        nslPrint("vector1:",vector1);
    }
}
```

This simple *print* method prints the values stored in *vector1*. To actually call the method we use the "dot" notation. For example, if we want to call the *print* method from within this or other class we would do the following:

```
MemoryCalc m();
m.print();
```

Similar to the **nslPrint** method NSLM also provides a wide number of methods for arithmetic calculations, file manipulation and other functionality as described in Appendix II.

Static Modifier

NSLM offers an additional **static** modifier affecting both attributes and methods. The modifier makes the previously defined *object attributes* and *object methods* become what is known as *class attributes* and *class methods* respectively. The difference between the two lies in that object attributes and methods are designed to be accessed by an object reference where every object from a particular class refer to different data (with similar or different values) for the same attribute. On the other hand, class attributes and methods are designed to be accessed by a class reference where all objects from a particular class refer to a common data with a unique value for the same attribute. In other words a class attribute is an attribute whose value is always the same to all objects instantiated from that class, i.e. each object does not have its own private copy of the attribute but a shared one with all other objects. For example, in code segment 6.7, we show how to define a class attribute and a class method for **MemoryCalc**.

```
nslClass MemoryCalc (int size) {
    private static int version;
    public static int print() {
        nslPrint("MemoryCalc");
    }
}
```

Code Segment 6.7
Example of the use of the static keyword

The method *print* is used to print the name of the class as opposed to the name of an object instance. The method is called using the class name as its reference

```
MemoryCalc.print();
```

This is quite useful in defining libraries that perform transformations dependent exclusively on data passed to it, such as with numerical functions. In this case no objects need to be instantiated from that class in order to execute the function. (In general objects are instantiated to store data for future use. In the case of simple transformation no "memory" is required and functions perform direct transformations based exclusively on arguments currently passed to it.)

6.5 Creation of New Module Types

Modules are the basis for processing and simulation in NSL. Modules are the most important NSL structure, distinguishing NSL from being "just another" object-oriented language. Modules are concurrent or *active* entities with the potential to be distributed[7] based on communication *ports* for sending and receiving data between modules. This is in addition to traditional object-oriented message passing between objects in the form of method invocations. Thus, modules are distinguished from object classes in that module methods are executed by the NSLM scheduler, whereas object methods have to be explicitly called by the user.

Template

The process of defining new modules is similar to that of object classes. A module *template* is defined having module attributes and methods similar to those defined for an object class in addition to specific module port attributes and simulation methods. In terms of syntax, modules use the special **nslModule** keyword instead of **nslClass**. The module definition template is shown in code segment 6.8.

```
nslModule module-name ( module-instantiation-spec ) module-
inheritance-spec
{
    module-attribute-spec
    module-method-spec
}
```

Code Segment 6.8
nslModule definition template.

The template section that appears outside the curly brackets corresponds to the module header, consisting of the following

- *module-name* is the name identifying the module.
- *module-instantiation-spec* defines instantiation arguments that must be passed when creating a new module instance.
- *module-inheritance-spec* defines class inheritance aspects for the module.

The template section that appears inside the curly brackets defines the actual structure and functionality of the module:

- *module-attribute-spec* defines the structure of the module in terms of primitive, object and module type variables, including ports necessary for external communication.
- *module-method-spec* defines the behavior of the module in terms of local functions or methods definitions, including simulation methods.

Header

The module-instantiation-spec within the header defines arguments that must be passed when instantiating a new module similar to class templates in NSLM. The specification is made of a list of type-name pairs separated by commas that may also be empty. For example, code segment 6.9 shows two instantiation parameters in **BasicModule**.[8]

```
nslModule BasicModule (int size, NslString0 c) module-
inheritance-spec
{
    module-attribute-spec
    module-method-spec
}
```

Code Segment 6.9
BasicModule header specification.

Inheritance

The *module-inheritance-spec* allows the module to inherit attributes and methods from a *base module class* or *super module*. Module inheritance is similar to that in regular classes except that all modules must inherit directly or indirectly from **NslModule** in order for modules to be correctly managed. If we want to define a new module type that inherits from one already created, then we must pass the required parameters to the super module class as shown in code segment 6.10. Since **BasicModule** requires both *size* and *c*, we pass them as parameters from **ExtendedModule**.

```
nslModule ExtendedModule (int size, NslString0 c, char ptype)
extends BasicModule(size,c)
{
    module-attribute-spec
    module-method-spec
}
```

If inheritance is not specified, as in code segment 6.11, the NSLM compiler automatically appends the code "**extends NslModule(charString** nslName, **NslModule** nslParent)" to the header.

```
nslModule BasicModule (int size, NslString0 c)
{

    module-attribute-spec
    module-method-spec
}
```

Also note that all modules inherit directly or indirectly from a class called **NslModule** in order to take advantage of attributes and methods such as getting the variable's name, getting the variable's parent, setting the script access to the variable, and printing the variable. Similar to class, NSL supports only single inheritance for modules.

Attributes

Attributes define the structure of the module. As in object classes, attributes may be either primitive, object or module types. For example, we add single input and output port to the **ExtendedModule** module structure, as shown in code segment 6.12.

```
nslModule ExtendedModule (int size, NslString0 c, char ptype)
extends BasicModule(size,c)
{

    public NslDinFloat1 din(size);
    public NslDoutFloat1 dout(size);
    module-method-spec
}
```

The attribute section consists of,

- **public NslDinFloat1** input port named *din*, with instantiation parameter *size* since it corresponds to a numeric vector.

- **public NslDoutFloat1** output port named *dout*, with instantiation parameter *size* since it corresponds to a numeric vector.

Methods

Modules are different from objects in their incorporation of simulation methods in addition to object type style methods. In this section we describe simulation methods followed by differential equation methods, of particular importance to modules.

Simulation

Simulation methods are executed during system runtime according to control parameters specified by the user from the script or window interpreter. Simulation methods, in addition to class methods, are inserted into *module-method-spec* section. In code segment 6.13, we define one protected method and three public methods. Two of these methods override two NSLM's predefined simulation methods, **initRun** and **simRun**, respectively.

(The **initRun** and **simRun** are discussed below; however, for a complete list of NslModule methods please see Appendix I, NSLM Methods.)

```
nslModule ExtendedModule (int size, NslString0 c, char ptype)
extends BasicModule(size,c)
{
    public NslDinFloat1 din(size);
    public NslDoutFloat1 dout(size);
    public double getVelocity(int deltax, int deltay) {
        //more code
    }
    public void initRun() {
        dout=0;
    }
    public void simRun(){
        //more code
    }
    protected NslDouble2 eyeMoveSpecial(int deltax, int deltay)
    {
        //more code
    }
}
```

Code Segment 6.13
Example of modules methods.

All simulation methods are defined in the class **NslModule** and are *overridden* by the user through similarly named methods in the new module. Note that many of these methods were given in chapter 3 together with examples. The following tables describe the available methods for *overriding* (all methods return a **void** type and have no arguments passed to them). table 6.19 shows the *connection* method.

Table 6.19
Connection method.

Connection Method	Description
makeConn	All connections and relabels between modules should be specified within this method.

Table 6.20 shows the *system* methods called once throughout the execution of the complete system.

System Methods	Description
initSys	This method should contain any initializations required for the complete system (one per module). This usually involves system variable initialziations.
endSys	It is the last method called before the end of the complete system simulation, for example to execute any summary type calculations.

Table 6.20.
System methods.

Table 6.21 shows the *module* methods called once during a complete module simulation.

Module Methods	Description
initModule	Initializes a module during every simulation, both training and run phases. For example, the number of simulation epochs or cycles per epoch may be set here.
endModule	Ends the complete simulation, both training and run phases. Performs any simulation post-processing.

Table 6.21 Module methods.

Table 6.22 shows the *train* methods called in relation to training aspects of the simulation.

Train Methods	Description
initTrainEpochs	Initializes variables that are needed for all train epochs.
endTrainEpochs	Summarizes the results from all train epochs.
initTrain	Initializes the training phase for all train cycles and is executed once per train epoch. Training variables are reset in this method.
simTrain	Contains training dynamics. Simulates the training phase for as many steps as specified or until reaching **trainEndTime** divided by **trainDelta**.
endTrain	Executes at the end of the training phase for a single step when the time step corresponds to **trainEndTime**. Usually used for compiling statistics and printing results after each train epoch.

Table 6.22 Train methods.

Table 6.23 shows the *run* methods called in relation to running aspects of the simulation.

Run Methods	Description
initRunEpochs	Initializes the variables that are needed for all run epochs.
endRunEpochs	Summarizes the results from all run epochs.
initRun	Initializes the run phase for al run cycles and is executed once per run epoch. Variables for the run are reset in this method.
simRun	Contains running dynamics. Simulates the run cycle for as many steps as specified or until reaching **runEndTime** divided by **runDelta**.
endRun	Executes at the end of the run phase for a single step when the time step corresponds to **runEndTime**. Usually used for compiling statistics from each run and printing some kind of results. It may include modifications on the simulation parameters.

Table 6.23 Run methods.

Note that it is not mandatory to redefine or override any of these methods. When not overridden, the default method within the direct superclass (or **NslModule** by default) will be called. Also, the simulation time in a **simTrain** phase or a **simRun** phase starts with time equal zero and changes by time equal **trainDelta** or **runDelta** after each cycle or step. The number of cycles and the number of epochs both start at one when time equals zero.

Since NSLM controls the scheduling of module methods, these should not be directly called from user-defined expressions or control statements.

Differential Equations

Differential equations are quite important in modeling neural networks. Simulation of neural networks as introduced in chapter 1 is based in NSL on the leaky integrator neural model specified by a first-order differential equation of the form

$$\tau \frac{dmp_t}{dt} = f(t, mp_t) \tag{6.1}$$

This first-order differential equation requires the use of numerical approximations to solve it. NSLM provides a general method for first-order differential equations defined as follows:

```
nslDiff(mp,τ,f(t,mp));
```

or

```
mp = nslDiff(mp,τ,f(t,mp));
```

where $f(t,mp)$ represents any mathematical expression, for example

```
f(t,mp) = -mp+s;
```

corresponds to the leaky integrator model where s represents to the neuron input. τ is a time constant having default value 1.0, and dt is the time delta. Since dt is not specified, its value is given from the script command interpreter.

While different numerical methods may be used to solve the equation, NSLM defines it in such a way that the actual neural network architecture and connections do *not* change when changing the aproximation method used. Different numerical methods may be more or less appropriate according to the desired numerical precision and the processing power of the computing machine. NSLM includes two approximation methods, *Euler* and 2nd order *Runge-Kutta*, specified by

```
setApproxMethod(method);
```

where *method* can be either the string **Euler** or **RungeKutta2**.

- The difference equation specified by the *Euler* approximation method is:

$$\frac{\tau(mp_{t+\Delta t} - mp_t)}{\Delta t} = f(t, mp_t) \tag{6.2}$$

and is modified to

$$mp_{t+\Delta t} = mp_t + \left(\frac{dt}{\tau}\right) f(t, mp_t) = mp_t + \left(\frac{dt}{\tau}\right)(-mp_t + s_t) \tag{6.3}$$

or expanding the equation for the leaky integrator,

$$mp_{t+\Delta t} = \left(1 - \frac{\Delta t}{\tau}\right) mp_t + \frac{\Delta t}{\tau} s_t \tag{6.4}$$

- The difference equation specified by the *Runge-Kutta2* approximation method is expanded into:

$$h = \frac{\Delta t}{\tau} \tag{6.5}$$

$$k_1 = hf(t, mp_t) \tag{6.6}$$

$$k_2 = hf\left(t + \frac{1}{2}h, mp_t + \frac{1}{2}k_1\right) \tag{6.7}$$

$$mp_{t+\Delta t} = mp_t + k_2 \tag{6.8}$$

or expanding the equation again,

$$mp_{t+\Delta t} = \left(1 - \frac{(\Delta t)^2}{4\tau^2}\right) mp_t + \frac{\Delta t}{2\tau} s_t \left(1 + \frac{\Delta t}{2\tau}\right) \tag{6.6}$$

Scheduling

NSL provides a multi-clock scheduler for each module during simulation. Every train cycle executes the **simTrain** method **trainDelta** times for as many cycles as specified by **numTrainEpochs**. Similarly, every run cycle executes the **simRun** method **runDelta** times for as many cycles as specified by **numRunEpochs**. The detailed order of execution including initializations is as follows:

1. For all modules execute **initSys**.
2. For all modules execute **makeConn**.
3. For all modules execute **initModule**.
4. Execute simulation cycles for as many epochs as specified, both train and run.
5. For all modules execute **endModule**.
6. For all modules execute **endSys**.

The controls these cycles by using either the menu commands from the NSL Executive window or the NSLS script commands in the script window (see chapter 5). However, **initSys**, **makeConn**, and **initModule** will all be called before the NSL Executive window and the script window appear. Figure 6.3 shows in more detail a flowchart corresponding to step 4: the train and run phases. (Usually the train phase is executed before the run phase.)

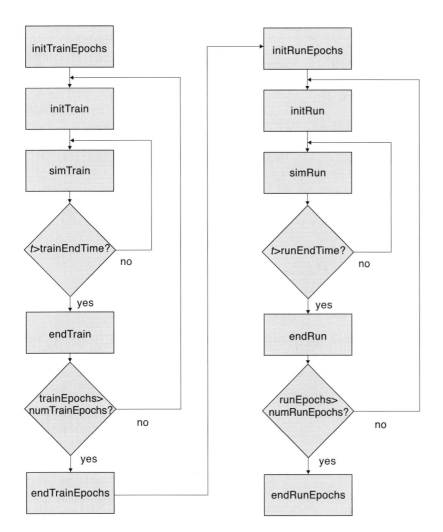

Figure 6.3
Flowchart showing train and run processing phases. Note that the outer loop is referred to as the "epoch" and the inner loop is referred to as the "cycle".

The scheduling described above is applied sequentially to all modules. In other words no module will execute a **simTrain** method unless all modules have previously executed an **initTrain** method. If a module does not define a particular method (say **initRun**), then that module will simply be skipped when its turn comes up for that phase of execution. The order in which modules are processed for a single method pass is **preorder** starting with the main model in the attribute reference tree hierarchy, as exemplified in figure 6.4. The simulation sequence is generated by going over all modules according to their initial instantiation specification, i.e. as soon a module is instantiated it is immediately put into the scheduling list. In figure 6.4, the scheduler would start from the top module **ModuleA** followed by its first child **ModuleB**. Since **ModuleB** has children, then the scheduling list continues with **ModuleC** and son on. The complete execution order in this example is alphabetical, i.e. **ModuleC** followed by **ModuleD** then followed by **ModuleE** and so on.[9] Note that the tree is implicitly built by NSL following the order of module instantiations by the user.

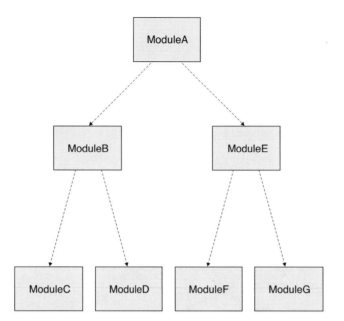

Figure 6.4
Dashed arrows in the frame
specify instantiation order,
starting with the top module
in preorder and depth first
fashion, in other words,
following names "alphabet-
wise."

The actual code to generate the tree shown in figure 6.14 is as follows (note the exact declaration order with the modules. The order of module definition templates is unimportant).

```
nslModule ModuleA ()
{
    ModuleB b();
    ModuleE e();
}
nslModule ModuleB ()
{
    ModuleC c();
    ModuleD d();
}
nslModule ModuleE ()
{
    ModuleF f();
    ModuleG g();
}
```

Code Segment 6.14
Module code definitions
generating the hierarchy tree
shown in figure 6.4. Note
however, that each module
must be declared in its own
file. Thus the above example
would take three files.

Buffering

To simulate concurrency in module execution NSL offers buffered ports as well as non-buffered (default) ports. In the default mode, ports are non-buffered and processing becomes sequential processing where new values from output ports are immediately sent to all ports connected to it. In this form, ports operate as a numeric object keeping values for internal and external use always the same. Concurrency is only simulated with buffered ports making processing order unimportant since all communication becomes buffered and output values are not immediately sent out from a module's output ports. With buffered ports, the buffer keeps temporary internal port values. After each simulation cycle the system copies the all buffered values into a second buffer used for communications with other modules. Since the default mode is set to non-buffered ports, the user may change a particular port to the buffering mode with the following command:

```
port.nslSetBuffering(true);
```

If instead of true the argument is **false** then the port becomes non-buffered. Additionally, NSL offers the following command to set all ports in a module to the buffered state:

```
module.nslSetBuffering(true);
```

To make all ports in all modules buffered the user may use the following command (again a **false** would reset this mode):

```
system.nslSetBuffering(true);
```

When dealing with buffered ports, the system internally executes a method named **nslUpdateBuffers** after each simulation cycle to update port buffers.

To get the current buffer setting we can call one of the following methods returning a *fg* boolean value:

```
fg=system.nslGetbuffering();
fg=module.nslGetBuffering();
fg=port.nslGetBuffering();
```

6.6 Creation of New Model Types

A *model* defines a complete program or application. Instead of having a "main" function as required in most programming languages, NSL applications require the existence of a *model* where execution begins. This *model* is unique to every NSL application. Its definition is somewhat similar to module definitions except in the use of the **nslModel** keyword (instead of nslModule) as shown in code segment 6.16. Note that NSLM does not allow any instantiation parameters nor a inheritiance specification for models.[10]

```
nslModel model-name ()
{
    model-attribute-spec
    model-method-spec
}
```

Code Segment 6.15
nslModel Definition
Template.

The template section that appears outside the curly brackets corresponds to the model header, consisting of the following

- m*odel-name* is the name identifying the model. This name is internally used by NSLM to implicitly instantiate the complete model.

The template section that appears inside the curly brackets defines the actual structure and functionality of the model:

- *model-attribute-spec* defines the structure of the model in terms of primitive, object and module type variables. With the exception of not having any port instantiations, this section is similar to that in modules.
- *model-method-spec* defines the behavior of the model in terms of local functions or methods definitions, including simulation methods.

For example, the **ExtendedModel** instantiates the **ExtendedModule** module as shown in code segment 6.17.

```
nslModel ExtendedModel ()
{
    public ExtendedModule em(10,"p1",'H');
}
```

Code Segment 6.16
nslModel example.

ExtendedModel is implicitly instantiated by NSL in order to execute the model.

6.7 Summary

In this chapter we have presented the key concepts and constructs needed to build a NSL model. Since NSLM is built on top of C++ and Java, we discussed the parts of the NSLM language that is shared with these two native languages. We also discussed the basic NSLM types and how to build NSLM modules and models. Finally, we presented a section on how to build your own NSLM classes and what restrictions one might encounter when doing this. Although this chapter described the NSL modeling language in more detail than that presented in chapter 3, to fully grasp the language we recommend that Appendix I, The NSLM Methods be reviewed.

Notes

1. We explain how to expand many of the NSLM constructs in the NSLM Parser Guide for Java and C++ technical report that can be found on the NSL web site. These expansions usually vary between Java and C++.

2. We use the terms *primitive* and *native* interchangeably in this document, although many languages make a distinction between these two terms. Native types in NSLM reflect the native types present in both C++ and Java except for charString and boolean which are special cases. We also refer to all other types as NSLM types.

3. Indexing in similar to C++ array indexing except for the fact that no pointer arithmetic is allowed. Additionally, Java allows one array to be assigned to another, in which case the reference of the array is copied between the two variables and not the elements. If we were to assign one native array to another native array, we would need to use the verbatim keyword described below.

4. A boolean array can be converted to an **int**, **float**, or **double** array.

5. In the current NSL version only 0 dimension **NslString** objects are supported although future NSL version will include additional dimension types.

6. We avoid the use of the *new* operator as in C++ or Java since C++ returns a pointer and Java returns a reference.

7. See some of our current work on distributed simulation discussed Appendix III— NSLC Extensions.

8. In addition to these two arguments, the NSLM compiler generates two more: "charString nslName" and "NslModule nslParent," where nslName is the name of the instance being instantiated and nslParent is the instance of the parent module instantiating this module instance. The parser adds these parameters when the module is instantiated as well.

9. Currently the order of execution of modules defaults to their hierarchical order and the order in which they were defined in the module. However, we expect to offer more control in the scheduling order in the future.

10. We expect to provide in the future instantiation parameters for models, analogous to the *args* parameters in Java.

7 The Scripting Language NSLS

In order to simulate a model created with NSLM it is necessary to specify the simulation interaction consisting of simulation control, model parameters, and visualization control. This can be done either by hard-coding the parameters within the model using NSLM, selecting the commands via the menu system, typing them in the Executive/Script window, or providing a script/batch file. While the NSLM language provides great expressive-ness, crucial for describing model architectures—and produces efficient code it requires the user to compile the models. To avoid re-compiling we provide the NSL script language known as NSLS which also provides a dynamic user control environment. With NSLS the user can interact very efficiently with a model during its simulation. Moreover, NSLS can be used to create a script/batch files to be executed over and over again. This is handy when the user is only interested in final results after a large number of iterations such as in the *Backpropagation* model (see chapter 3). NSLS contributes the following functionality:

- model parameter assignment
- input specification
- simulation control
- file control
- graphics control

Additionally, the NSL script interpreter interacts with the well-known scripting language TCL, the Tool Command Language (Ousterhout 1994) and Jacl, the Java Command Language extension to TCL (Scriptics 1999), thus providing NSL and TCL functionality. We refer to the combined language as NSLS and to individual commands as belonging to TCL or to NSL. An important characteristic of NSLS is that TCL and NSL commands may be combined as part of single more powerful commands, one of the advantages of having the two. In particular, NSLS commands may be applied to TCL primitive types and NSLM object types (NslFloat0, etc.) but unfortunately we cannot access the NSLM primitive types (float, etc.) from the Script Language. NSLS commands include assigning and retrieving NSLM object values as well as instantiating new NSLM objects from NSLS.

As introduced in chapter 2, when NSL is originally launched from the operating system, it brings up the NSL Executive window.[1] The top part of this window, the executive panel, contains menu buttons that let the user execute many of the NSLS control commands. The bottom part of the executive window, the script window, is where NSLS commands can be interactively typed.

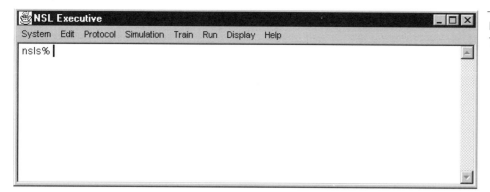

Figure 7.1
The NSL Executive Window

In the rest of this chapter we describe how parameters, simulation control, and visualization control are interactively specified using the NSLS language.

7.1 Overview
We give an overview of general aspects to NSLS.

General Conventions
There are a number of general conventions we shall be using throughout this chapter:

- **Bold** letters indicate key words or commands and *italics* indicate variables or parameters to be provided by the user.

- Names for classes, modules and models start with upper case letters, e.g., **ModuleX**.

- Names for objects, module instances, model instances, and methods start with lower case letters, e.g., **moduleX**.

- Names of files storing NSLS simulation scripts should end with a ".nsl" extension.

- The script (interpreter) window provides a main prompt of "nsls%" and a secondary prompt of ">". The secondary prompt is used when a command is unfinished and continued on the next line.

- Either a carriage return or a semicolon marks the end of line in NSLS.

- A hash sign '#' precedes comments. If there is a comment at the end of a line, then a semi-colon must appear before the comment, i.e. ";#".

- To continue a command on more than one line a backslash "\" must be used at the end of every line except the last one. No characters may appear after the backslash, including empty spaces. The only exception is a statement involving an open bracket being closed on a different line.

- Spaces are very significant in NSLS (as in TCL). For example, $m(1,1)$ is not the same as $m(1, 1)$ (the latter has a space and generates two separate expressions instead of one).

- TCL commands do not have any particular prefix, they follow directly with the *command*,

```
nsls% command
```

- All NSL commands must have a **nsl** prefix followed by the actual *command*,

```
nsls% nsl command
```

- Variable names must begin with an alphabetic character either upper, lower case or an underscore.

- In terms of graphics, all frame and canvas names should start with a lower case letter.

Help

NSL provides extensive on-line information from the NSL web page at **http://www-hbp.usc.edu** or **http://cannes.rhon.itam.mx**. NSLS script related information is also available by typing one of the following commands in the Executive/Script window:

```
nsls% nsl help
```

or specific information on a command can be retrieved by typing:

```
nsls% nsl help command
```

Exit

To terminate the script interpreter and close all windows, type the following command in the Executive/Script window:

```
nsls% nsl exit
```

Note that the TCL **exit** command can also be used, but does not handle the termination as nicely as **nsl exit**. The **nsl exit** command calls **endModule** and **endSystem** as well as closing all files before exiting.

7.2 TCL Primitives Types

We briefly describe some of the more important commands on *primitive* types in TCL with relation to NSLS (for a complete language description please refer to Ousterhout (1994)). TCL primitive types are made primarily of numbers and characters and do not have any relation with primitive types defined in NSLM. In general, TCL is considered a *non-typed* language since variables do not involve an explicit type declaration but instead have their type implicitly specified according to initial value assignment. While there is some TCL support for *objects* types, such as with TK graphic objects, we will concentrate only in TCL basics, primarily variables, arrays, expressions, control statements and procedures.

Variables

TCL variables may be assigned values directly from TCL or indirectly from NSLM objects. TCL variables are assigned values as they are initialized using the *set* command as follows

```
set var value
```

For example, to set the value of *i* to 0 we would do

```
set i 0
```

TCL variable values can be obtained by preceding the variable name with a "$" sign, e.g. *$var*. For example, to set the value of a new variable *j* to the value of *i*:

```
set j $i
```

The values of TCL variables may then be used to set values to other TCL variables or NSLM objects attributes, the latter being of particular interest in NSLS.

Arrays

Arrays in TCL are somewhat different in both semantics and syntax from traditional programming language arrays. Arrays in TCL are actually *associative* arrays, in that elements are associated with a particular element name instead of index number. Arrays are only single sized but multiple dimensions can be simulated with names containing multiple commas. Arrays are defined using the **set** command together with parenthesis grouping elements. For example:

```
set vararray(one) 1
```

Multiple dimension arrays are simulated as follows,

```
set vararray(1,1) 30
set vararray(1,2) 99
set vararray(1,3) 7
```

where *vararray*(1,1) simulates the first row and column. Note that *vararray* is not really double sized in TCL but instead each vector element is associated with a "*x,y*" style name. Thus, you should be careful not to add additional letters to the element name such as spaces, since "*x, y*" (extra space character) would specify a different string and thus a different element name.

Expressions and Control Statements

TCL supports a number of expressions on numerical and character variables. These include numerical operators as well as commands and functions applied to both numeric and character sets. Brackets are quite particular in TCL in that they separate all kinds of expressions. In terms of control statements, TCL provides with the following (note the space between bracket sections):

- **for** control statement. For example

```
for {set x 0} {$x<10} {incr x} {
    puts "x is $x"
}
```

where curly brackets separate sections in the **for** loop, **incr** increments *x* while **puts**, which can also print to a file, prints to the screen.

- **while** control statement. For example

```
set x 0
while {$x<10} {
    puts "x is $x"
    incr x
}
```

which performs the same computation as the previous **for** loop.

- **if-else-then** control statement. For example

```
if { x > 0 } {
    set y 1
} elseif { x = 0 } {
set y 0 }
} else { set y -1 }
```

where there may be any number of **elseif** sections and both the **elseif** and **else** section are optional.

* **switch** control statement. For example

```
switch $x {
    abc {set b $y }
    hij {set b $z}
    default {set b $v}
}
```

where *x* is a string being compared to the different string options. If the string matches one of the options, then the corresponding execution statements within the curly brackets are executed.

Procedures

TCL procedures are helpful in reusing script code. For example, we define a *testHopfiledNet* procedure to run the *Hopfield* model with different input sets (the nsl set and run commands are described in section 7.3),

```
proc testHopfiledNet { input {distortion 0} } {
    puts "Testing with distortion $distorion"
    nsl set hopfieldModel.distortion $distortion
    nsl set hopfieldModel.in.pat $input
    nsl train
}
```

The procedure receives two parameters, *input* and *distortion*, the latter with default of 0. We can then generate a variable a set to simulate a double array of positive or negative ones. Note how array elements are specified in different (brackets) sections in variable *a*.

```
set a {
{ -1 -1 1 1 -1 -1 }
{ -1 1 -1 -1 1 -1 }
{ -1 1 1 1 1 -1 }
{ -1 1 1 1 1 -1 }
{ -1 1 -1 -1 1 -1 }
{ -1 1 -1 -1 1 -1 }
}
```

We call the procedure with *a* and 10 and obtain back the "puts" string.

```
testHopfieldNet $a 10
```

Testing with distortion equal 10, we call all call the procedure with only a single parameter, obtaining back the default value of 0 in this case.

```
testHopfieldNet $a
```

Testing with distortion equal 0.

Note that procedure parameters are always local to that procedure and are passed by value. If we want to pass variables by reference, we should use the TCL command **upvar**. If we want to use a non-local variable, we will have to let the procedure know the global variables by using the TCL **global** command.

System Commands

TCL offers a number of commands to interact with the external system environment. Of particular interest are the following commands,

```
cd
```

that changes the current relative directory to a new one. This is particularly important when the user wants to load script files from that directory and even more important when script files themsleves load additional files from that directory. Without doing a "cd" these latter files would not be found. Another useful command is,

```
pwd
```

checking the current working directory.

7.3 NSL Objects, Modules and Model Types

Besides TCL primitive type, NSLS can process object, module and model type variables as defined in NSLM. Sharing of variables between NSLM and NSLS is quite important since without it the user would not be able to have a good control over the model during its simulation. In general there are some limitations on how much can be accessed from NSLM in NSLS. For example, NSLM variables can be accessed from NSLS but the other way around is not possible. In the following sections we describe in more detail this sharing and how it is achieved.

Access

Accessing NSLM variables from NSLS is exclusively done by variable name and as long as the corresponding NSLM protection allows. Protections are set within NSLM via the **nslSetAccess** method where three options can be specified: "N" for no access, "R" for read access and "W" for write (and read) access, with the default being "W". (We hope to change the default access to "R" in a future version.)

```
public void initModule() {
    hv.nslSetAcccess('W');
}
```

Recall that **initModule** is the method where module variables are initialized. In chapter 2 we showed how to modify the offset, **hu**, from the scripting window. To do this, **hu**, must have **write access** which can be set with **nslSetAccess**. Since variables are not global in NSLM but local within some branch of a particular model hierarchy tree, to access a particular variable we must know its exact location within the tree, similar to referencing variables within NSLM.

Reference Tree for Model Variables

Variables are referenced using the "dot" notation similar to that in NSLM. The exception is that visibility for accessing NSLM objects is controlled *by name* and not by the variable's visibility modifier, i.e. *public, protected* or *private*. Referencing can be either *absolute* or *relative* as in NSLM referencing.

Absolute referencing starts always from **system** when accessing system variables or from a particular model name when accessing model variables. For example, the absolute reference to an object named *obj111* would be as follows

```
model.obj1.obj11.obj111
```

Relative referencing starts from a current location in the tree hierarchy using the path variable. For example, we could set the special variable called **varpath** that acts as a "bookmark" of where we are:

```
nsl set varpath model.obj1.obj11
```

Once this is set, we can use *relative* referencing from then on. The relative reference for *obj111* would simply be:

```
obj111
```

Expressions

NSLS provides two basic methods, **set** and **get**, to access NSLM attribute variables.

Set

Objects can be assigned data values using the **set** command, analogous to the *assignment* operator in NSLM.

To assign data,

```
nsl set object-name value
```

where *object-name* is the name of an existing object and *value* corresponds to a matching attribute type value.

For example, to set the value of "1" to a scalar object found in *model.obj1.obj11* would be use:

```
nsl set model.obj1.obj11 1
```

In general, the number of elements typed in *value* will correspond to the dimension defined for the object. The exception is to set all of the values in an *object* to a unique *value* corresponding to a single element. According to the object type and corresponding dimension NSL uses the following format:

- For **Nsl*Type*0** corresponding to single elements, for example, we set a scalar as

```
nsl set tu 1.0
```

assigning 1.0 to a zero dimension *tu* object.

- For **Nsl*Type*1** corresponding to a list or vector, for example, we set a 9-element vector as

```
nsl set s { 0 0 0 0 1 0 2 0 0 }
```

The expression assigns the nine integer values to a one dimension *s* object: 1 to $s[4]$ and 2 to $s[6]$, and the rest 0. (Remember that indices start with 0 and spaces must be left between brackets and other characters.) Objects can be assigned single element values by using parenthesis around element indices. For example:

```
nsl set s 0
nsl set s(4) 1
nsl set s(6) 2
```

is equivalent to the initial example.

- For **Nsl*Type2*** corresponding to a two-dimensional list or matrix, we set the values of a 2x9 matrix using:

```
nsl set s {{ 0 0 0 0 1 0 2 0 0 }
         { 3 0 0 0 0 0 0 0 0 }}
```

The expression assigns integer values to a two dimensional s object: 1 to $s(0,4)$ 2 to $s(0,6)$, 3 to $s(0,1)$ and the rest 0. We can also type the above all on one line. (Notice that if an interactively specified command is incomplete then the ">" prompt will appear. When the command is complete the prompt will change back to "nsls%".)

Matrices can be assigned single element values by using parenthesis around element indices. For example

```
nsl set s 0
nsl set s(0,4) 1
nsl set s(0,6) 2
nsl set s(1,0) 3
```

is equivalent to the initial example.

- For **Nsl*Type3*** corresponding to a three-dimensional list or vector of matrices, we set the values of a 2x2x9 array using:

```
nsl set s {{{ 0 0 0 0 1 0 2 0 0 } { 3 0 0 0 0 0 0 0 0 }}
         {{ 0 0 0 0 4 0 5 0 0 } { 6 0 0 0 0 0 0 0 0 }}}
```

The expression assigns integer values to a three dimension s object: 1 to $s(0,0,4)$ 2 to $s(0,0,6)$, 3 to $s(0,0,1)$, 4 to $s(1,0,4)$ 5 to $s(1,0,6)$, 6 to $s(1,0,1)$ and the rest 0. Again we can assign single element values by using parenthesis around element indices. For example

```
nsl set s 0
nsl set s(0,0,4) 1
```

and so forth.

- For **Nsl*Type4*** corresponding to a four-dimensional list or a vector of three-dimensional matrices, for example, we set a 2x2x2x9 array as

```
nsl set s {{{{ 0 0 0 0 1 0 2 0 0 }{ 3 0 0 0 0 0 0 0 0 }}
         {{ 0 0 0 0 4 0 5 0 0 }{ 6 0 0 0 0 0 0 0 0 }}}
         {{{ 0 0 0 0 7 0 8 0 0 }{ 9 0 0 0 0 0 0 0 0 }}
         {{ 0 0 0 0 10 0 11 0 0 }{ 12 0 0 0 0 0 0 0 0 }}}}
```

The expression assigns integer values to a four dimensional s object: 1 to $s(0,0,0,4)$ 2 to $s(0,0,0,6)$, 3 to $s(0,0,0,1)$ and so forth. Again we can assign single element values by using parenthesis around element indices. For example

```
nsl set s 0
nsl set s(0,0,0,4) 1
```

and so forth.

Get

The **get** command is somewhat similar to the **set** command. The main difference lies in that it retrieves the value instead of setting it. Since NSLS does not let the user create new NSLM variables, the result from a get command must be stored into a TCL variable. We use the following TCL substitution format to retrieve values with the NSLS **get** command into a TCL variable command (notice the brackets below):

```
set tclvar [nsl get object-name]
```

where *tclvar* is the name of the TCL variable storing the resulting value, *object-name* is the name of an existing object. For example,

```
set s [nsl get model.obj1.obj11]
```

Since TCL expressions always return a string, the "[**nsl get** object-name]" will return a string as well, setting the value of *s* to the corresponding return value. For example, if "*model.obj1.obj11*" was a two dimensional 2x2 matrix containing integer values, then "*model.obj1.obj11*" might return the string "{{ 9 5 }{7 4 }}".

If the user tries the "**nsl get** *object-name*" command without assigning the returning string to a variable, a TCL script error will occur. TCL would not know how to interpret the resultant string and would print an "invalid command name" message.

According to the object type and corresponding dimension NSL uses the following format:

- For **Nsl*Type*0** corresponding to single elements, for example, we get a scalar as

```
nsl get tu
```

would return the value stored in *tu*, for example 1.0.

- For **Nsl*Type*1** corresponding to a list or vector, for example, we get a 9-element vector as

```
nsl get s
```

The expression returns a one dimension vector, for example { 0 0 0 0 1 0 2 0 0 }. Using parenthesis around element indices can retrieve single values. For example

```
nsl get s(4)
```

would return 1.

- For **Nsl*Type*2** corresponding to a two-dimensional list or matrix, for example, we get a 2x9 matrix as

```
nsl get s
```

The expression returns a two dimension matrix, for example {{ 0 0 0 0 1 0 2 0 0 }{ 3 0 0 0 0 0 0 0 0 }}. Using parenthesis around element indices can retrieve single values. For example

```
nsl get s(0,4)
```

would return 1.

- For **Nsl*Type*3** corresponding to a three-dimensional list or array of matrices, for example, we get a 2x2x9 array as

```
nsl get s
```

The expression returns a three dimension array, for example {{{ 0 0 0 0 1 0 2 0 0 }{ 3 0 0 0 0 0 0 0 }}{{ 0 0 0 0 4 0 5 0 0 }{ 6 0 0 0 0 0 0 0 }}}. Using parenthesis around element indices can retrieve single values. For example

```
nsl get s(0,0,4)
```

would return 1.

- For **Nsl*Type*4** corresponding to a four-dimensional list or two-dimensional array of matrices, for example, we get a 2x2x2x9 array as

```
nsl get s
```

The expression returns a four dimensional array, for example {{{{ 0 0 0 0 1 0 2 0 0 }{ 3 0 0 0 0 0 0 0 }}{{ 0 0 0 0 4 0 5 0 0 }{ 6 0 0 0 0 0 0 0 }}}{{{ 0 0 0 0 7 0 8 0 0 }{ 9 0 0 0 0 0 0 0 }}{{ 0 0 0 0 10 0 11 0 0 }{ 12 0 0 0 0 0 0 0 }}}}. Using parenthesis around element indices can retrieve single values. For example

```
nsl get s(0,0,0,4)
```

would return 1.

Another useful function is the **-dim** option. We can use **-dim** to get the sizes of the dimensions from a NSL type object:

```
nsl get s -dim
```

returns {2 2 2 9} for the four dimensional array mentioned above.

Simulation Methods

NSLS enables the user to call all NSLM simulation methods described in chapter 6 in controlling the overall simulation sequence. Starting with table 7.1 we describe simulation methods that may be called from NSLS as control commands together with additional one. These commands may involve optional parameters and most of these commands can be called from the executive window menus as well (see chapter 5), all requiring the "nsl" prefix in the script. table 7.1 shows the *connection* command called once throughout the execution of the complete system.

Connection Command	Optional Parameters	Description
makeConn	none	Execute the **makeConn** simulation method for all modules in the model.

Table 7.1 Connection command.

Table 7.2 shows the *system* commands called once throughout the execution of the complete system.

System Command	Optional Parameters	Description
initSys	none	Execute the **initSys** simulation method for all modules in the model.
endSys	none	Execute the **endSys** simulation method for all modules in the model.

Table 7.2 System commands.

Table 7.3 shows the *module* commands called once during a complete module simulation.

Module Command	Optional Parameters	Description
initModule	none	Execute the **initModule** simulation method for all modules in the model.
endModule	none	Execute the **endModule** simulation method for all modules in the model.

Table 7.3 Module commands.

Table 7.4 shows the basic **train** commands called in relation to training aspects of the simulation.

Train Command	Optional Parameters	Description
initTrainEpochs	none	Execute the **initTrainEpochs** simulation method for all modules in the model.
endTrainEpochs	none	Execute the **endTrainEpochs** simulation method for all modules in the model.
initTrain	none	Execute the **initTrain** simulation method for all modules in the model.
simTrain	*trainEndTime*	Execute the **simTrain** simulation method for all modules in the model. Simulation starts at *t*=0 until *trainEndTime* (a real number) or until *system.trainEndTime* is reached. The actual number of steps is specified by *trainEndTime* divided by *trainDelta*.
endTrain	none	Execute the **endTrain** simulation method for all modules in the model.

Table 7.4 Basic train commands.

Table 7.5 shows additional **train** commands called in relation to training aspects of the simulation.

Train Command	Optional Parameters	Description
train	*trainEndTime*	Execute **initTrain** once, followed by **simTrain** starting at *t*=0 until reaching *trainEndTime* or *system.trainEndTime* followed by **endTrain** at the end. Simulation takes place for all specified epochs.
doTrainEpochTimes	*numTrainEpochs*	Execute the previous **train** command for *numTrainEpochs* times.
breakEpochs	none	Stop the simulation in between two epochs.
stepEpochs	*numTrainEpochs*	According to the current state of the simulation, execute either the train phase or run phase for all modules in the model *numTrainEpochs*, or once if not specified. If a **breakEpochs** was previously called then start from the next epoch.
contEpochs	*lastTrainEpoch*	According to the current state of the simulation, execute either the train phase or run phase for all modules in the model until *lastTrainEpoch* or until all epochs have been processed. If a **breakTrainEpochs** was previously called then start from the next epoch.
breakCycles	none	Stop the simulation in between two cycles.

Table 7.5 Additional train commands.

Train Command	Optional Parameters	Description

Table 7.5 *(continued)*

Train Command	Optional Parameters	Description
contCycles	*trainEndTime*	Execute **simTrain** method starting at *t=trainTime* (current training time) until reaching *trainEndTime* (a real number) or *system.trainEndTime* if not specified.
stepCycles	*numTrainCycles*	Execute the **simTrain** method for *numTrainCycles* (an integer). If *numTrainCycles* is not specified, it steps one cycle only.
breakModules	none	Stop the simulation in between modules.
stepModules	*numTrainModules*	According to the current state of the simulation, execute the **simTrain** method for all modules in a model *numTrainModule* times, or once if not specified. If a **breakModule** was previously called then start from the next module.
contModules	*lastTrainModule*	According to the current state of the simulation, execute the **simTrain** for all modules in the model until *numTrainModule*, or until all modules have been processed. If a **breakModule** was previously called then start from the next module.

Table 7.5
Additional **train** commands.

Table 7.6 shows the basic **run** commands called in relation to running aspects of the simulation.

Run Command	Optional Parameters	Description
initRunEpochs	none	Execute the **initRunEpochs** simulation method for all modules in the model.
endRunEpochs	none	Execute the **endRunEpochs** simulation method for all modules in the model.
initRun	none	Execute the **initRun**simulation method for all modules in the model.
simRun	*runEndTime*	Execute the **simRun** simulation method for all modules in the model. Simulation starts at *t*=0 until *runEndTime* (a real number) or until *system.runEndTime* is reached. The actual number of steps is specified by *runEndTime* divided by *runDelta*.
endRun	none	Execute the **endRun** simulation method for all modules in the model.

Table 7.6
Basic **run** commands.

Table 7.7 describes additional **run** commands called in relation to running aspects of the simulation.

Command	Optional Parameters	Description
run	*runEndTime*	Execute **initRun** once, followed by **simRun** starting at *t*=0 until reaching *runEndTime* or *system.runEndTime* followed by **endRun** at the end. Simulation takes place for all specified epochs.
doRunEpochTimes	*numRunEpochs*	Execute the previous **run** command for *numRunEpochs* times.
breakEpochs	none	Stop the simulation in between two epochs for all modules in the model.
stepEpochs	*numRunEpochs*	According to the current state of the simulation, execute either the train phase or run phase for all modules in the model *numRunEpochs*, or once if not specified. If a **breakEpochs** was previously called then start from the next epoch.
contEpochs	*lastRunEpoch*	According to the current state of the simulation, execute either the train phase or run phase for all modules in the model until *lastRunEpoch* or until all epochs have been processed. If a **breakEpochs** was previously called then start from the next epoch.
breakCycles	none	Stop the simulation in between two cycles.
contCycles	*runEndTime*	Execute **simRun** method starting at *t=runTime* (current run time) until reaching *runEndTime* (a real number) or *system.runEndTime* if not specified.
stepCycles	*numRunCycles*	Execute the **simRun** method for *numRunCycles* (an integer). If *numRunCycles* is not specified, it steps one cycle only.
breakModules	none	Stop the simulation in between modules.
stepModules	*numRunModules*	According to the current state of the simulation, execute the **simRun** method for all modules in a model *numRunModule* times, or once if not specified. If a **breakModules** was previously called, then start from the next module.
contModules	*lastRunModule*	According to the current state of the simulation, execute the **simRun** for all modules in the model until *numRunModule*, or until all modules have been processed. If a **breakModules** was previously called, then start from the next module.

Simulation Parameters

There are a number of simulation parameters that can be specified affecting the overall simulation. These values can be overriden by paremeters passed to the simulation methods as described in the previous section. These parameters are applied to all modules at once when setting them at the system level as follows,

```
nsl set system.parameter value
```

where *parameter* is the corresponding system parameter.

Table 7.7
Additional NSL run commands

These attributes may also be set by module by specifying the following

```
nsl set module.parameter value
```

These parameters will be described in terms of "train", "run" and "integration" parameters.

Train

The system train parameters are described in table 7.8.

Parameter	Default Value	Description
trainDelta	1.0	Training delta (step size) for the entire system.
trainEndTime	1.0	Training end time for the entire system.
numTrainEpochs	1	Training epochs for the entire system.

For example, to set the value to 5.0 of **trainEndTime** for all modules in the system do the following:

Table 7.8
System Train Parameters

```
nsl set system.trainEndTime 5.0
```

Run

The system run parameters are described in table 7.9.

Parameter	Default Value	Description
runDelta	1.0	Run delta (step size) of the entire system.
runEndTime	1.0	Run end time of the entire system.
numRunEpochs	1	Number of runs (analogous to epochs) for the entire system

For example, to set the value to 5.0 of **runEndTime** for all modules in the system do the following:

Table 7.9
System Run Parameters

```
nsl set system.runEndTime 5.0
```

Integration Approximation Methods

As discussed in chapter 6, NSL provides numerical methods for integration. The involved parameters may be set at the system level or per module. The parameters are described in the following statements, and they are set as follows,

```
nsl set system.approximation.parameter value
```

or for a particular module,

```
nsl set module.approximation.parameter value
```

Table 7.10
System Approximation
Parameters

where *parameter* represents the corresponding integration parameter as shown in table 7.10.

Parameter	Default Value	Description
method	Euler	NSL offers the following two numerical method options: **Euler** or **RungeKutta2**.
delta	1.0	The user specifies the approximation step or delta for the complete system.

7.4 Input Output

There are a number of input and output commands dealing with script and data files.

Script Files

Script files store NSLS style command files. These files may be loaded to avoid writing single commands at a time. Additionally, the user may store a complete window interaction (a "log") to be loaded at a alter time without having to duplicate it again. In general, multiple script files can be associated with a single model.

Source

Script files are loaded into the simulator with following command:

```
nsl source file-name
```

(File names must be either relative to the current directory or require an absolute path to the desire file. Additionally, NSL uses the file "SCS_LIBRARY_PATHS" located in at the user's home directory to also search for these files.

Data Files

Besides script files, NSLS also supports reading and writing data as "open format" **ascii text**—text that would need to be read or written in a specific format for the particular model—from/to files or the screen ("standard output"). In particular, it is quite useful to read and store data generated by the simulation into files. Data stored in files can be used as input to new simulations, such as when saving training weights as with *Backpropagation*, or simply as a means of analyzing the simulation output later on in numerical detail. Note that for simplicity these files may actually follow the NSLS script format although NSL gives the user this "open format" added flexibility. Note also that script files are usually loaded (read) all at once while data files are read line by line since only the user knows its particular format. For this reason NSL provides with a number of commands to manipulate files.

Open

Opens a file using a particular access type: read (r), write (w) and append (a) having as default read.

```
open file-name file-access
```

If the file is successfully opened, the command will return a file descriptor that can be saved into a TCL variable using for example

```
set f [open input.dat r]
```

Gets

The *gets* command retrieves the next line from the file associated with the file descriptor passed as an argument. If the file has reached its end, it returns the empty string. For example

```
nsl set hopfieldModel.in.pat [gets $f]
```

Puts

The *puts* command passes a string as argument to the file associated with the file descriptor. It adds a new line character at the end of the string, for example

```
puts $f [nsl get hopfieldModel.hopfield.weights]
```

Eof

The *eof* command tells you if the file associated with the file descriptor has reached its end. If this is true, it returns 1, otherwise 0.

```
while {![eof $f]} {
    nsl set hopfieldModel.in.pat [gets $f]
    nsl run
}
```

Close

The *close* command closes the file associated with the file descriptor passed as an argument.

```
close $f
```

Monitor

The *monitor* command is similar to the "puts" command; however, it continuously "puts" the value of the variable being monitored into the file or screen until specified otherwise and returns a monitor descriptor. To enable an object specified by name to be written into a file do:

```
nsl monitor object-name -file file-descriptor
```

If *file-descriptor* is not specified, then "standard output" is taken as the output file name, which sends the data to the script window, (or where the standard output was redirected):

```
nsl monitor object-name
```

Additional parameters may be included in the monitor command.

```
nsl monitor -parameter value
```

These parameters are given in table 7.11.

parameter	default	description
start	Current time	Start time in the user's specified units of time (usec, msec, seconds, etc).
stop	End time	Stop time in the user's specified units of time.
freq	Delta	Frequency is the number of cycles until the next reporting period. One means report every cycle, two means report every other cycle, etc.

All visible NSL objects in a module may be enabled for monitoring by using an asterisk, "*", for example

```
nsl monitor model.module.*
```

Table 7.11
Parameters for the Monitor Command—start parameter, stop parameter, freq parameter.

In the case of NSL types of 0 dimension, the object data will be written in a single line. In the case of NSL array types, the object data will be written in row major format.

To "unmonitor" a particular variable we can type:

```
nsl unmonitor object-name
```

7.5 Graphics Displays

Another important functionality of NSLS is to support interactive graphical display generation. This is achieved both using the script window and script files. In chapter 5 we discussed how to build the window interface and graphical displays using the NSLM language and how to interact with them from the menu interface. In this chapter we will discuss how to interact using the NSLS language.

Reference Tree for Canvases

In NSLS as in TCL, all windows spring from one parent window—the root window—denoted by ".nsl". In addition to **varpath** (section 7.3), NSLS also provide the **displaypath** variable that acts just like **varpath** but is used to reduce the amount of typing when specifying a display path, for example

```
nsl set displaypath .nsl.frame1.canvas12
```

Create and Configure

NSLS uses a general format in creating new windows and configuring already created ones. Window properties or attributes can be set during their creation or modified afterwards.

To create a new window where initial attributes are specified using the "*-attribute value*" format,

```
nsl create window window-name -attribute value
```

To configure an already created window with attributes specified by the "*-attribute value*" format,

```
nsl configure window window-name -attribute value
```

Note many any attributes may be changed in a single command using multiple "*-attribute value*" pairs in the same line.

NslExecutiveWindow

The first window in the graphics interface is always the **NSL Executive/Script** instantiated by the system and window shown in figure 7.1. This is the root window or console in the NSL window hierarchy and denoted by ".nsl". Each additional window/frame added to the screen should append its name to this executive window name. Since the **executive** window is already instantiated, we can only modify its attribute values shown in table 7.12.

parameter	type	default	description
width	int	100	width in pixels
height	int	100	height in pixels
x0	int	0	left position in x in pixels
y0	int	0	top position in y in pixels

Table 7.12
Executive Window Parameters—width parameter, height parameter, x0 parameter, y0 parameter.

For example, we could change the size of the **NslExecutiveWindow** window by specifying the following

```
nsl configure .nsl -width 400 -height 200
```

NslOutFrame

The user may instantiate multiple **NslOutFrames** representing independent windows on the screen, analogous to the **NslExecutiveWindow**. **NslOutFrames** are used to display **NslOutCanvas** (to be described in the next section) holding actual graphical output. To create a new **NslOutFrame** we can type

```
nsl create NslOutFrame .nsl.frame-name
```

where *frame-name* is used to reference the newly instantiated frame object. This name can then be used for further configuration. The **NslOutFrame** attribute list is shown in table 7.13

parameter	type	default	description
display	charString		frame name
title	charString	display name	any string name to appear in the frame label
rows	int	1	the number of rows
column	int	1	the number of columns
x0	int	0	position in x direction in pixels
y0	int	0	position in y direction in pixels
width	int	100	frame width in pixels
height	int	100	frame height in pixels
font	charString		font used
background	charString		background color
foreground	charString		foreground color
freq	int	1	graphics update frequency in relation to simulation step. Default is 1 corresponding to simulation step

Note that NSL can display the output data with frequencies different to those used by the simulator in performing the actual variable updates. Since displaying data may become very slow, modifying this frequency can significantly speed up the overall time or "wall clock time" of the simulation. The only restriction on frequency is that all the variables within an output frame must have the same output display frequency.

Table 7.13
NslOutFrame Attributes.

To create an output frame named *diddayOut* with width 100 and height 200, we would type:

```
nsl create NslOutFrame .nsl.diddayOut -width 100 -height 200
```

For example, if we later want to change the foreground color to white we would type:

```
nsl configure .nsl.diddayOut -foreground white
```

NslOutCanvas

NSL can instantiate multiple **NslOutCanvas** inside a single independent **NslOutFrame** window. Canvases are not independent windows on the screen, but are always part of a **NslOutFrame**. To instantiate a new **NslOutCanvas** the user has to specify besides a *canvas-name* a variable name "**–var** *var-name*" specifying the particular variable being output in addition to attribute values. For example, the following line instantiates a new canvas in an existing frame,

```
nsl create NslOutCanvas .nsl.frame-name.canvas-name \
    -var var-name -attributes value
```

Note that the variable name is a required parameter. The **NslOutCanvas** parameter list is given in table 7.14.

parameter	type	default	description
display	charString		frame name
title	charString	display name	canvas label
var	Object type		NSL object to be display in the canvas. Required.
graph	charString		graph type—see table 5.2.
position	charString		position in output frame: first, next, previous, and last.
wymin	float double		low variable value in y direction
wymax	float double		high variable value in y direction
wxmin	float double		low value in the x direction—for temporal plots this is time zero.
wxmax	float double		high value in the x direction—for temporal plots this is the max time.
freq	int		the frequency or time step used for collecting data from the simulation thread
drawcolor	charString		draw color
drawstyle	charString		draw style
xlabel	charString		label placed along x axis
ylabel	charString		label placed along y axis
option	charString		re-scale or shift
grid	boolean	true	grid is drawn

Table 7.14
NslOutCanvas Parameters.

As a general example, to create a display canvas *s* inside an output frame named *maxSelector* with an area level graph displaying the values between -1 and 2 for layer variable *"s"* we would type

```
nsl create NslOutCanvas .nsl.maxSelector.s -var didday.s \
    -wymin -1 -wymax 2 -graph Area
```

When can change for example the **NslOutCanvas** minimum and maximum values as follows:

```
nsl configure .nsl.maxSelector.s -wymin -10 -wymax 20
```

Note that the order in specifying parameters is irrelevant.

NslInFrame

The user may instantiate multiple **NslInFrames**, similar to the **NslOutFrames**. **NslInFrames** are used to display **NslInCanvases** where the user may interact with the simulation by providing input or by changing values as the simulation is running. To isntantiate a new **NslInFrame** we type

```
nsl create NslInFrame .nsl.frame-name
```

where *frame-name* is used for referencing the newly created frame. The NslInFrame attribute list is shown in table 7.15

parameter	type	default	description
display	charString		frame name
title	charString	display name	any string name to appear in the frame label
rows	int	1	the number of rows
column	int	1	the number of columns
x0	int	0	position in x direction in pixels
y0	int	0	position in y direction in pixels
width	int	100	frame width in pixels
height	int	100	frame height in pixels
font	charString		font used
background	charString		background color
foreground	charString		foreground color
freq	charString	1	graphics update frequency in relation to simulation step. Default is 1 corresponding to simulation step

Table 7.15
NslInFrame Attributes.

To create an input frame named *diddayIn* with width 100 and height 200, we would type:

```
nsl create NslInFrame .nsl.diddayIn -width 100 -height 200
```

For example, to change the foreground color to white we would do

```
nsl configure .nsl.diddayIn -foreground white
```

NslInCanvas

NSL can instantiate multiple **NslInCanvases** inside a **NslInFrame** in order to generate graphical input from the simulation. Similar to **NslOutCanvases**, **NslInCanvases** are not independent windows on the screen, but are always part of a **NslInFrame**. To instantiate a new **NslInCanvas** the user has to specify besides a *canvas-name* a variable name "**–var** *var-name*" specifying the particular variable being used for input in addition to attribute values.

```
nsl create NslInCanvas .nsl.frame-name.canvas-name \
    -var var-name -attributes value
```

Note that the variable name is a required parameter. The parameter list is shown in table 7.16

parameter	type	default	description
display	charString		frame name
title	charString	display name	canvas label
var	Object Type		NSL object to be display in the canvas. Required.
graph	charString		graph type—see specified list below
position	charString		position in output frame: first, next, previous, and last.
wymin	float double		low variable value in y direction
wymax	float double		high variable value in y direction
wxmin	float double		low value in the x direction—for temporal plots this is time zero.
wxmax	float double		high value in the x direction—for temporal plots this is the max time.
freq	float double		the frequency or time step used for collecting data from the simulation thread
drawcolor	charString		draw color
drawstyle	charString		draw style
xlabel	charString		label placed along x axis
ylabel	charString		label placed along y axis
option	charString		rescale or shift
grid	boolean	true	grid is drawn

Input graph types may be specified with one of the following strings: **InputImage** and **NumericEditor** as described in chapter 5.

Table 7.16
NslInCavas Attributes.

As a general example, to create a display canvas *s* inside an output frame named *maxSelector* with an inputImage graph displaying the values between 0 and 1 for layer variable *"s"* we would type

```
nsl create NslInCanvas .nsl.didday.s -var maxSelector.s \
    -wymin 0 -wymax 1 -graph inputImage
```

When can change for example the **NslInCanvas** minimum and maximum values as follows:

```
nsl configure .nsl.maxSelector.s -wymin -10 -wymax 20
```

Print

The user can print graphical windows to a file using the PostScript format. The command to do this is:

```
nsl print -name displayname -filename -filename
```

Note that the name parameter can be either a whole frame or a single canvas. The parameters for the **print** command are given in table 7.17.

Parameter	type	default	description
name	charString		Display name: either "screen", ".ex", fully extended frame name, or fully extended canvas name
size	int, int	8.5" by 11"	width and height in pixels
position	int, int	centered	x and y position in pixels
orientation	charString	portrait	landscape or portrait

7.6 Summary

The NSLS scripting language is a very powerful language whereas we have only described its basics. We showed how to use TCL commands to manipulate values of NSLM variables and how to provide control structure to scripts (*if*, *while*, *for*, and *switch*). We also saw how to get data from NSLM variables and store the information in NSLS variables. A very popular use of the NSLS language is in controlling the simulation with commands such as "nsl trainAndRunAll", "nsl stepTrain", "nslBreakCycle", etc. Finally, we documented how to create new **NslOutFrames** and **NslInFrames**, as well as how to add **NslOutCanvases** and **NslInCanvases** to them.

Notes

1. Note that NSL can be executed in **noDisplay** mode in which case no executive window is brought up.

Table 7.17
Print Command Parameters.

8 Adaptive Resonance Theory

T. Tanaka and A. Weitzenfeld[1]

8.1 Introduction

The adaptive resonance theory (ART) has been developed to avoid the stability-plasticity dilemma in competitive networks learning. The stability-plasticity dilemma addresses how a learning system can preserve its previously learned knowledge while keeping its ability to learn new patterns. ART architecture models can self-organize in real time producing stable recognition while getting input patterns beyond those originally stored.

ART is a family of different neural architectures. The first and most basic architecture is ART1 (Carpenter and Grossberg, 1987). ART1 can learn and recognize binary patterns. ART2 (Carpenter and Grossberg, 1987) is a class of architectures categorizing arbitrary sequences of analog input patterns. ART is used in modeling such as invariant visual pattern recognition (Carpenter et al 1989) where biological equivalence is discussed (Carpenter and Grossberg 1990).

An ART system consists of two subsystems, an attentional subsystem and an orienting subsystem. The stabilization of learning and activation occurs in the attentional subsystem by matching bottom-up input activation and top-down expectation. The orienting subsystem controls the attentional subsystem when a mismatch occurs in the attentional subsystem. In other words, the orienting subsystem works like a novelty detector.

An ART system has four basic properties. The first is the self-scaling computational units. The attentional subsystem is based on competitive learning enhancing pattern features but suppressing noise. The second is self-adjusting memory search. The system can search memory in parallel and adaptively change its search order. Third, already learned patterns directly access their corresponding category. Finally, the system can adaptively modulate attentional vigilance using the environment as a teacher. If the environment disapproves the current recognition of the system, it changes this parameter to be more vigilant.

There are two models of ART1, a slow-learning and a fast-learning one. The slow learning model is described by in terms of differential equations while the fast learning model uses the results of convergence in the slow learning model. In this chapter we will not show a full implementation on ART1, instead an implementation of the fast learning model will be more efficient and sufficient to show the ART1 architecture behavior.

8.2 Model Description

ART1 is the simplest ART learning model specifically designed for recognizing binary patterns. The ART1 system consists of an attentional subsystem and an orienting subsystem as shown in figure 8.1.

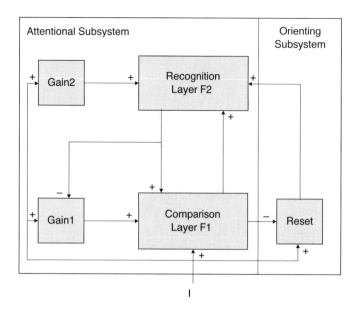

Figure 8.1
ART1 consists of an attentional subsystem and an orienting subsystem. The attentional subsystem has two short term memory (STM) stages, *F1* and *F2*. Long term memory (LTM) traces between *F1* and *F2* multiply the signal in these pathways. Gain control signals enable *F1* and *F2* to distinguish current stages of a running cycle. STM reset wave inhibits active *F2* cells when mismatches between bottom-up and top-down signals occur at *F1*.

The attentional subsystem consists of two competitive networks, the comparison layer *F1* and the recognition layer *F2*, and two control gains, Gain 1 and Gain 2. The orienting subsystem contains the reset layer for controlling the attentional subsystem overall dynamics.

The comparison layer receives the binary external input passing it to the recognition layer responsible for matching it to a classification category. This result is passed back to the comparison layer to find out if the category matches that of the input vector. If there is a match a new input vector is read and the cycle starts again. If there is a mismatch the orienting system is in charge of inhibiting the previous category in order to get a new category match in the recognition layer. The two gains control the activity of the recognition and comparison layer, respectively.

A processing element x_{1i} in layer *F1* is shown in figure 8.2.

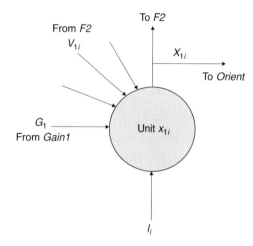

Figure 8.2
A processing unit x_{1i} in *F1* receives input from: pattern I_i, gain control signal G_1 and V_{1i} equivalent to output X_{2j} from *F2* multiplied by interconnection weight E_{21ij}. The local activity serving also as unit output is X_{1i}.

The excitatory input to x_{1i} in layer *F1* comes from three sources: (1) the external input vector I_i, (2) the control gain G_1 and (3) the internal network input V_{1i} made of the output from *F2* multiplied appropriate connections weights. There is no inhibitory input to the neuron. The output of the neuron is fed to the *F2* layer as well as the orient subsystem.

A processing element x_{2j} in layer $F2$ is shown in figure 8.3.

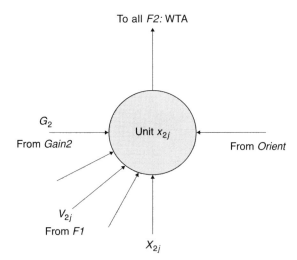

Figure 8.3
A processing element x_{2j} in $F2$ receives input from: gain control signal G_2 and V_{2j} equivalent to output X_{1i} from $F1$ multiplied by interconnection weight W_{12ji}. The local activity is also the unit output X_{2j}.

The excitatory input to x_{2j} in $F2$ comes from three sources: (1) the orient subsystem, (2) the control gain G_2 and (3) the internal network input V_{2j} made of the output from $F1$ multiplied appropriate connections weights. There is no inhibitory input to the neuron. The output of the neuron is fed to the $F1$ layer as well as the Gain 1 control.

The original dynamic equations (Carpenter and Grossberg 1987) handle both binary and analog computations. We shall concentrate here on the binary model. Processing in ART1 can be divided into four phases, (1) recognition, (2) comparison, (3) search, and (4) learning.

Recognition

Initially, in the recognition or bottom-up activation, no input vector I is applied disabling all recognition in $F2$ and making the two control gains, G_1 and G_2, equal to zero. This causes all $F2$ elements to be set to zero, giving them an equal chance to win the subsequent recognition competition. When an input vector is applied one or more of its components must be set to one thereby making both G_1 and G_2 equal to one.

Thus, the control gain G_1 depends on both the input vector I and the output X_2 from $F2$,

$$G_1 = \begin{cases} 1 & \text{if } I \neq 0 \text{ and } X_2 = 0 \\ 0 & \text{otherwise} \end{cases} \tag{8.1}$$

In other words, if there is an input vector I and $F2$ is not actively producing output, then $G_1 = 1$. Any other combination of activity on I and $F2$ would inhibit the gain control from exciting units on $F1$.

On the other hand, the output G_2 of the gain control module depends only on the input vector I,

$$G_2 = \begin{cases} 1 & \text{if } I \neq 0 \\ 0 & \text{otherwise} \end{cases} \tag{8.2}$$

In other words, if there exists an input vector then $G_2 = 1$ and recognition in $F2$ is allowed.

Each node in $F1$ receiving a nonzero input value generates an STM pattern activity greater than zero and the node's output is an exact duplicate of input vector. Since both X_{1i} and I_i are binary, their values would be either 1 or 0,

$$X_1 = I, \text{ if } G_1 = 1 \tag{8.3}$$

Each node in *F1* whose activity is beyond the threshold sends excitatory outputs to the *F2* nodes. The *F1* output pattern X_1 is multiplied by the LTM traces W_{12} connecting from *F1* to *F2*. Each node in *F2* sums up all its LTM gated signals

$$V_{2j} = \sum_i X_{1i} W_{12ji}$$ (8.4)

These connections represent the input pattern classification categories, where each weight stores one category. The output X_{2j} is defined so that the element that receives the largest input should be clearly enhanced. As such, the competitive network *F2* works as a winner-take-all network described by.

$$X_{2j} = \begin{cases} 1 & \text{if } G_2 = 1 \cap V_{2j} = \max_k \{V_{2k}\} \forall k \\ 0 & \text{otherwise} \end{cases}$$ (8.5)

The *F2* unit receiving the largest *F1* output is the one that best matches the input vector category, thus winning the competition. The *F2* winner node fires, having its value set to one, inhibiting all other nodes in the layer resulting in all other nodes being set to zero.

Comparison

In the comparison or top-down template matching, the STM activation pattern X_2 on *F2* generates a top-down template on *F1*. This pattern is multiplied by the LTM traces W_{12} connecting from *F2* to *F1*. Each node in *F1* sums up all its LTM gated signals

$$V_{1i} = \sum_j X_{2j} W_{21ij}$$ (8.6)

The most active recognition unit from *F2* passes a one back to the comparison layer *F1*. Since the recognition layer is now active, G_1 is inhibited and its output is set to zero.

In accordance with the "2/3" rule, stating that from three different input sources at least two are required to be active in order to generate an excitatory output, the only comparison units that will fire are those that receive simultaneous ones from the input vector and the recognition layer. Units not receiving a top down signal from *F2* must be inactive even if they receive input from below. This is summarized as follows

$$X_{1i} = \begin{cases} 1 & I_i \cap V_{1i} = 1 \\ 0 & \text{otherwise} \end{cases}$$ (8.7)

If there is a good match between the top-down template and the input vector, the system becomes stable and learning may occur.

If there is a mismatch between the input vector and the activity coming from the recognition layer, this indicates that the pattern being returned is not the one desired and the recognition layer should be inhibited.

Search

The reset layer in the orienting subsystem measures the similarity between the input vector and the recognition layer output pattern. If a mismatch between them, the reset layer inhibits the *F2* layer activity. The orienting systems compares the input vector to the *F1* layer output and causes a reset signal if their degree of similarity is less than the vigilance level, where ρ is the vigilance parameter set as $0 < \rho \leq 1$.

The input pattern mismatch occurs if the following inequality is true,

$$\rho < \frac{|X_1|}{|I|}$$ (8.8)

If the two patterns differ by more than the vigilance parameter, a reset signal is sent to disable the firing unit in the recognition layer $F2$. The effect of the reset is to force the output of the recognition layer back to zero, disabling it for the duration of the current classification in order to search for a better match.

The parameter ρ determines how large a mismatch is tolerated. A large vigilance parameter makes the system to search for new categories in response to small difference between I and X_2 learning to classify input patterns into a large number of finer categories. Having a small vigilance parameter allows for larger differences and more input patterns are classified into the same category.

When a mismatch occurs, the total inhibitory signal from $F1$ to the orienting subsystem is increased. If the inhibition is sufficient, the orienting subsystem fires and sends a reset signal. The activated signal affects the $F2$ nodes in a state-dependent fashion. If an $F2$ node is active, the signal through a mechanism known as gated dipole field causes a long-lasting inhibition.

When the active $F2$ node is suppressed, the top-down output pattern X_2 and the top-down template V_1 are removed and the former $F1$ activation pattern X_1 is generated again. The newly generated pattern X_1 causes the orienting subsystem to cancel the reset signal and bottom-up activation starts again. Since $F2$ nodes having fired receive the long-lasting inhibition, a different $F2$ unit will win in the recognition layer and a different stored pattern is fed back to the comparison layer. If the pattern once again does not match the input, the whole process gets repeated. .

If no reset signal is generated this time, the match is adequate and the classification is finished.

The above three stages, that is, recognition, comparison, and search, are repeated until the input pattern matches a top-down template X_1. Otherwise a $F2$ node that has not learned any patterns yet is activated. In the latter case, the chosen $F2$ node becomes a learned new input pattern recognition category.

Learning

The above three stages take place very quickly relative to the time constants of the learning equations of the LTM traces between $F1$ and $F2$. Thus, we can assume that the learning occurs only when the STM reset and search process end and all STM patterns on $F1$ and $F2$ are stable.

The LTM traces from $F1$ to $F2$ follow the equation

$$\tau_1 \frac{dW_{12ij}}{dt} = \begin{cases} \left(1-W_{12ij}\right)L - W_{12ij}\left(|X_1|-1\right) & \text{if } V_{1i} \text{ and } V_{1j} \text{ are active} \\ -|X_1|W_{12ij} & \text{if only } V_{1j} \text{ is active} \\ 0 & \text{if only } V_{1j} \text{ is inactive} \end{cases} \quad (8.9)$$

where τ_1 is the time constant and L is a parameter with a value greater than one. Because time constant τ is sufficiently larger than the STM activation and smaller than the input pattern presentation, the above is a slow learning equation that converges in the fast learning equation

$$W_{12ij} = \begin{cases} \dfrac{L}{L-1+|X_1|} & \text{if } V_{1i} \text{ and } V_{1j} \text{ are active} \\ 0 & \text{if only } V_{1j} \text{ is active} \\ \text{no change} & \text{if only } V_{1j} \text{ is inactive} \end{cases} \quad (8.10)$$

The initial values for W_{12ij} must be randomly chosen while satisfying the inequality

$$0 < W_{12ij} < \frac{L}{L-1+|M|} \tag{8.11}$$

where M is the input pattern dimension equal to the number of nodes in $F1$.

The LTM traces from $F2$ to $F1$ follows the equation,

$$\tau_2 \frac{dW_{21ji}}{dt} = X_{2j}\left(-W_{21ji} + X_{1i}\right) \tag{8.12}$$

where τ_2 is the time constant and the equation is defined to converge during a presentation of an input pattern. Thus, the fast learning equation of the for W_{21ji} is

$$W_{21ji} = \begin{cases} 1 & \text{if } V_{1i} \text{ and } V_{1j} \text{ are active} \\ 0 & \text{if only } V_{1i} \text{ is inactive} \end{cases} \tag{8.13}$$

The initial value for W_{21ji} must be randomly chosen to satisfy the inequality

$$1 \geq W_{21ji}(0) > C \tag{8.14}$$

where C is decided by the slow learning equation parameters. However, all $W_{21ji}(0)$ may be set 1 in the fast learning case.

Theorems

The theorems describing ART1 behavior are described next with proofs given in Carpenter and Grossberg (1987). These theorems hold in the fast learning case with initial LTM traces satisfying constraints (10) and (14). If parameters are properly set, however, the following results also hold in the slow learning case.

(Theorem 1) Direct Access of Learned Patterns

If an $F2$ node has already learned input pattern I as its template, then input pattern I activates the $F2$ node at once.

The theorem states that a pattern that has been perfectly memorized by an $F2$ node activates the node immediately.

(Theorem 2) Stable Category Learning

This theorem guarantees that the LTM traces W_{12ij} and W_{21ji} become stable after a finite number of learning trials in response to an arbitrary list of binary input patterns. The V_{1j} template corresponding to the jth $F2$ node remains constant after at most M-1 times.

In stable states, the LTM traces W_{12ij} become $L/(L-1+M)$ if the ith element of the top-down template corresponding to the jth $F2$ node is one. Otherwise, it is zero. The LTM traces W_{21ji} become one if the ith element of the template of corresponding to the jth $F2$ node is one. Otherwise, it is zero.

However, theorem 2 doesn't guarantee that a perfectly coded input pattern by an $F2$ node will be coded by the same $F2$ node after presentation. The $F2$ node may forget the input pattern in successive learning, though the template of the $F2$ node continues to be a subset of the input pattern.

(Theorem 3) Direct Access after Learning Stabilizes

After learning has stabilized in response to an arbitrary list of binary input patterns, each input pattern I either directly activates the $F2$ node which possesses the largest subset template with respect to I, or I cannot activate any $F2$ node. In the latter case, $F2$ contains no uncommitted nodes.

This theorem guarantees that a memorized pattern activates an *F2* node at once after learning and that all *F2* nodes have been already committed if any input patterns cannot be coded. If an input pattern list contains many different input patterns and *F2* contains fewer nodes, all input patterns cannot be coded with ρ close to 1.

However, the theorem doesn't guarantee that an input pattern having activated an *F2* node during learning should have been coded. If there are many input patterns with respect to the number of *F2* nodes, input patterns which have smaller $|X_1|$ tend to be coded while input patterns with larger $|X_1|$ tend to be coded by their subsets or not coded at all after learning.

8.3 Model Implementation

The complete model incorporates the Attentional and Orient Subsystem into a single **Art** module, as shown in figure 8.4, together with the **ArtModel** instantiating the **Art** module with the appropriate sizes for its layers.

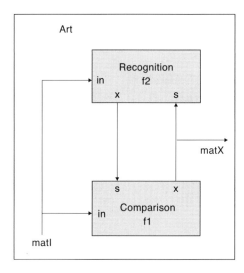

Figure 8.4
ART module containing the F2 and F2 submodules incorporating the functionality of both the Attentional and Orienting subsystems.

Art Module

Due to the limited process complexity of some of the components of the model only two submodules **F1** and **F2** are defined within the Art module. These two submodules correspond to layers *F1* and *F2* in the Attentional subsystem and include their respective gains. Also considering the simplicity of the orienting subsystem structures, it is incorporated directly into module F1.

Every simulation run initialization, corresponding to the beginning of a new epoch, a new input pattern is sent to the F1 and F2 input vector ports `in`. Since the input ports in is a vector and `matI` is a matrix we do a corresponding conversion between the two.

```
public void initRun() {
    matrixToVector(matI,in);
}
```

After completing a simulation run the **endRun** method is called, in this case we want to update the `matX` array in order to display to the user the letter output in a visually appropriate form.

```
public void endRun() {
    vectorToMatrix(x,matX);
}
```

Comparison Module

The Comparison module contains the corresponding data structure for the F1 layer including gain 1. Input layer s and activity layer x are both initialized to 0 while weights are initialized 1.0. This is all done in the **initModule** method. The **initTrain** method resets the active elements. Simulation processing is specified in the **simTrain** method as follows

```
public void simTrain() {
    if (resetActive == 1) { // input vector G1 condition, eq
(8.1)
            resetActive = 0;
        active = -1;
        x = in;
    }
    else { // eq (8.7)
       if (s.nslMax() > 0)
          s.nslMax(active);
          v = w*s; // eq (8.6)
    // this is a step function: x=nslStep(in+s,1.99)
       for (int i = 0;i < in.getSize();i++) {
            if (in[i] + v[i] >= 1.99)
                x[i] = 1.0;
            else
                x[i] = 0.0;
       }
    }
}
```

This module executes the bottom-up activation, the top-down template matching, and the STM reset and search. The activation cycle is repeated until matching is complete.

After running a complete simulation for a single pattern the **endTrain** method gets called. The module changes the LTM traces F12 and F21 after the system reaches stable responding to an input pattern. This modifies bottom-up and top-down traces F12 and F21 by the fast learning equations. The LTM learning module may be turned off when learning is unnecessary.

```
public void endTrain() {
    s.nslMax(active); // eq. (8.9)

    for (int i = 0;i < w.getRows();i++) {
       if (x[i] == 1.0)
             w[i][active] = 1.0;
       else
             w[i][active] = 0.0;
    }
}
```

Recognition Module

The Recognition module contains the corresponding data structures for the F2 layer. Simulation variables are initialized in the **initModule** method as follows:

```
public void initModule() {
// initialization of all LTM weights // eq (8.10)
    float max_value = l.getData()/(l.getData() - 1.0 +
    in.getSize());
    for (int xi = 0; xi < w.getRows(); xi++) {
        for (int yi = 0; yi < w.getCols(); yi++) {
                w[xi][yi] = uniformRandom(float(0.0),max_value);
        }
    }
}
```

The **initTrain** method resets the active elements. Simulation processing is specified in the **simTrain** method where LTM traces are multiplied to the input from F1 and F2 activation x is computed. The F2 unit that receives the biggest input from F1 that has not been reset is activated while the other units are deactivated.

```
public void simTrain() {
    if (s.nslSum() / in.nslSum() < rho.getData()) { // eq (8.8)
        resetY[active] = -1.0;
        active = -1;
    }
    if (active >= 0) {
        nslPrintln("Matching is passed");
        system.breakCycle();
        return;
    }
    v = w*s; // eq (8.6)
    num_type  maxvalue;
    int    i;
    active = -1;
    x = 0.0;
    float  BIG_MINUS = -1.0; // the smallest value in this
    program
    // To exclude units which have been already reset
    for (i = 0;i < resetY.getSize();i++) {
        if (resetY[i] == -1.0) {
                v[i] = BIG_MINUS;
        }
    }
    // search for the unit which receives maximum input
    maxvalue = v.nslMax();
    // In the case that there is no available unit
    if (maxvalue == BIG_MINUS) {
        active = -1;
        nslPrint("An error has occured");
        system.breakCycle();
        return;
    }
```

```
// To find the maximum input // eq (8.5)
for (i = 0;i < v.getSize();i++) {
    if (v[i] == maxvalue) {
            x[i] = 1.0;
            active = i;
            break;
    }
}
// For the error
if (i >= v.getSize()) {
        nslPrintln("An error has occured");
        system.breakCycle();
        return;
}
if (active < 0) {
        nslPrintln("There are no available units");
        system.breakCycle();
        return;
}
}
```

After running a complete simulation for a single pattern the **endTrain** method gets called.

```
public void endTrain() {
    nslPrintln("Top-Down Template Unit:" ,active);
    if (active < 0) {
        nslPrintln("There are no units for this input");
        system.breakCycle();
        return;
    }
    float val = l.getData() / (l.getData() - 1.0 + s.sum()); //
    eq (8.11)
    for (int i = 0; i < w.getCols(); i++) {
        if (s[i] == 1.0)
            w[active][i] = val;
        else
            w[active][i] = 0.0;
    }
}
```

8.4 Simulation and Results[2]

The ART1 model simulation will be illustrated with character recognition example (Carpenter and Grossberg, 1987). The NSLS command file ART1.nsls contains NSL command to set parameters and prepare graphics. The parameters to be set are only the vigilance parameter and the weight initialization parameter besides the usual simulation steps specification.

```
nsl set art.f2.rho 0.7
nsl set art.f2.l 2.0
```

The system may run without learning by setting the epoch steps to 0.

A window frame with two windows inside corresponding to the input vector and *F1* activation pattern *X*, both shown as a square pattern, are opened in the simulation. A second frame with a single window shows the F2 activation pattern *X*. The latter layer is shown as a vector representing a group of classified categories.

Execution

A typical ART1 simulation session is as follows;

1. **Loading ArtModel.nsl:** "nsl source artModel.nsl."
2. **Initialization:** Execute the NSL command "nsl init." This initializes LTM traces and variables.
3. **Setting character:** Characters may be interactively fed by the user or read from a script file. For example read the "nsl source patI1.nsl" file for a single letter.
4. **Activation and Learning:** Type "nsl train" to train a single cycle of the Art model. After either the maximum number of simulation steps are executed or X_2 stabilizes, **endTrain** is executed. Learning may be disabled, only by setting the epoch step number to 1.

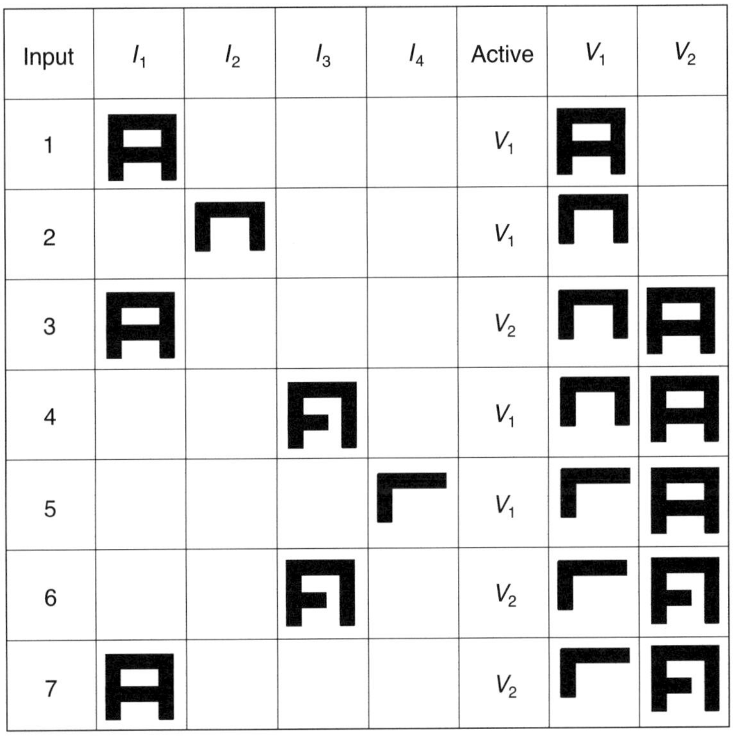

Figure 8.5
Four two-dimensional 5 by 5 (I_1, I_2, I_3 and I_4) patterns are presented to the ART1 system. The correct output is specified by the active *V* element.

Output

We give a simple simulation example in this section. Four input patterns are presented to the model for a total of seven times. The input patterns, the *F2* nodes activated by them, and top-down template of the activated *F2* nodes are shown in figure 8.5.

5. An input pattern I_1 is given in the first presentation. Because no patterns have been memorized yet, the input pattern is completely learned by an *F2* node n_1 and the top-down template of n_1 is I_1 after learning.
6. An input pattern I_2 is then given. Because I_2 is a subset of I_1, I_2 directly activates the same *F2* node n_1, and I_2 becomes a new template of n_1.

7. The input pattern I_1 is presented again in the third trial. The $F2$ node n_1 is activated at first, but it is reset because its template pattern I_2 and the input pattern I_1 are very different. Thus, another $F2$ node n_2 is activated and I_1 becomes its template.

8. An input pattern I_3 is given in the fourth presentation. Though I_3 looks closer to I_1 than I_2, I_3 directly accesses n_1 and the activated pattern on $F1$ is I_2. The top-down template of n_1 doesn't change and it is still I_2.

9. The next input pattern I_4 activates n_1 because I_4 is a subset of the current template I_2 of n_1. Then, the template of n_1 becomes I_4 instead of I_2.

10. Next, the input pattern I_3 is given again. It activates n_1 at first, but it is reset because its current template I_4 and I_3 are very different. Thus, I_3 activates the $F2$ node n_2 at the second search, and it becomes the template of the node.

11. Finally, the input pattern I_1 is given again. It directly activates the $F2$ node n_2 and the activated pattern on $F1$ is I_3.

The NSL simulation displays for the V elements are shown in figure 8.6.

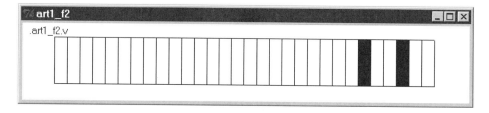

Figure 8.6
V elements in the recognition module of the ART1 system.

The NSL simulation displays comparing the letter input to the corresponding output is shown in figure 8.7. The above example illustrates some of the features of the model:

- An F2 node that memorizes an input pattern will not necessarily keep memorizing it. Though the F2 node n1 first memorizes the input pattern I1 in the above simulation, for example, the node doesn't respond to I1 in the final presentation. This means that the final stable state of the model may be largely different from early stages.

- Simpler patterns which have smaller |I|'s tend to be learned. Thus, when the number of the F2 nodes are limited, complex patterns may not be learned. Skilled adjustment of a vigilance parameter is indispensable for balanced learning.

- The criterion to classify input patterns is not intuitive. For example, the input pattern I3 is judged closer to I2 than I1.

- The previous top-down template n presented as an input pattern is not necessarily the final activation pattern on F1. This means that the model cannot restore pixels erased by noise though it can remove pixels added by noise.

- These features may be flaws of the model, but they can be taken also as good points.

8.5 Summary

Though we chose a simplified way to simulate ART1 on NSL, some interesting features of ART1 have been made clear. Different extensions can be made to the NSL implementation of ART1:

- The first extension would be a full implementation of ART1 original dynamic equations, in particular the inclusion of membrane potential equations of $F1$ and $F2$ nodes and the slow learning equations.

- The second extension would be to improve ART1. Some features present in our simulation are not desirable for many applications. We believe some improvements of the learning equations and matching rules would extend to further applications while keeping the basic structure of ART.

The third extension would be the implementation of other ART models. ART is a theory applying to many models, such as ART2, FUZZY-ART (Carpenter et al 1991), besides various practical applications.

A good exercise here would be to use the *Maximum Selector* model instead of the simple WTA used in ART.

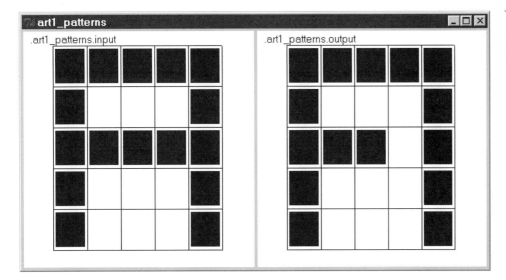

Figure 8.7
Sample letter input and output in the ART1 system.

Notes

1. A. Weitzenfeld developed the NSL3.0 version from the original NSL2.1 model implementation written by T. Tanaka as well as contributed Section 8.3 and part of Section 8.4 to this chapter.

2. The Art model was implemented and tested under NSLC.

9 Depth Perception

A. Weitzenfeld and M. Arbib

9.1 Introduction

Depth Perception enables us to see the world in terms of objects located at various distances from us. From a single eye at a single time we can determine the direction in space of various features of the world. Different techniques are available to locate where the feature is in depth along the given direction (see Arbib 1989 for further details):

- *Stereopsis* uses cues provided by correlating visual input to two spatially separated eyes.
- *Optic flow* uses the information provided to the eye at different times.
- *Accommodation* works by determining what focal length will best bring an object into focus.
- *Convergence* is based on how the eyes must turn to fixate the object in question.

A three dimensional scene presented to the left eye differs from that presented to the right eye. A single point projection on each retina corresponds to a whole ray of points in space, but points on two retinae determine a single point in space, the intersection of the corresponding rays (figure 9.1).

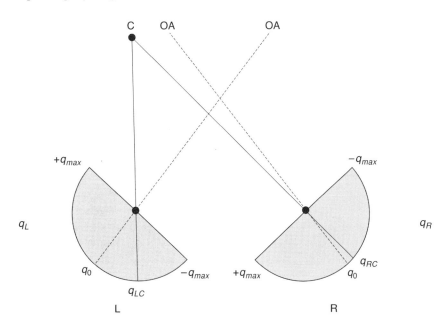

Figure 9.1
Points on a single ray (projector) match to a single point on each retina. The inter-section of two rays, a ray for each retina, determines a single point in space. In this example, *C* projects to q_{RC} on the right retina and q_{LC} on the left retina, respectively. *OA* defines the *optic axis*.

In *stereopsis*, depth computation is based on the disparity or displacement between the projection of corresponding points on the two retinae. For example, from figure 9.1, the disparity generated by the projection of point C in the two retinae is defined as the spatial displacement between q_{RC} and q_{LC}. This is calculated by $(q_{RC}-q_0) - (q_{LC}-q_0) = q_{RC} -q_{LC}$.

In order to visualize the relationship between disparity d and retinal angle q, the mapping of the right eye coordinate system onto a Cartesian grid is shown in figure 9.2. Radial lines are at equal angular increments q and arcs are lines of constant disparity d spaced at equal increments of disparity. Disparity increases as the arcs get closer to the retina, where depth resolution becomes finer for closer objects.

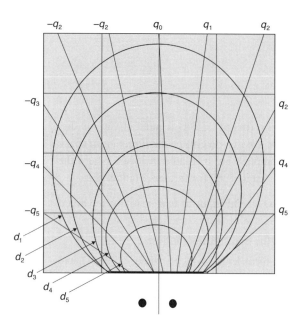

Figure 9.2
Mapping of the right eyed coordinate system onto a Cartesian grid. The two disks under the grid represent the two eyes. Arcs correspond to disparity d, increasing as objects get closer to the retinae. Disparity resolution increases as well, as the arcs get closer to the eyes. Angular position q corresponds to the rays emanating from the retina at constant angular increments.

An problem arising from *stereopsis* is the ambiguity created by pairs of points generating similar retinal projections (figure 9.3),

$$q_{RA} = q_{RD}, q_{LA} = q_{LC}, q_{RB} = q_{RC}, q_{LB} = q_{LD}$$

The generated disparities are:

$$d_A = q_{RA} - q_{LA}, d_B = q_{RB} - q_{LB}, d_C = q_{RC} - q_{LA}, d_D = q_{RD} - q_{LD}$$

giving rise to the following ambiguity:

$$d_A + d_B = d_C + d_D$$

where one pair of points would be the be correct one, while the second pair corresponds to "ghost" points emerging from the disparity maps. In this situation there is no way of knowing which pair is the "true" pair of points.

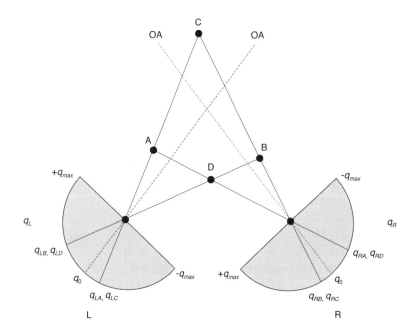

Figure 9.3
There is an ambiguity generated by projections of pairs of points. Stimuli B and C project to the same point on the right retina, similarly A and D. The same happens on the left retina, where A and C match to the same point, similarly to B and D. While one of the pairs may be the true pair, there is no way to distinguish it from the second ghost pair since their projection is exactly the same.

Two depth perception models resolving this ambiguity are described here: (1) The disparity model by Dev (1975), based exclusively on disparity cues, and (2) the disparity and accommodation model by House (1985), using accommodation cues cooperatively with disparity cues to improve depth estimates.

9.2 Model Description: Disparity

To remove the ambiguity problem Dev (1975) developed a cooperative computational model for building the depth map "guided by the plausible hypothesis that our visual world is made up of relatively few connected regions." This model used neurons whose firing level represented a degree of confidence that a point was located at a corresponding position in three-dimensional space. The neurons were so connected via inhibitory interneurons that cells that coded for nearby directions in space and similar depths should excite each other, whereas cells that corresponded to nearby directions in space and dissimilar depths should inhibit each other. The model is shown in figure 9.4: (1) an excitatory manifold M indexed by retina position q and disparity d, where nearby cells excite each other, and cells for a given q and differing d inhibit each other via (2) an inhibitory interneuron U indexed only by retinal position q. Competition along the d dimension ensures that for each q, a cell (q,d) will be active for at most one d; cooperation along the q dimension encourages groups of active cells for a nearby q to have similar d, thus yielding a segmentation of the image. (See Amari and Arbib 1977 for more detail).

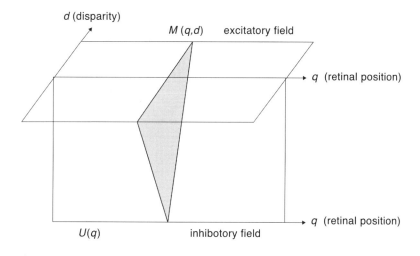

Figure 9.4
The Dev disparity model incorporates an excitatory manifold M indexed by retina position q and disparity d, and an inhibitory interneuron U indexed only by retinal position q.

The model contains a **Dev** disparity module (figure 9.5):

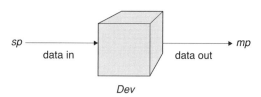

Figure 9.5
The Dev disparity module contains an input port sp that receives external data and an output port mp that generates output data.

The **Dev** module is implemented by a neural network described by the following equations, where m corresponds to the excitatory field, u corresponds to the inhibitory field and s corresponds to the input from the retina (figure 9.6):

$$\tau_m \frac{\partial m_{ij}}{\partial t} = -m_{ij} + w_m * f\left(m_{ij}\right) - w_u * g\left(u_j\right) - h_m + s_{ij} \tag{9.1}$$

$$\tau_u \frac{\partial u_j}{\partial t} = -u_j + \sum_i f\left(m_{ij}\right) - h_u \qquad (9.2)$$

$$f\left(m_{ij}\right) = step\left(m_{ij}, k\right) \qquad (9.3)$$

$$g\left(u_j\right) = ramp\left(u_j\right) \qquad (9.4)$$

Input s is computed by calculating disparity between left r_L and right r_R retina mappings. $r_L(q)$ is set to 1 if some object projects to point q on the left retina, $r_L(q)$ is set to 0 otherwise; and similarly for $r_R(q)$. Stereo input is then defined as

$$s_d(q) = R_L(q)\, R_R(q+d) \qquad (9.5)$$

which is 1 only if there is an object at position q on the left retina as well as at $q+d$ on the right retina, and is otherwise 0. In the present section, we simply present the computed s-array to the Dev module; in the second half of the chapter we will present a Retina module that explicitly computes the s-array (and an accommodation array) from the activity on the 2 retinas. (Note that a more subtle version of the model would require similar local features, rather than mere presence of an object, at q_L and $(q+d)_R$. However, the modular design of NSL would come to the rescue here, since the input s, rather than being computed by the above formula, would then be supplied by a module computing feature-based disparities instead.)

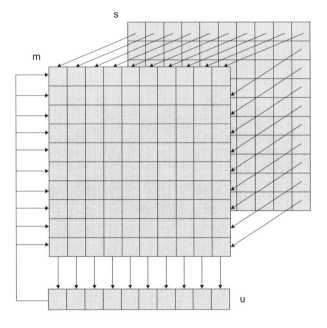

Figure 9.6
The **Dev** module consists of layers *m* corresponding to the excitatory field and *u* corresponding to the inhibitory field and *s* to the input from the retina.

9.3 Model Implementation: Disparity

There exist a number of possible different designs when building the model in NSLM. Different neural layers may be assigned to different modules, or a number of them may be part of a single module. In the design presented here, the second approach is taken, where the **Dev** and **DevModel** implementation in NSLM are as shown below:

Dev

The **Dev** module has the following definition:

```
nslModule Dev (int sizeX, int sizeY) {
```

Input layer $s(d,q)$, corresponds to the s layer. The excitatory layer $m(d,q)$ and inhibitory layer $u(q)$ are each defined by a membrane potential array (mp and up) and a firing array (mf and uf).

```
private NslDinFloat2 s(sizeX, sizeY);
private NslDoutFloat2 mf (sizeX, sizeY);
private NslFloat2 mp(sizeX, sizeY);
private NslFloat1 up (sizeY);
private NslFloat1 uf(sizeY);
```

Following, constants are declared. tm and tu are time constants, hm and hu are threshold constants. ksm, kmu, and kum are connectivity constants; k is used as a step function parameter; and wm is used as an excitatory convolution mask.

The **initRun** procedure reinitializes all layers for each simulation run:

```
public void initRun () {
    mp = 0;
    mf = 0;
    up = 0;
    uf = 0;
}
```

The **simRun** procedure defines the dynamic equations:

```
public void simRun () {
    mp  = nslDiff(mp, tm, -mp + ks*s -
        kum*nslExpandRows(uf,mp.getRows())+ wm@mf + hm);
    mf = nslStep(mp, k);
    up  = nslDiff(up,tu, -up + kmu*nslReduceRows(mf) + hu);
    uf = nslRamp(up);
}
```

DepthModel

The **DepthModel** module is used to instantiate the **Dev** module. No connections are required between the two modules since no information is passed. The **Dev** module produces output but does not receive input from other modules. (Input port sp is actually not used, but is defined for future extensibility.)

```
nslModel DepthModel () {
```

Constant sizes for arrays are:

```
private int sizeX = 10;
private int sizeY = 8;
```

The assemblage consists of the following module:

```
private Dev dev(sizeX, sizeY);
```

9.4 Simulation and Results: Disparity

The NSLS script for the Dev model contains system simulation parameter assignments. Three of these parameters are time step, simulation end time, and the approximation method:

```
nsl set system.simDelta 0.1
nsl set system.simEndTime 10.0
nsl set system.diff.approximation euler
```

The **Dev** module parameters are then assigned. Connectivity constants are assigned to 1.0. *tm* and *tu* need a common value, as well as *hm* and *hu*. *wm* is assigned five elements between 0 and 1.0. (These constants could have been assigned values directly in NSLM, but can be overridden by the script language.):

The parameters within the Dev module are set as follows:

```
nsl set devModel.kum 1.0
nsl set devModel.kmu 1.0
nsl set devModel.ks 2.0
nsl set devModel.wm 0.4 0.6 1.0 0.6 0.4
nsl set devModel.tm 1.0
nsl set devModel.tu 1.0
nsl set devModel.hm -1.2
nsl set devModel.hu -0.7
nsl set devModel.k 0.75
```

Input data is directly generated into *s*, mapping real points as well as "ghosts" (points with value 1). In the present example, we have followed the scenario of figure 9.3 where 2 "real" points generate a set of disparities that is also consistent with 2 "ghost" points, yielding a total of 4 "initial candidates" in the array below.

```
nsl set devModel.s {
{ 0 0 0 0 0 0 0 0 }
{ 0 0 0 0 0 0 0 0 }
{ 0 0 0 0 1 0 0 0 }
{ 0 0 0 0 0 0 0 0 }
{ 0 0 1 0 1 0 0 0 }
{ 0 0 0 0 0 0 0 0 }
{ 0 0 1 0 0 0 0 0 }
{ 0 0 0 0 0 0 0 0 }
{ 0 0 0 0 0 0 0 0 }
{ 0 0 0 0 0 0 0 0 }}
```

Graphics is specified by first creating a frame to contain the desired display windows:

```
nsl create DisplayFrame .depth
```

In each frame we reproduce three windows containing a layer activity each: on top the input *s* staying the same throughout the simulation, in the middle the main layer activity *mp* and in the bottom the main layer activation *mf*. The three display windows are created using the default layout where each new window is added beneath the previous one:

```
nsl create DisplayWindow  s -width 500 -height 200
    -graph areaLevel -wymin -1.0 -wymax 2.0
nsl create DisplayWindow mp -width 500 -height 200
    -graph areaLevel -wymin -3.0 -wymax 3.0
nsl create DisplayWindow mf -width 500 -height 200
    -graph areaLevel -wymin 0.0 -wymax 1.0
```

Simulation results during time steps 0 and 2, corresponding to the network building up internal values, are shown in figure 9.7.

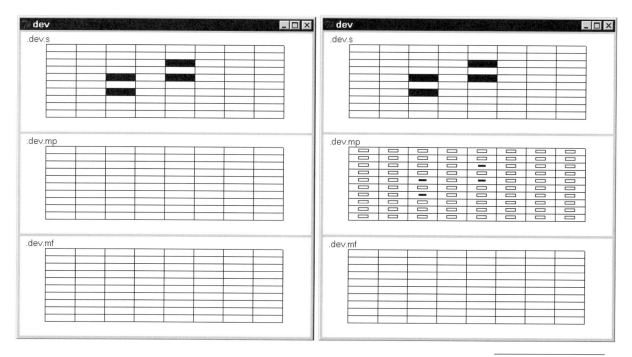

Simulation results during time steps 4 and 6, corresponding to the network completing building up internal values and solving the ambiguity, are shown in figure 9.8.

Figure 9.7
The Dev model simulation steps 0 and 2.

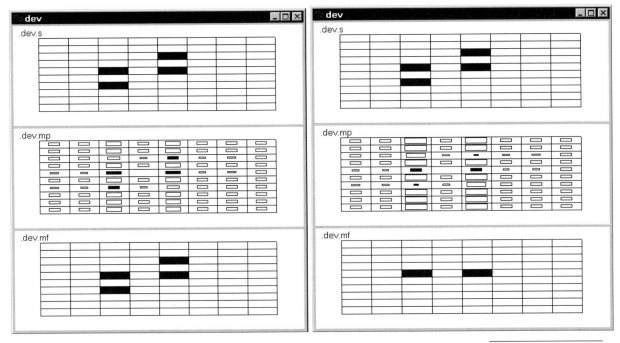

Returning to the situation shown in figure 9.3, the reader will note that the Dev model favors targets *A* and *B* as the "real" targets, and exorcises *C* and *D* as "ghost targets", even though we had noted that the retinal data were neutral as to the choice of (*A,B*) versus (*C, D*). This is because the design of the Dev model meets the constraint that the world is made up of surfaces, and thus favors a choice consistent with nearby points of similar disparity over other choices. We now turn to an architecture which exploits accommodation as well as disparity cues. Although we do not show this explicitly, the reader can check that if *C* and *D* are the "real" inputs, then the new model will verify this, whereas the Dev model will not.

Figure 9.8
The Dev model simulation steps 4 and 6.

9.5 Model Description: Disparity and Accommodation

In many cases, depth perception models depending entirely on disparity cues will converge to an adequate depth segmentation of the image. However, such a system may need extra cues. The ambiguity resulting from matching a number of points in space to the same retina coordinate can be reduced by the use of vergence information to give the system an initial depth estimate. Another method is to use accommodation information to provide the initial bias for a depth perception system. It is the latter approach that we adopt here.

The cue interaction model (House 1985) uses two systems, each based on Dev's stereopsis model, to build a depth map. One is driven by disparity cues, the other by accommodation cues, while corresponding points in the two maps have excitatory cross-coupling. The model is sketched in figure 9.9. *M* is an accommodation driven field; it receives information about accommodation and—left to its own devices—sharpens up that information to yield depth estimates. *S* is the disparity driven-field, corresponding to Dev's original system: it receives disparity information and suppresses (what may be) ghost targets. Moreover, the systems are intercoupled so that a point in the accommodation field *M* excites the corresponding point in the disparity field *S*, and viceversa. Thus, a high confidence in a particular (direction, depth) coordinate in one layer will bias activity in the other layer accordingly. The model is so tuned that binocular depth cues predominate where available, but monocular accommodative cues remain sufficient to determine depth in the absence of binocular cues.

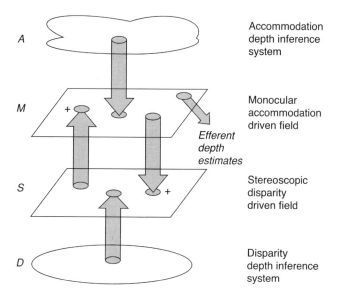

Figure 9.9
The cue interaction model
for depth mapping uses
cross-coupling between an
accommodation-driven
system and a disparity-
driven system.

The model is composed of the following modules (figure 9.10):

- **Dev2**: There are two instances of an extended Dev module, now called Dev2, one processing disparity information and the other accommodation information. Each consists of an input port a, receiving data from the **Retina**, a second input port s, receiving input from the other Dev2 module, and an output port mf, delegating its output back to Stereo.

- **Retina**: The Retina module processes retina information. It contains an input port in, delegated from Stereo, and two output ports, d and a, for disparity and accommodation, respectively.

- **Stereo**: The Stereo assemblage provides composition and encapsulation for the entire model. It delegates its processing to the Retina and two Dev2 modules. The Stereo module consists of two external ports, input port in and output port out.

- **Visin**: The Visin module generates the external stimuli. It contains an out output port connected to the Stereo module.

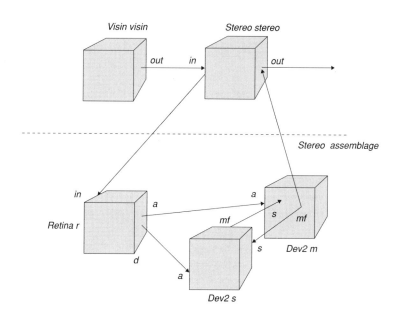

Figure 9.10
Disparity and Accommodation
model modules: A Visin input
module, a Stereo assemblage,
a Retina module, and two
Dev2 modules.

Note, the two Dev2 modules are implemented by neural networks similar to those defined in the original Dev module. These equations are extended to enable cross-coupling between Dev modules, where m and s correspond to the excitatory fields, u and v to the inhibitory fields and a and d are the input from the retina (figure 9.11). Consistent with the definition of Stereo below, you must make the Dev2 modules identical—we have 2 instances of the same module, and we will show how we connect them to yield their differential function. The variables internal to each instance must be identical, only connections and relabelings distinguish them:

- Disparity (**Dev2** s):

$$\tau_s \frac{\partial s_{ij}}{\partial t} = -s_{ij} + w_s * f\big(s_{ij}\big) + w_t * f\big(t_{ij}\big) - w_v * g\big(v_j\big) - h_s + d_{ij} \tag{9.6}$$

$$\tau_v \frac{\partial v_j}{\partial t} = -v_j + \sum_i f\big(s_{ij}\big) - h_v \tag{9.7}$$

$$f\big(s_{ij}\big) = sigma\big(s_{ij}\big) \tag{9.8}$$

$$g\big(v_j\big) = ramp\big(v_j\big) \tag{9.9}$$

- Accommodation (**Dev2** m):

$$\tau_m \frac{\partial m_{ij}}{\partial t} = -m_{ij} + w_m * f\big(m_{ij}\big) + w_t * f\big(t_{ij}\big) - w_u * g\big(u_j\big) - h_m + a_{ij} \tag{9.10}$$

$$\tau_u \frac{\partial u_j}{\partial t} = -u_j + \sum_i f\big(m_{ij}\big) - h_u \tag{9.11}$$

$$f\big(m_{ij}\big) = sigma\big(m_{ij}\big) \tag{9.12}$$

$$g\big(u_j\big) = ramp\big(u_j\big) \tag{9.13}$$

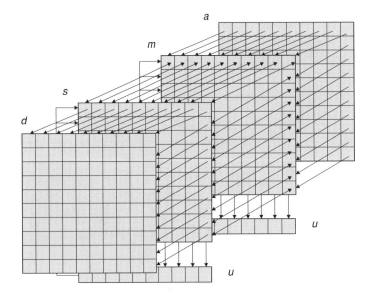

Figure 9.11
Two **Dev** neural networks consisting of m and s corresponding to the excitatory fields, u and v to the inhibitory fields, and a and d are the input from the retina.

9.6 Model Implementation: Disparity and Accommodation[1]

The model is composed of the following modules: **Dev2**, **Retina**, **Stereo**, and **Visin**:

Dev2

The **Dev2** module is defined as before:

```
nslModule Dev2 (int sizeX, int sizeY) {
```

Input layer $s(d,q)$, corresponds to the s layer. An additional layer t is used for cross-coupling between **Dev2** modules.

```
public NslDinFloat2 a(sizeX,sizeY);
public NslDinFloat2 s(sizeX,sizeY);
public NslDoutFloat2 mf(sizeX,sizeY);
private NslFloat2 mp(sizeX,sizeY);
private NslFloat1 up(sizeY);
private NslFloat1 uf(sizeY);
```

Following, constants are declared similar to the original Dev module. *wm* is the convolution mask, with size 3, and instead of a step function, a saturation function is used; thus instead of k, $x1$ and $x2$ are used as parameters.

```
private NslFloat0 ksm();
private NslFloat0 kmu();
private NslFloat0 kum();
private NslFloat0 ktm();
private NslFloat1 wm(3);
private NslFloat0 tm();
private NslFloat0 tu();
private NslFloat0 hm();
private NslFloat0 hu();
private NslFloat0 x1();
private NslFloat0 x2();
```

The **initRun** procedure reinitializes all layers to 0 for each simulation run:

```
public void initRun () {
    mp = 0;
    mf = 0;
    up = 0;
    uf = 0;
}
```

The **simRun** procedure defines the dynamic equations. They are similar to the Dev equations except for the addition of t in the expression:

```
public void simRun () {
    mp = nslDiff(mp, tm, -mp + ksm*s -
        kum*nslExpandRows(uf,mp.getRows())+ ktm*t + wm@mf + hm);
    mf = nslSigmoid(mp,x1,x2);
    up = nslDiff(up,tu, -up + kmu*nslReduceRows(mf) + hu);
    uf = nslRamp(up);
}
```

Retina

The **Retina** module is defined as follows (detailed processing for this assemblage is described in House (1985)):

```
nslModule Retina (int sizeX, int sizeY, int sizeR) {
```

The external data arrays are: world input *in* and output retina vector *r*:

```
private NslDinFloat2 in(sizeX, sizeY);  // world input
private NslDoutFloat2 a(sizeX, sizeY); // accommodation layer
private NslDoutFloat2 d(sizeX, sizeY); // disparity layer
private NslFloat1 rr(sizeR);       // right retina
private NslFloat1 rl(sizeR);       // left retina
```

Following, constants are declared:

```
private NslFloat0 w(); // 1/2 of interpupillary distance (cm)
private NslFloat0 yf();// intersection of optical axes
    (0,yf) (cm)
private NslFloat0 l(); // interpupillary line distance from
    origin (cm)
private NslFloat0 dmax();  // maximum disparity
private NslFloat0 sigma(); // spread parameter
```

The **initRun** procedure produces the retina mapping (since images are static, there is no need for a **simRun** procedure):

```
public void initRun()
{
    view_to_right_retina(rr,in,w,yf,l);
    view_to_left_retina(rl,in,w,yf,l);
    retina_to_accommodation(a,in,rr,w,yf,l,dmax,sigma);
    retina_to_disparity(d,rr,rl);
}
```

Stereo

The **Stereo** assemblage is defined as follows:

```
nslModule Stereo (int sizeX, int sizeY, int sizeR) {
```

The assemblage consists of the following modules:

```
private Retina r(sizeX, sizeY, sizeR);
private Dev2 m(sizeX, sizeY), s(sizeX, sizeY);
```

Input and output ports are defined as follows:

```
public NslDinFloat2 in(sizeX, sizeY);
public NslDoutFloat2 out(sizeX, sizeY);
```

Connections and relabels are as follows:

```
public void makeConn () {
    nslConnect (r.a,m.a);
    nslConnect (r.d,s.a);
    nslConnect (m.mf,s.s);
    nslConnect (s.mf,m.s);
    nslRelabel (in,retina.in);
    nslRelabel (s.mf,mf);
}
```

Visin

The **Visin** module is defined as follows:

```
nslModule Visin (int sizeX, int sizeY) {
```

The external data array is: world input *in*:

```
private NslDoutFloat2 out(sizeX, sizeY);
```

DepthModel

The **DepthModel** model instantiates the **Visin** and **Stereo** modules. A connection is made between ports in these two modules.

```
nslModel DepthModel () {
```

Constant sizes for arrays are:

```
private int sizeX = 11; // 81;
private int sizeY = 11; // 81;
private int sizeR = 21; // 161;
```

The assemblage consists of the following modules:

```
private Visin visin(sizeX, sizeY);
private Stereo stereo(sizeX, sizeY,sizeR);
```

Connections and relabels are as follows:

```
public void makeConn () {
    nslConnect (visin.out, stereo.in);
}
```

9.7 Simulation and Results: Disparity and Accommodation[2]

The NSLS code for the House model involves system simulation parameter assignments, including time steps, simulation end time, and the integration method to be used by all differential equations:

```
nsl set system.simDelta 0.05
nsl set system.simEndTime 2.0
nsl set system.diff.approximation euler
nsl set system.diff.delta 0.05
```

Retina parameters,

```
nsl set DepthModel.stereo.r.w 3.0
nsl set DepthModel.stereo.r.yf -10.0
nsl set DepthModel.stereo.r.l 22.0
nsl set DepthModel.stereo.r.dmax 0.25
nsl set DepthModel.stereo.r.sigma 0.25
```

Dev2 disparity parameters,

```
nsl set DepthModel.stereo.s.tu 0.1
nsl set DepthModel.stereo.s.tm 0.3
nsl set DepthModel.stereo.s.hu 0.0
nsl set DepthModel.stereo.s.hm 0.0
nsl set DepthModel.stereo.s.x1 0.1
nsl set DepthModel.stereo.s.x2 1.1
nsl set DepthModel.stereo.s.wm 0.25 0.68 0.25
nsl set DepthModel.stereo.s.kmu 1.0
nsl set DepthModel.stereo.s.kam 0.5
nsl set DepthModel.stereo.s.kum 0.6
nsl set DepthModel.stereo.s.ks 0.8
```

Dev2 accommodation parameters,

```
nsl set DepthModel.stereo.m.tu 0.1
nsl set DepthModel.stereo.m.tm 0.3
nsl set DepthModel.stereo.s.hu 0.0
nsl set DepthModel.stereo.s.hm 0.0
nsl set DepthModel.stereo.m.x1 0.1
nsl set DepthModel.stereo.m.x2 1.1
nsl set DepthModel.stereo.m.wm 0.25 0.68 0.25
nsl set DepthModel.stereo.m.kmu 1.0
nsl set DepthModel.stereo.m.kam 0.5
nsl set DepthModel.stereo.m.kum 0.6
nsl set DepthModel.stereo.m.ks 0.8
```

Input to the model, **Visin** module, is

```
nsl set DepthModel.visin.out{35,41} 1.0
nsl set DepthModel.visin.out{45,55} 1.0
```

Graphics is specified as follows:

```
nsl create DisplayFrame .fw0
nsl create DisplayWindow vis.out -width 450 -height 600 -graph
    areaLevel \-wymin 0.0 -wymax 1.0
nsl create DisplayFrame .fw1
nsl create DisplayWindow st.m.mf -width 450 -height 300 -graph
    spatial3 \   -wymin -1.0 -wymax 1.0 -x0 20 -x1 80 -y0 35
    -y1 50 -sz 100 nsl create DisplayWindow st.s.mf -width 450
    -height 300 -graph spatial3 \
    -wymin -1.0 -wymax 1.0 -x0 20 -x1 80 -y0 35 -y1 50 -sz 100
```

Simulation input (time step 0) is shown in figure 9.12. Input array *in* and output arrays *a* and *d*, all read from the **Retina**.

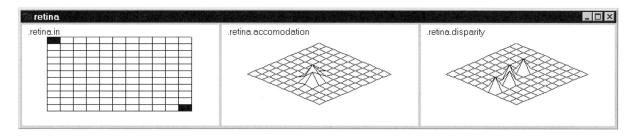

Simulation for disparity *s* and accommodation *m* corresponding to the two **Dev2** modules, is shown in figure 9.13, during time 0.25.

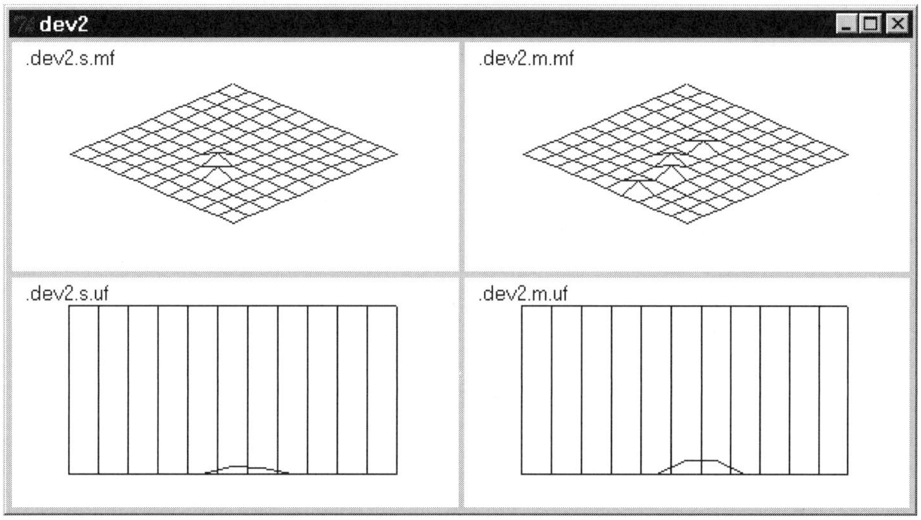

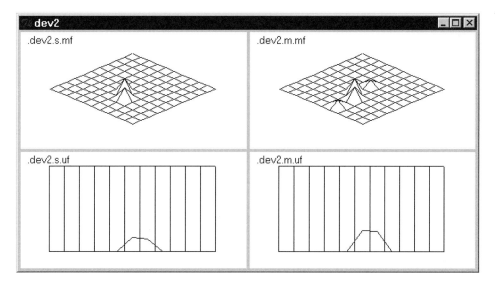

Figure 9.12
World input for processing: Input array *in* and output arrays *a* and *d*, from the **Retina**.

Figure 9.13
Disparity *s* and accommodation *m* corresponding to the two **Dev2** modules, during time 0.25.

Simulation for disparity *s* and accommodation *m* corresponding to the two **Dev2** modules, is shown in figure 9.14, during time 0.50.

Figure 9.14
Disparity *s* and accommodation *m* corresponding to the two **Dev2** modules, during time 0.50.

Simulation for disparity *s* and accommodation *m* corresponding to the two **Dev2** modules, is shown in figure 9.15, during time 0.75.

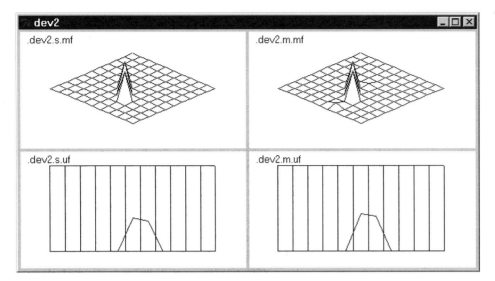

Figure 9.15
Disparity *s* and accommodation *m* corresponding to
the two **Dev** modules,
during time 0.75.

9.8 Summary

We have shown how to take advantage of the features in NSLM to modularly extend the original Dev disparity model into the House depth perception model. The ability to extend models makes NSL a very powerful simulation language. There are other modular decompositions alternative to the one presented in this model. When to choose one decomposition versus another one, depends on the complexity of the model and how much extensibility is desired. For example, we could further decomposing the retina module into an assemblage made of a left and right retina and disparity and accommodation components as shown in figure 9.16. This would require further refinement of the model equations and would be useful as far as we can actually assign separate code to each box. We leave this to the user as an exercise.

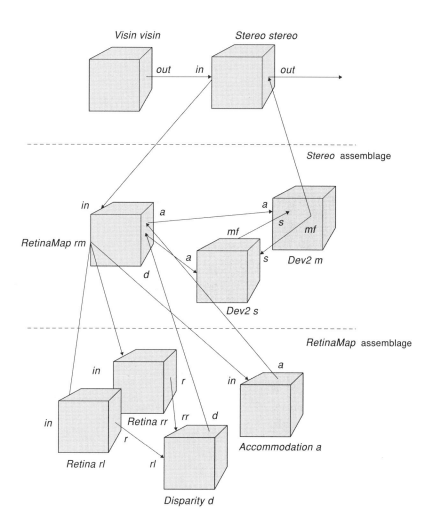

Figure 9.16
Additional depth model decomposition by making the Retina module a RetinaMap assemblage composed of two retina submodule (left and right) and separate accommodation and disparity submodules.

Notes

1. The Depth Perception model was implemented and tested under NSLC.
2. The Depth Perception model was implemented and tested under NSLC.

10 Retina[1]

F. J. Corbacho and A. Weitzenfeld[2]

10.1 Introduction

Teeters and Arbib (1991) (Teeters and Arbib 1991) presented a model of the anuran retina which qualitatively accounts for the characteristic response properties used to distinguish ganglion cell types in anurans. Teeters et al. (1993) tested the model's ability to reproduce quantitatively tabulated data on the dependency on stimulus shape and size, with a new implementation of the model in the neural simulation language NSL. Data of Ewert & Hock (1972) relating toad R2, R3, and R4 ganglion cell responses to moving worm, antiworm, and square-shaped stimuli of various edge lengths are used to test stimulus shape and size dependency. Gaillard et al. (1998) submitted the model to the whole battery of physiological experiments to validate the performance under different stimulation conditions. We stress here the importance of a populational approach to the models. We place more emphasis on the variation of response properties in a population of neurons of the *same* class, rather than questing for *the* neuron of a given type.

10.2 Model Description

The anuran retina model of Teeters et al. (1993) accounts for the qualitative characteristic response properties used to classify anuran ganglion cell types as well as for the quantitatively determined ganglion cell responses dependent on stimulus size and shape. The structure of the model is shown in figure 10.1.

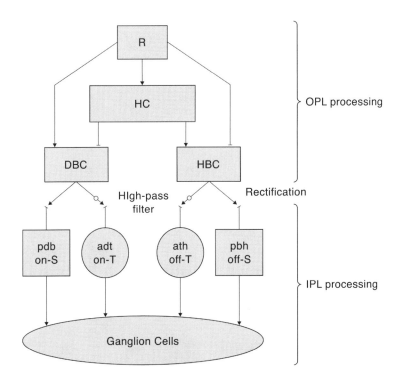

Figure 10.1

Overview of model structure. Cell types are: R - Receptors; HC - Horizontal cells, DBC and HBC - Depolarizing and Hyperpolarizing bipolar cells; PBD and PBH - positive part of bipolar cell potentials; ATD and ATH - transient amacrine cells from DBC and HBC channel; OPL - outer plexiform layer. IPL - inner plexiform layer.

The top part shows the layers of cells that feed all the ganglion cells, while the bottom part shows the specific inputs for each ganglion cell type. Each single cell in these diagrams represents a layer of cells in the formal model. We summarize the different layers of the model in table 10.1 and the equations for the model in table 10.2. We will present possible improvements as the exposition progresses.

Abbreviation	Description
R	Receptor cell
H (HC)	Horizontal Cell
R0 - R4	Retinal ganglion cell types: classes 0 to 4
HBC	Hyperpolarizing Bipolar Cell
DBC	Depolarizing Bipolar Cell
PBH	Positive component of the Hyperpolarizing Bipolar Cell
PBD	Positive component of the Depolarizing Bipolar Cell
ATH	Hyperpolarizing Transient Amacrine
ATD	Depolarizing Transient Amacrine
ERF	Excitatory Receptive Field
IRF	Inhibitory Receptive Field

Table 10.1
Neural layers.

Neuron Layer	Equations		
Receptor	$R = 1 - I$		(10.1)
Horizontal	$\tau_H \, dH/dt = H_0 - H$, $H_0 = 0$ ambient light, 1 ambient dark; $\tau_H = 0.1$		(10.2)
	Off channel	**On channel**	
Bipolars	HBC = R - H (10.3) $PBH = \max(HBC, 0)$ (10.5)	DBC = H - R (10.4) $PBD = \max(DBC, 0)$ (10.6)	
Amacrines	$\tau_a \, dHBX/dt = HBC - HBX$, $\tau_a = 0.3$ (10.7) $ATH_t = \max$ $(HBC\text{-}HBX, ATH_{t-1} \, e^{-t/\tau_a})$ (10.8)	$\tau_a \, dDBX/dt = DBC - DBX$ (10.9) $ATD_t = \max$ $(DBC\text{-}DBX, ATD_{t-1} \, e^{-t/\tau_a})$ (10.10)	
R0 Cells	$R0 = k0*ATD - k1 * ((3 \cdot ATH) + ATD)$ with k0 = mask(4, 1.8, 1), k1 = mask(15.5, 3.7, 0.8)		(10.11)
R1 Cells	$R1 = k0 * (PBD+PBH+ATD+ATH) - k1 * (ATD+ATH)$ with k0 = mask(3, 2.3, 1), k1 = mask(19.5, 4.6, 3)		(10.12)
R2 Cells	$R2 = g \cdot ((k0*PBH) + tc)$ where tc = k0*ATH - k1 * (ATH+ATD), and g = pos(tc) where pos(x) = 1 if x > 0, 0 otherwise with k0 = mask(4, 2.4, 1), k1 = mask(19.5, 4.6, 3)		(10.13)
R3 Cells	$R3 = k0*a - (k1*a)_{delayed}$ where a = p $\cdot$ ATD + ATH with p = 0.4, k0 = mask(8, 2.4, 1), k1 = mask(19.5, 4.6, 1.4) while $(s)_{delayed}$ = signal s delayed by 40 milliseconds.		(10.14)
R4 Cells	$R4 = k0 * (ATH - x \cdot ATD)$ with x = 1, k0 = mask(15.5, 3.5, 1).		(10.15)

Table 10.2
Algorithms for receptors through ganglion cells in the model.

Receptors (R) convert light energy into neural potentials. The hyperpolarizing response to light is modeled by setting the receptor potential to the inverse of light intensity (I) that ranges from 0 (dark) to 1 (light). Adaptation and other complexities are not included in the model. Note that in the case of R2, the model uses two temporary variables *tc* and *g* where *tc* is the total transient input to the cell and *g* is a gate which is set to 1 if the net transient excitation is larger than the inhibition.

Horizontal cells (H) form the surround receptive field of both bipolar cell types. They are modeled so that they are only sensitive to the background illumination of the surround (H_0 in table 10.2) and are spatially invariant (uniform potential model) through the infinite spread of the activation within the cells. This simple interpretation of horizontal cell function ignores the effect of presentation of a local stimulus and suggests that their main function is to bias the bipolar cells so they operate in their region of maximal sensitivity.

Bipolar cells (HBC, DBC) are computed as a difference between receptor and horizontal cell activity. Hyperpolarizing bipolar cells (HBC) hyperpolarize in response to light, depolarizing bipolar cells (DBC) depolarize in response to light. **PBH** and **PBD** are the positive components of the HBC and DBC responses.

Transient **Amacrine Cells (ATH, ATD)** convert the sustained bipolar outputs into transient signals. The transient amacrines are modeled as pseudo differentiators which operate by subtracting the leaky-integrated bipolar potential from the sustained bipolar potential, and then amplifying the difference if it is above threshold. We modeled the Bipolars and Amacrines to have one-to-one connections from the preceding layers based on the following assumptions: (i) horizontal cells in this model have a uniform potential which in effect makes the spatial connection properties mostly irrelevant, and (ii) dendritic tree diameters of the Bipolars and Amacrines are smaller than those of the ganglion cells.

The model input to the ganglion cells (receptors through bipolar and amacrine) ignores optics, different receptor types, light adaptation, and distinctions between other subtypes of horizontal, bipolar, and amacrine cells. It is not our claim that this simplification exhausts the functionality of these cells. Rather, we seek to emphasize that only those properties analyzed in this paper are essential for understanding the range of ganglion cell properties described here. In fact, the Teeters and Arbib (1991) implementation of the horizontal and bipolar cells does not really affect the outcome of the stimulus shape and size discrimination tasks. Nevertheless we need the horizontal and bipolar cells to account for other phenomena caused by changes in whole field illumination.

Ganglion cells (R0 – R4) receive input from bipolar and amacrine cells. Unlike the bipolar and amacrine cells which have one-to-one connections to their preceding layers, each ganglion cell input is composed of a central ERF (Excitatory Receptive Field), and a wider IRF (Inhibitory Receptive Field). The spatial properties of the ERF and IRF are specified as two-dimensional Gaussians. The notation "*mask(dia, sig, wgt)*" in table 10.2 denotes a 2-dimensional Gaussian with standard deviation *sig* (in visual degrees) which is truncated with diameter *dia* (so that the Gaussian values are replaced by 0 for points more distant than *dia*/2, also in visual degrees, from the center), and which is normalized so that the sum of all elements is equal to *wgt* (for a more detailed description see Appendix I). The ERF extent is modeled as arising from ganglion cell dendritic tree topology that is narrowly spread, whereas the IRF arises from a more widely spread topology. The corresponding diagrams are shown in figure 10.2.

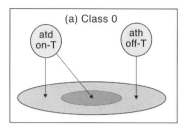
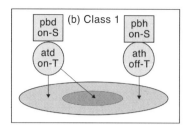

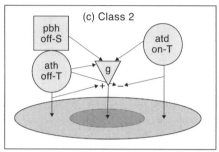

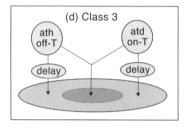
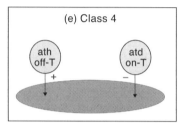

Figure 10.2
Ganglion cells R0 through R4. The receptive field for ganglion cells type R0 through R3 is composed of a small excitatory receptive field (ERF) and an overlapping larger inhibitory receptive field (IRF). The ERF and IRF in the R4 model are the same size. Input to both ERF and IRF are from bipolar and amacrine cells (pbd, phb, ath, atd). Spatial connections and other details of the algorithms are not shown here but are given in the text. (From Teeters and Arbib 1991.)

Stimulus Shape and Size Dependency

In general, the average response of anuran ganglion cells to a moving stimulus depends on stimulus configuration, size, and velocity—a long thin bar moving in the direction of its long axis (a "worm" stimulus) will normally give a different response than the same sized stimulus moving perpendicular to its long axis ("antiworm"). Likewise, a square shaped stimulus will often generate a different response than do worm or antiworm stimuli. The response dependence on the edge length of moving worm, antiworm, and square-shaped stimuli has been determined in the toad (Ewert and Hock, 1972; Ewert, 1976) and in the frog (Schürg-Pfeiffer and Ewert, 1981). The data sets are quite different even though the same anuran cell types are recorded. In the frog data, only the R3 cell shows a distinct difference in response to worm, antiworm, and square stimuli. Although Teeters and Arbib (1991) mainly tuned the ganglion cell models to frog data, this paper will use the toad data because toad ganglion cells show a much better ability to differentiate between stimulus types.

Ewert (personal communication) only used a cell's response to the *leading edge* of the stimulus to calculate the average response (nevertheless, our temporal graphs show both the leading and the trailing edge). In accordance to this methodology, we relied on the leading edge response to calculate the average response—in all the cases the leading edge responses are clearly discernible from the residual responses. Our ability to match these data (and those analyzed by Teeters and Arbib (1991)) suggests that the model is indeed robust enough to serve as a valid "front end" for *Rana computatrix* (Arbib, 1987).

A brief qualitative analysis of the model responses to various stimulus shapes and sizes could offer some useful guidelines for further tuning of the base model. An instantaneous response of a ganglion cell is the result of summation of ERF induced excitatory response and the IRF induced inhibitory response. The inputs to ERF and IRF could be of different combinations of channels (PBH, PBD, ATH, ATD) depending on the ganglion cell types. For instance, R2 receives PBH and ATH channels for its ERF, ATH and ATD channels for its IRF. However, sustained bipolar channel (PBH, PBD) responses and transient amacrine channel (ATH,ATD) responses present different spatial characteristics. For example, the PBH bipolar channel layer forms an activation profile identical to the size and shape of the dark stimulus. The Teeters and Arbib (1991) model uses a high pass filter to represent the amacrine cells as they convert sustained bipolar signals into transients. The resulting amacrine cell layer forms an exponentially decaying surface starting from the edges of the moving stimulus: the ATH layer forms such a surface starting from the leading edge of a dark moving surface, and the ATD layer from the trailing edge.

If the shapes of the stimulus classes are restricted to rectangles and if each bipolar and amacrine cell has maximum instantaneous firing rate of 1, overall activities of PBH and ATH on their layers are:

$$PBH_{sum} = lh \tag{10.15}$$

$$ATH_{sum} = h \int_{x=0}^{1} e^{-x/v\tau} dx \tag{10.16}$$

where x is the distance between the amacrines corresponding to the leading edge and the position of amacrines the stimulus has passed over. Obviously, PBH_{sum} is a function of both stimulus length (l) and height (h) while ATH_{sum} is only dependent on height of the stimulus for given velocity (v) and time constant (τ). Thus, while the activation pattern on the PBH layer directly reflects stimulus shape and size, ATH layer activation pattern produces identical firing patterns for worm, antiworm and square so long as they have the same height. These different spatial firing patterns of bipolars and amacrines will form the basis of the shape dependence of ganglion cells.

The average response of anuran ganglion cells usually increases with stimulus size smaller than the ERF. Assuming that response durations are about equal for a given velocity, the increase in ganglion cell response in our model stems from the fact that as stimulus size increases, it excites a larger area of receptors and thus bipolars and amacrines. This increases the instantaneous ganglion cell response that is proportional to the sum of activation of amacrines and/or bipolars within the ERF. However, bipolar and amacrine contributions to the response growth will be different in that bipolar channel contributions will increase proportional to the stimulus area but the amacrine channel contribution will increase proportional to the height. As the stimulus size increases beyond the ERF and into the IRF region, the IRF-contributed inhibition takes effect and reduces the total response.

Due to size limitations, in this chapter we will focus on R3 cells for a detailed analysis. A similar analysis is provided in Teeters et al. (1993) for the rest of the ganglion cells.

10.3 Model Implementation

The model implementation consists at the top level of a **RetinaModel** and a **Retina** module. The **Retina** module contains a Visin module for generating synthetic visual input, the Receptors, Horizontal Cells, Bipolar Cells, Amacrine Cells and Ganglion Cells, R2, R3 and R4, each organized into its own module, as shown in figure 10.3.

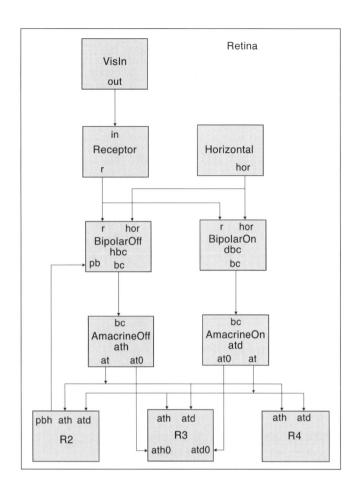

Figure 10.3
Retina module consisting of the following submodules interconnected between them: Stimulus, Receptors, Horizontal Cells, Bipolar Cells (on and off channel), Amacrine Cells (on and off channels) and ganglion cells R2, R3 and R4

Note that we use the same module definition for both on and off channel bipolars and Amacrines.

Visin

The Visin module uses a special input structure to simulate visual input (see Appendix III for details). Different kinds of moving (or static) stimuli may be defined interactively. In the **simRun** function the model simply needs to specify the in.run() function call for the actual computation to take place. Note that we initialize *in* to 0 previously to reset the visual input.

```
public void simRun()
{
    in = 0;   // need to reset all values first
    in.run(); // compute stimulus position according to pars
        set in file
    out = in; // export
}
```

Receptor

The Receptor module contains an input port *in* receiving visual input, while an output port *r* sends output to the following modules in the data path. The **initRun** method initializes *r* to 0. The **simRun** method sets the receptor *r* value to the input stimulus while time is less than 7.0 in order to stop it in the ERF. After that its value is sustained from its last value staying constant.

```
public void simRun()
{
    if (system.getSimTime() <= 7.0)
        r = in;
}
```

Horizontal Cells

The horizontal cells get their input from the ambient light through *hLevel*. The **Horizontal** module has only a single output port *hor*. The **initRun** method initializes *hor* to 0. The **simRun** method computes a differential equation corresponding to a leaky integrator model for the horizontal cells

```
public void simRun()
{
    nslDiff(hor,tm,hLevel - hor);
}
```

Bipolars

Bipolar cells receive input from both the receptors and the horizontal cells. We describe a single Bipolar module for both the on and off channel cells. The distinction is made in terms of an *on_off* instantiation parameter. If "1" the cells are considered *Hyperpolarizing Bipolars* and if "-1" they are considered Depolarizing Bipolars. The **initRun** method initializes *bc* and *pb* to 0. The **simRun** method computes the bipolar cell activity *bc* as a difference between the values of the receptors and horizontal cells, with its sign depending on whether they are on or off channel cells. An additional output to the module is *pb* corresponding rectified value from the cell activity.

```
public void simRun()
{
    bc = on_off*(r - hor);
    pb = nslMax(bc,0);
}
```

Amacrines

Amacrine cells receive input from the bipolar cells. We describe a single Amacrine module for both the on and off channel cells. The distinction is made this time in terms of whether it receives input from an on or off channel bipolar cell. The **initRun** method initializes all variables to 0 and gets the value of the system delta to be used for numerical approximation (dt = system.getRunDelta()). The **simRun** method computes the amacrine cell activity *at* through an average exact method instead of the leaky integrator method.

```
public void simRun()
{
    // nslDiff(ax,tm, bc - ax);        // Euler method.
    ax = diff_ae(ax,bc,old_bc,tm);     // Average Exact Method.
    at1 = 5*(bc - ax);
    at2 = nslExp(-dt/tm.getData())*at;     // compute from
        previous at value
    at = nslMax(at1,at2);
    old_bc = bc;                       // keep old bc
}
```

The following average exact approximation method is used,

```
private NslFloat2 diff_ae(NslFloat2 v,NslFloat2 s,NslFloat2
    prev,NslFloat0 tm)
{
    float dt,tc,temp;
    int vmax = v.getRows();  // Size of the matrices.

    NslFloat2 term1(vmax,vmax);
    NslFloat2 term2(vmax,vmax);

    dt = system.getSimDelta();
    tc = tm.getData();

    if (dt != 0 && tc != 0){
        temp = exp(-dt/tc);
        term1 = (NslFloat2) ((1 - temp) * s + temp * v);
        term2 = (NslFloat2) ((s - prev) * (temp * (tc + dt) -
            tc) / dt);
    }
    return (term1 + term2);
}
```

Ganglion Cell R2

We model only ganglion cells R2, R3 and R4. All of them receive input from both the on and off channel amacrine cells. R2 in particular also receives input from the rectification of the on channel bipolar cell. The R2 module thus includes three input ports without any output port. It includes both an excitatory receptive field (ERF) and an inhibitory receptive field (IRF). The **initRun** method initializes the cell activity to 0. It also calculates the excitatory and inhibitory receptive fields through a Gaussian function. R2 in particular calculates the difference of gaussians (DOG) between *erf* and *irf* in *rf*.

```
public void initRun()
{
    r2 = 0; r2f = 0;
    nslGaussian(erf,erf_dia,erf_sig,erf_wgt); // Gaussian ERF
kernel
    nslGaussian(irf,irf_dia,irf_sig,irf_wgt); // Gaussian IRF
        kernel
    rf = erf - irf;            // DOG for the r2 ganglion cells
}
```

The **simRun** method computes a sustained *erf* (*sust_erf*) and *irf* (*sust_irf*) values from the *erf* and *irf* rectified bipolar cell input convolution, respectively. The cell activity *r2* is computed from a convolution of *r2* with the amacrine cell input. The output *r2f* is computed by a ramp function.

```
public void simRun()
{
    sust_erf = newconv(erf, pbh_erf * pbh); // sustained erf
        input
    sust_irf = newconv(irf, pbh_irf * pbh); // sustained irf
        input
    sust = sust_erf - sust_irf;                      // sustained
        input

    temp = ath + trailing * atd; // trailing is the effect of
        the trailing
                            // edge set to 0 to get Ewert's data
    r2 = newconv(rf, temp) + sust; // New convolution and No
        Leaky Integ.
    r2f = k*nslRamp(r2);
}
```

The following convolution method returning a 2d matrix of different size (in this example 1x1) is used:

```
private NslFloat2 newconv(NslFloat2& a, NslFloat2& b)
// a is the Mask and b is the input layer.
{
  int saimax = a.getRows();
  int sajmax = a.getCols();
  int sbimax = b.getRows();
  int sbjmax = b.getCols();

  int leftbound = 1;    // 32; for the 72x72
  NslFloat2 c(1,1); // Make this variable size // c(8,8) for
    72x72

  for (int i = 0; i < leftbound; i = i+4) {
    for (int j = 0; j < leftbound; j = j+4){
      float val = 0.0;
      for (int m = 0; m < saimax; m++)
        for (int n = 0; n < sajmax; n++)
          val = val + a[m][n] * b[i+m][j+n];
      c[i/4][j/4] = val;
    }
  }
  return c;
}
```

Ganglion Cell R3

The ganglion cells R3 are similar to R2 in that they receive input from both the on and off channel amacrine cells. The R3 module includes two input ports without any output port. It includes both an excitatory receptive field (ERF) and an inhibitory receptive field (IRF). The **initRun** method initializes the cell activity to 0. It also calculates the excitatory and inhibitory receptive fields through a Gaussian function.

```
public void initRun()
{
    r3 = 0; r3f = 0;
    nslGaussian(erf,erf_dia,erf_sig,erf_wgt); // Gaussian ERF
        kernel
    nslGaussian(irf,irf_dia,irf_sig,irf_wgt); // Gaussian IRF
        kernel
}
```

The **simRun** method computes an *all* input value from both amacrine cells for its *erf* while storing old values for its *irf*. The cell activity *r3* is computed from a convolution of *r3* with the amacrine cell input from *all* by its *erf* and *old* for its *irf*. The output *r3f* is computed by a ramp function.

```
public void simRun()
{
    all = p * atd + ath;
    old = p * old_atd + old_ath;

    r3 = newconv(erf, all) - newconv(irf, old);
    r3f = k*nslRamp(r3);
}
```

Ganglion Cell R4

The ganglion cells R4 are similar to R2 and R3 in that they receive input from both the on and off channel amacrine cells. The R4 module includes two input ports without any output port. It includes only an excitatory receptive field (ERF). The **initRun** method reinitializes the cell activity to 0. It also calculates the excitatory receptive field through a Gaussian function.

```
public void initRun()
{
    r3 = 0; r3t = 0; r3f = 0;
    nslGaussian(erf,erf_dia,erf_sig,erf_wgt); // Gaussian ERF
        kernel
}
```

The **simRun** method computes the cell activity *r4* by a convolution with the amacrine cell input difference by its *erf*. The output *r4f* is computed by a squashing function on *r4t* computed as a ramp function on *r4*.

```
public void simRun()
{
r4 = newconv(erf, (ath - atd));
    r4t = nslRamp(r4);
    r4f = k*r4t/(r4t+0.2); // Squashing function
}
```

10.4 Simulation and Results[3]

As previously mentioned, we do quantitative modeling of Anuran retina responses for stimulus shape and size dependency. In this simulations we test the model's ability to reproduce quantitatively tabulated data on the dependency on stimulus shape and size

(Ewert 1976). The goal has been to match Ewert's quantitative data on the Toad's retinal ganglion cells. Input to the model is Light on the receptors (40X40 to simulate the receptive field of a single ganglion cell of each type). The model also simulates "simple" Horizontal and Bipolar cells. The output of the model represents the temporal firing rate of a Ganglion cell of each type (R2, R3, R4). Note that there is no trailing-edge effect since Ewert computed his data with only the response to the leading edge. Furthermore, no Leaky Integrators we used for the Ganglion Cells.

Simulation Parameters

The simulation parameters include the *delta* and *endTime*

```
nsl set system.runDelta 0.066 ;# Simulation Time Step = 66
    msec.
nsl set system.runEndTime 7.0 ;# Total simulation time = 7 sec
```

Model Parameters

Model parameters are set for the different modules.

Horizontal Cell parameters:

```
nsl set retinaModel.retina.hor.tm 0.1
nsl set retinaModel.retina.hor.hlevel 0   ;# Uniform horizontal
    cell potential
          ;# 0 if the background is bright, 1 if dark.
```

Amacrine Cell parameters:

```
nsl set retinaModel.retina.ath.tm 0.3
nsl set retinaModel.retina.atd.tm 0.3
```

Ganglion Cell R2 parameters:

```
nsl set retinaModel.retina.r2.pbh_erf 0.3
nsl set retinaModel.retina.r2.pbh_irf 0

nsl set retinaModel.retina.r2.trailing 0 ;# Effect of trailing
    edge on R2.
nsl set retinaModel.retina.r2.k 43.8 ;# Scaling Factors for
    ganglion cells.

nsl set retinaModel.retina.r2.erf_dia 4.0 ;# R2 ERF diameter.
nsl set retinaModel.retina.r2.irf_dia 19.5
nsl set retinaModel.retina.r2.erf_sig 2.4 ;# R2 ERF sigmoid
    (for the Gaussian)
nsl set retinaModel.retina.r2.irf_sig 4.0
nsl set retinaModel.retina.r2.erf_wgt 1.0 ;# R2 ERF weight
nsl set retinaModel.retina.r2.irf_wgt 2.3
```

Ganglion Cell R3 parameters:

```
nsl set retinaModel.retina.r3.p 0.5  ;# Effect of trailing
    edge on R3
nsl set retinaModel.retina.r3.k 44.0
nsl set retinaModel.retina.r3.erf_dia 8.0
nsl set retinaModel.retina.r3.irf_dia 19.5
nsl set retinaModel.retina.r3.erf_sig 2.0
nsl set retinaModel.retina.r3.irf_sig 10.0
nsl set retinaModel.retina.r3.erf_wgt 1.15
nsl set retinaModel.retina.r3.irf_wgt 2.38
```

Ganglion Cell R4 parameters:

```
nsl set retinaModel.retina.r4.k 37.5
nsl set retinaModel.retina.r4.erf_dia 15.5
nsl set retinaModel.retina.r4.erf_sig 3.5
nsl set retinaModel.retina.r4.erf_wgt 1.0
```

Input Stimulus

Visual input stimulus plays an important role in the Retina model. To simulate this input the model uses the NSL input library which generates arbitrary sized 2D rectangles moving on the visual field as explained in Appendix III. To be able to incorporate this input the modeler needs to specify mapping parameters between the input and the receptor layer.

In the Retina model, the user has to choose among different types of stimuli. There are 15 options among Worms, Antiworms and Squares of 2, 4, 8, 16 and 32 visual degrees. These sizes are used in order to reproduce Ewert's data on presentation of Squares, Worms and Antiworms from 2 to 32 visual degrees. A particular concern on stimulus presentation relates to single cone receptors in the retina. While they have a density of about 5 to 30 cells per visual degree depending on their location (Carey, 1975) simulation tests have shown that a density of only 2 cells per visual degree allows sufficient accuracy for modeling responses to the stimuli considered here. When the stimulus edge partially covers a receptor, we set the receptor inputs to values proportional to the area covered by the actual (analytical/continuous) stimulus. The error from the edge effect is then about 4% relative to the analytical solution (Teeters, 1989).

We allow an arbitrary size and shape bitmap to represent our stimulus. In the simulations for the size and shape dependence of the ganglion cells, the velocity of the stimulus was set to 7.6°/sec so that the stimulus moves approximately 15 pixels in the grid each simulated second.

The following code in the "retina.nsl" file contains specification parameters for the visual input. The first values to be set are the distance between adjacent array elements in the receptor in mapping to the visual input coordinates (dx and dy) together with the origin of the coordinate system (xz and yz). Instead of 0.5°/cell we specify here 2°/cell for visualization purposes. This will affect the sizes of stimuli chosen in that we will make them 4 times as big to compensate for the enlargement.

```
nsl set retinaModel.retina.visin.input.dx 2
nsl set retinaModel.retina.visin.input.dy 2
nsl set retinaModel.retina.visin.input.xz 0
nsl set retinaModel.retina.visin.input.yz 20
```

For each stimulus we want to simulate on the visual field we choose its size and initial position. In the retina model, the user will choose among three types of stimuli with varying sizes, consisting of 5 sizes starting with 2 degrees. In table 10.3 we show three different experiments for the Retina model.

Stimulus	Initial Center Location (*xc,yc*)	Size (*dx,dy*)	Speed (*vx,vy*)
Antiworm	(-1,0)	(2,16)	(7.6,0)
Worm	(-8,0)	(16,2)	(7.6,0)
Square	(-8,0)	(16,16)	(7.6,0)

Table 10.3

Algorithms for the model of ganglion cells

Since we will be scaling values, as previously explained, by 4, we provide a corresponding *scale* variable as follows,

```
set scale 4
```

For a WORM stimulus we load the "worm.nsl" file:

```
set dx [expr 16*$scale]  ;# Size, 2 4 8 16 32
set dy [expr 2*$scale]   ;# CTE
set vx [expr 7.6*$scale] ;# Speed, number of squares per
    second, 7.6 deg/sec.
nsl create BlockStim stim -layer retinaModel.retina.visin.in \
    -spec_type center -xc [expr -$dx/2] -yc 0 -dx $dx -dy $dy -
        vx $vx
```

Note how we create a rectangle or "BlockStim" whose size is given by "dx" and "dy", its speed by "vx", all scaled by the *scale* factor, and whose initial center position is given by "-xc" and "-yc". The resulting temporal output for the three ganglion cells for a 16x2 worm is shown in figure 10.4.

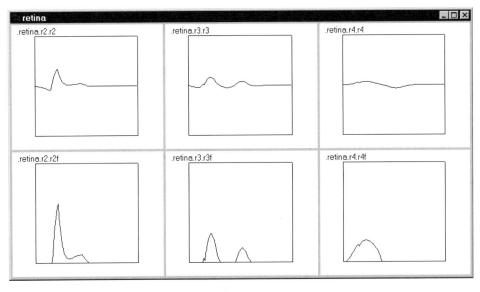

Worm: 16x2

Figure 10.4

These graphs display cell activity (top level) and firing rate (bottom level) versus time in seconds for a 16x2 moving worm. Columns specify different types of ganglion cells, R2, R3 and R4.

For ANTIWORM as the stimulus we need to load the "antiworm.nsl" file:

```
set dx [expr 2*$scale]
set dy [expr 16*$scale]   ;# Size, 2 4 8 16 32
set vx [expr 7.6*$scale] ;# Speed, number of squares per
    second, 7.6 deg/sec.
nsl create BlockStim stim -layer retinaModel.retina.visin.in \
    -spec_type center -xc [expr -$dx/2] -yc 0 -dx $dx -dy $dy -
    vx $vx
```

Again we create a rectangle or "BlockStim" whose size is given by "dx" and "dy", its speed by "vx", all scaled by the *scale* factor, and whose initial center position is given by "-xc" and "-yc". The resulting temporal output for the three ganglion cells for a 2x16 antiworm is shown in figure 10.5.

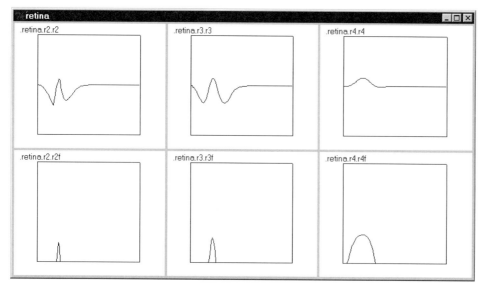

Antiworm: 2x16

Figure 10.5

These graphs display cell activity (top level) and firing rate (bottom level) versus time in seconds for a 2x16 moving antiworm. Columns specify different types of ganglion cells, R2, R3 and R4.

For a SQUARE as the stimulus we need to load the "square.nsl" file:

```
set dx [expr 16*$scale]   ;# Size, 2 4 8 16 32
set dy [expr 16*$scale]   ;# Size, 2 4 8 16 32
set vx [expr 7.6*$scale] ;# Speed, number of squares per
    second, 7.6 deg/sec.
nsl create BlockStim stim -layer retinaModel.retina.visin.in \
    -spec_type center -xc [expr -$dx/2] -yc 0 -dx $dx -dy $dy -
        vx $vx
```

The resulting temporal output for the three ganglion cells for a 16x16 square is shown in figure 10.6.

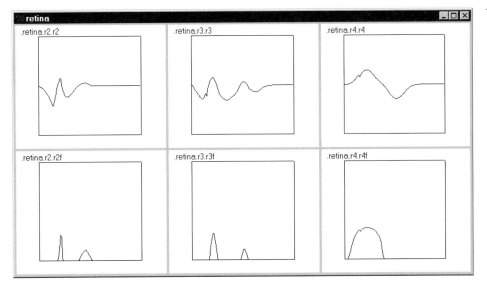

Figure 10.6
These graphs display activity (top level) and firing rate (bottom level) versus time in seconds for a 16x16 moving square. Columns specify different types of ganglion cells, R2, R3 and R4.

Square 16x16

To allow comparison between the model behavior and tabulated data, the temporal responses of the ganglion cells generated by the model are converted to an average response that is then scaled. The average response is calculated as the area under the above threshold curve divided by the time from first to last above threshold response to the leading edge of the stimulus (or, in other cases, from the beginning of the leading edge response to the end of the trailing edge response):

$$\sum_{t=T_0}^{T_0} \frac{R(t)}{T_n - T_0} \tag{10.17}$$

where T_0 is the time for the first such response and T_n is the time for the last. If the response decays in an exponential manner and is not actively abolished, the response duration will be infinitely long. For that reason the threshold used is not zero but a small positive number (0.001).

The analogous experimental average is equal to the total number of spikes divided by the time from first to last spike during this period. Scaling is achieved by multiplying all calculated average responses by a "scaling constant" so that the scaled average response to a 2x2 square moving at 7.6°/second matches that found experimentally by Ewert (1976).

10.5 Summary

The essential features of the models presented in this paper enabling a close match to the stimulus shape and size dependency data were also used by several earlier models that attempted to explain those properties in anurans.

For example, the DOG center-surround structure was used to account for response in the R2 and R3 cells by an der Heiden & Roth (1987, 1989), Ewert & von Seelen (1974, also reported in Ewert 1976), and by Grüsser & Grüsser-Cornehls (1973). Variations in the temporal filter characteristics of retinal elements have been used by Eckmiller (1975), Grüsser (1967) and Grüsser et al. (1968) to account for variations in the velocity exponent. However, where the previous models were specialized to account for only particular phenomena, the models in this paper are not only able to account for the dependence on stimulus shape and size, but also able to account for the generation of characteristic ganglion cell response properties despite additional constraints applied to the ganglion cell models developed by Teeters and Arbib (1991). For the R2, R3 and R4 cell models given in Teeters and Arbib (1991), the response dependence on stimulus shape and size was tested in two parts. First, the original unmodified model was tested. Second, parameter adjustments and in some cases algorithm modifications, were made in an attempt to "tune" the model to attain a closer match to the experimental data on stimulus shape and size dependence. While the original untuned models did not quantitatively match the data, they were qualitatively correct.

Stimulus Size Dependence of R3 Cells

The Teeters and Arbib (1991) model does not match the data very well because the response to worms decreases with increasing edge length and there is a separation of the square and antiworm responses for large stimuli. Both of these effects are due to the inclusion of the slight trailing edge response generated by the model to long square and worm stimuli when calculating the average response.

Only minor changes are needed to tune the model. Excluding the trailing edge (and relying only on the leading edge) response for the calculation of the average responses (Ewert, personal communication) allows a good match to the data, although the response to the 32° square and antiworm is too large. Further, increasing the weight and the standard deviation of the IRF Gaussian mask and a little decrease in standard deviation of ERF mask allows a better match. This suggests that the IRF receptive field is essentially like a plateau, with a very small decay with distance, while the ERF receptive field is like a sharp peak. Comparison with the R2 temporal responses (Teeters et al., 1993) reveals that the main differences lie in (i) R2 responses show a sustained component for the long worm and a sustained rebound for the large square stimuli, while (ii) R3 responses show transient responses for both the leading and the trailing edges of the long worm and large square stimuli. The simulated temporal responses of R2 and R3 for the different stimuli approximate observed experimental data (Gaillard, personal communication) fairly well.

Predictions Based on the Modified Model Behavior

We now consider two important questions in detail: how do the changes made to the models here affect their ability to account for characteristics addressed by Teeters and Arbib (1991), and what predictions result from the changes?

- **R2 cell**: Characteristic R2 responses as identified by Maturana, Lettvin, McCulloch & Pitts (1960), and Grüsser & Grüsser-Cornehls (1976) are a lack of response to a diffuse light change, a lack of response to a moving antiworm longer than 10°, a prolonged response to a moving stimulus that stops in the ERF, a sensitivity to movement, a cessation of sustained response following a transient off of the general illumination, and a stronger response to small objects than to large objects. All of these characteristic responses but one are found in the toad R2 cells studied by Ewert & Hock—toad R2's respond to antiworm stimuli up to 16° in length. The tuning performed in this paper does not destroy the ability of the R2 model to account for these properties. Specifically, reduction in the IRF weighting to the R2 model will not allow response to full field flashes because the total IRF weighting is still larger than that of the ERF. Sensitivity to movement is preserved because the modified R2 cell receives input from transient amacrine cells that respond only to change. However, inclusion of PBH input to IRF leads to:

- **Prediction 1**: For R2 cells tested by Ewert & Hock (1972), while the average response to squares and antiworms of the same height may be almost identical, the temporal responses (spike trains) will be different as shown in figure 10.4.

Future Refinements of the Retina Model

The shape/size tuned retinal model could be tested against other qualitative and quantitative data such as the average response as a function of velocity, adaptive state, etc. (Grüsser & Grüsser-Cornehls, 1976). In order to account for these data, we should probably incorporate more detailed physiological and morphological facts. Some of the most obvious ingredients could be:

1. A more detailed Horizontal cell model that is sensitive to the presentation of local stimuli.

2. Feedback loops among some layers (e.g., feedback from the amacrines to the bipolars).

3. Multi-compartmental dendritic processing and axonal transmission properties.

Also we have to note that the modeling of transient amacrine cells was based on phenomenological observations rather than on detailed physiological data on these cells. It might be possible to express the comparatively more responsive synaptic transfer process of R3s by, for instance, decreasing the amacrine time constant.

Teeters (1989) comments that the high-pass filter transient amacrine is unsuitable for the R4 cell model. This points out the need for an improved transient generating mechanism in the R4 cell. In retrospect, this is not surprising, because other properties of R4 cells, such as rhythmical bursting and delayed response to illumination decreases also cannot be accounted for easily by the high pass filter mechanism used in the model. Rhythmical bursting also occurs in some R3 cells (Maturana et al., 1960), suggesting that a high pass filter may also be inadequate to explain all of their response properties. Some type of negative feedback, with time delays or voltage dependent activation, is an obvious candidate mechanism that could generate oscillations in the neural potentials leading to bursting type response patterns. Further simulations will be needed to determine if such a mechanism can be made to simultaneously account for the characteristic R4 properties, the velocity exponent, rhythmic bursting, and the long response duration to a decrease in illumination. However, some of the characteristic R4 properties such as prolonged response to a stationary dark object and to the general illumination decrease can be achieved by incorporating the off channel bipolar inputs. In fact, Lee (1986) uses the sustained amacrine channel, PBH in our model, as the sole input to his R4 cells. It may also be possible to model the R4's large time constant for a moving object with the proper formulation of spatially sensitive horizontal cells.

Providing a Flexible Framework for Modeling Anuran Retina

In summary, our current retina model cannot match all the experimental data, but does show how a relatively simple model can explain a wide range of ganglion cell properties. It also makes clear how, by changing parameter values of different inputs to the ganglion cells, the response properties of the ganglion cells will in turn change. For instance, when the weight of the input from the PBH to the IRF of R2 cells is increased, the previously described average response of the cell will diminish as well as the strength of the sustained response.

We should also note that retinal ganglion cells of the "same" type show a population of responses, as is elegantly shown in Gaillard's (personal communication, 1991) experiment on R3 type cells. Gaillard's result shows surprisingly large variances in ERF size, temporal activation patterns, etc., among the R3 cells. Similarly, we can expect that bipolars and amacrines will also form statistical distributions of responses. It may be that during embryogenesis a connection pattern from amacrines to a ganglion cell will be basically homogeneous, but that during postnatal development certain connections are strengthened while some are weakened thus giving the diversity among ganglion cells of the same type. The fact that reciprocal connections exist between the bipolar cells and amacrines gives some hope that a similar connectivity may exist between amacrines and ganglion cells, which could provide information paths for selective strengthening and weakening required for diversity.

In our current model the amacrine population is represented by a layer of cells that share exactly the same properties. This has proven enough to match the experimental data described in this paper. But it is certain that the real retina contains several kinds of amacrine cells showing different properties, and this could promote higher variability in the response profiles of the ganglion population whose response depend on amacrine input. For instance, in our preliminary studies on the velocity dependence of ganglion cells we found it beneficial to decrease the high pass filter (amacrine) time constant from 300ms to 50ms for the R3 and R4 ganglion cells to yield a better fit to the quantitative data. This suggests that the amacrine time constant may be better represented as forming a statistical distribution such as a normal distribution centered at a "typical" value and that the amacrines feeding into the R3 consists mostly of the values in the lower spectrum. The populational approach could also be applied to the ganglion cells. Thus, we are led to place more emphasis on the variation of response properties in a population of neurons of the "same" class, rather than questing for "the" neuron of a given type.

One question that could arise when considering the populational approach is whether there exists an ill-defined boundary or just a "continuum" between different classes of ganglion cells. Should we construct a model so that it is possible for one category of cells to jump to another simply by, for instance, adjusting the "power" of a sustained input or the transient input? Gaillard (personal communication) has found "R3-like" units whose characteristic responses are similar to R3 units but whose velocity dependence is closer to that found in R2 ganglion cells. Their response profiles are stronger in intensity and temporally more extended than those of typical R3 units. R3s differ from R2s in that (i) their ERFs are larger, (ii) their ERFs receive no sustained input channel, and (iii) they have delayed IRF-inhibition. We believe the significance of these differences increases in the order listed above. We also think the more important a characteristic is, the less flexible are the parameters that make the characteristic. Notice that the "discrimination curves" of R2 and R3 cells to different stimuli are surprisingly similar. The main difference lies in a shift of the optimal length of the square (S) and the antiworm (A) from 4° (R2 units) to 8° (R3 units) and consequently in a shift of the crossing point between Worm (W), S, and A curves. This difference can be accounted for by a simple difference in the R3's ERF size and therefore we may predict that some R3 cells may have smaller ERFs so that their responses to dynamic visual stimuli are similar to R2 responses.

Notes

1. Preparation of this paper was supported in part by award number IBN-9411503 for Collaborative Research (M.A. Arbib and A. Weerasuriya, co-Principal Investigators) from the National Science Foundation.

2. A. Weitzenfeld developed the NSL3.0 version from the original NSL2.1 model implementation written by F. Corbacho as well as contributed Section 10.3 and part of section 10.4 to this chapter.

3. The Retina model was implemented and tested under NSLC.

11 Receptive Fields[1]

F. Morán, J. C. Chacón, M. A. Andrade and A. Weitzenfeld

11.1 Introduction

The visual nervous system in higher mammals shows a high degree of organization in which different selectivity properties are found. However, the necessary quantity of information for specifying that connectivity is much higher than the information stored in the genetic code (von der Malsburg 1987). Some organizing processes have been found which could explain this fact.

In an early stage of the development of the mammal embryo, the nervous fibers coming from the ganglion cells grow from retina to brain establishing connections into the visual cortex. Once a primary gross connection is reached, a self-organizing process, dependent on neural activity, takes place and the connections are pruned, which gives functional characteristics to the visual system (Linsker 1990; Singer 1987; Stryker 1986; von der Malsburg and Singer 1988). This mechanism permits several superposed mappings to appear in the visual cortex (Fregnac and Imbert 1984; Orban 1984; Tootell et al 1981).

The receptive field is a characteristic organization of the visual system (Hubel and Wiesel 1963; Orban 1984). A receptive field of a neuron is the compact region of the visual space that affects the activity of that neuron. A well-known example is the on-off or Mexican-hat shaped receptive field, with circular symmetry. If the center area is stimulated, an activatory response is produced in the target neuron, whereas the stimulation in the neighborhood produces inhibition.

Based on neurophysiological knowledge, some models that explain visual cortex organization during development have been proposed (Erwin et al 1995). Most of them use neural network architectures and activity dependent rules (Linsker 1986; Miller et al 1989; von der Malsburg 1990).

The self-organizing network presented in this chapter shows how *diffusion of synaptic activity, competitive synaptic growth* and *synaptic evolution* can explain the development of variable sized on-off receptive fields in a developmental stage of a mammal embryo prior to visual experience. Synaptic activity is driven by either *activity correlation* or *activity anti-correlation* (i.e., Hebbian (Hebb 1949) or anti-Hebbian (Carlson 1990; Földiak 1990) learning rules, respectively).

11.2 Model Description

The model presented in this chapter is based on the classical work of von der Malsburg (Häussler and von der Malsburg 1983), that has been previously proposed elsewhere (Andrade and Moran 1996). The architecture of the network is schematically represented in figure 11.1.

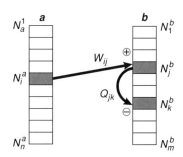

Figure 11.1

The model consists of two neuron layers: (1) an input layer *a* (corresponding to LGN - Lateral Geniculate Nucleus) and (2) an output layer *b* (corresponding to Primary Visual Cortex). These two layers are fully interconnected by excitatory connections, $W_{ij} > 0$ ($i = 1,...,n$; $j = 1,...,m$), while the output layer is fully interconnected by lateral inhibitory connections, $Q_{jk} > 0$, ($j,k = 1,...,m$).

The evolution of the system connectivity starts with an initial random state that will converge into a final state by processing the following differential equations:

$$\frac{dW_{ij}(t)}{dt} = \alpha + \beta W_{ij}(t)(F_{ij}^{a}(t) - \gamma W_{ij}^{2}(t))$$

$$\frac{dQ_{jk}(t)}{dt} = \alpha + \beta Q_{jk}(t)(F_{jk}^{b}(t) - \gamma Q_{jk}^{2}(t))$$

(11.1)

where α is a positive constant that accounts for the generation of new synaptic connections, and parameter β accounts for the rate of change of the established connections.

The terms, $W_{ij}(t)F_{ij}^{a}(t)$ and $Q_{jk}(t)F_{jk}^{b}(t)$, represent a *growth factor* whose value depends on the temporal correlation of the signals connecting the neurons. The growth factor describes the increase (or decrease) of a particular synapse depending on the *global* state of all the network synapses. F_{ij}^{a} and F_{jk}^{b} are the growth factors of synaptic weights W and Q, respectively. Growth factor F_{ij}^{a} uses a Hebbian rule, since it increases the value of an excitatory connection when correlation grows, as described in previous models for the development of retinotopic connectivity (Häussler and von der Malsburg 1983) and ocular domains (Andrade and Moran 1996). However, growth factor F_{jk}^{b} one uses an anti-Hebbian rule (Carlson 1990; Földiak 1990), since the inhibitory connection is increased.

The decaying terms $W_{ij}(t)\gamma W^{2}{}_{ij}(t)$ and $Q_{jk}(t)\gamma Q^{2}{}_{jk}(t)$ are cubic weight terms multiplied by a constant γ controlling their respective contribution. These terms account for the *individual* growth restrictions for each synaptic connection.

The growth factors are a function of the neurons activity correlation (Andrade and Moran 1997; Häussler and von der Malsburg 1983):

$$F_{ij}^{a}(t) \propto <A_{i}^{a}(t), A_{j}^{b}(t) > t$$

$$F_{jk}^{b}(t) \propto <A_{j}^{b}(t), A_{k}^{b}(t) > t$$

(11.2)

where $A_{i}^{a}(t)$ represents the activity of the input layer neurons N_{i}^{a} (for $i = 1,...,n$), and $A_{j}^{b}(t)$ represents the activity of the output layer neurons N_{j}^{b} (for $j = 1,...,m$).

Initially, the only source of activity is spontaneous activity from the photoreceptors (layer a in this model), since the visual system does not receive any coherent visual signal from the environment. Therefore, the spontaneous and non-correlated activity $f_{i}(t)$ will be the only source of activity in layer a. Moreover, due to the lateral propagation of activity in that layer, the resulting neuron output will depend on its own activity as well as on its neighboring neurons, modulated by a cushioning diffusion term,

$$D_{ij}^{a} = G^{a}(|i - j|)$$

(11.3)

where G^{a} is a function of the distance between the neurons assumed to be Gaussian:

$$G^{a}(x) = \frac{h_a}{s_a}\exp\left(-(x/s_a)^2/2\right)$$

$$G^{b}(x) = \frac{h_b}{s_b}\exp\left(-(x/s_b)^2/2\right)$$

(11.4)

where s_a and s_b are positive constants describing the Gaussian width, and h_a and h_b indicate the surface under the curve, with $x = |i - j|$.

In other words, the output activity of the neuron is given by:

$$A_{i}^{a}(t) = \sum_{k=1}^{n} f_k(t)D_{ki}^{a}$$

(11.5)

This activity is transmitted to the output layer by means of the excitatory connections W_{ij}. In output layer b, the signal received by each neuron is modified by two different effects: lateral excitatory diffusion of the signal and lateral inhibitory transmission of the signal, Q_{jk}. The two combined effects lead to the following expression describing activity in the output neurons:

$$A_j^b(t) = \sum_{q=1}^{n} \sum_{p=1}^{n} \sum_{o=1}^{m} f_q^a(t) D_{qp}^a W_{po}(t) \left(D_{kj}^b - \sum_{l=1}^{m} D_{ol}^b Q_{lj}(t) \right) \tag{11.6}$$

Since the input layer activity is spontaneous, there is no correlation between the activity of two neurons, that is to say:

$$< f_i(t), f_j(t) > t = \begin{cases} 1 \text{ if } i = j \\ 0 \text{ if } i \neq j \end{cases} \tag{11.7}$$

Or what amounts to:

$$< f_i(t), f_j(t) > t = \delta_{ij} \tag{11.8}$$

where δ is Kronecker's delta. Taking this into account, we can rewrite expression (11.1) as follows (for a more detailed description see (Andrade and Moran 1997)):

$$\frac{dW_{ij}(t)}{dt} = \alpha + \beta W_{ij}(t) \left[\sum_{q=1}^{n} D_{qi}^a E_{qj}(t) - \gamma W_{ij}^2(t) \right]$$
$$\frac{dQ_{jk}(t)}{dt} = \alpha + \beta Q_{jk}(t) \left[\sum_{q=1}^{n} E_{qj}(t) E_{qk}(t) - \gamma Q_{ij}^2(t) \right] \tag{11.9}$$

where

$$E_{ij}(t) = \sum_{k=1}^{n} D_{ik}^a \sum_{p=1}^{m} W_{kp}(t) \left(D_{pj}^b - \sum_{l=1}^{m} D_{pl}^b Q_{lj}(t) \right) \tag{11.10}$$

It should be noted that a side effect of these correlation functions is that all spontaneous activity has been *explicitly* eliminated from the two equations. Among other considerations, this results in a much easier numeric integration.

11.3 Model Architecture

The model is implemented by a **Recfield** instantiated by the **RecfieldModel** at the top level. The **Recfield** module contains four modules, **LayerA**, **LayerB**, **ConnectW** and **ConnectQ** as shown in figure 11.2.

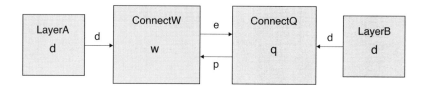

The **Recfield** module instantiates its four submodules as follows (note the different parameters passed to each),

Figure 11.2
The Recfield module is composed of LayerA module sending data *d* to the excitatory connection module ConnectW and LayerB module send data *d* to inhibitory connection module ConnectQ. Module *ConnectW* send data *e* to *ConnectQ*. *ConnectQ* module sends data *p* to *ConnectW*.

```
nslModule Recfield (int x1, int y1, int x2, int y2)
{
    private LayerA a(x1, y1);
    private LayerB b(x2, y2);

    private ConnectW w(x1, y1, x2, y2);
    private ConnectQ q(x1, y1, x2, y2);
}
```

In our model all parameters passed to **Recfield**, *x1*, *y1*, *x2* and *y2*, have a size of 5.

LayerA Module

LayerA module defines the diffused activation *da* with the help of a gaussian distribution function,

```
nslModule LayerA (int x1, int y1)
{
    public NslDoutFloat4 d(x1, y1, x1, y1);   // (da), to w

    private NslFloat0 s(); // gaussian spread (sa)
    private NslFloat0 h(); // gaussian height (ha)
}
```

The **initRun** method computes *d* value. Note that a user defined external function is applied,

```
public void initRun()
{
    nslGaussian(d,h,s);
}
```

The gaussian function is defined as a library (it will also be used by **LayerB**).

```
private void nslGaussian(NslFloat4 g, NslFloat0 h, NslFloat0 s)
{
    int       i, j, k, l;      // loops
    float     dist,dx,dy;
    int x1 = g.getRows();
    int y1 = g.getCols();
    for (i = 0; i < x1; i++)
      for (j = 0; j < y1; j++)
        for (k = 0; k < x1; k++)
          for (l = 0; l < y1; l++) {
    dx = nslAbs(i - k);
    if (dx > (x1 / 2))
    dx = x1 - dx;
    dy = nslAbs(j - l);
    if (dy > (y1 / 2))
    dy = y1 - dy;
    dist = nslSqrt (dx*dx + dy*dy);
    g[i][j][k][l] = (h/s)*nslExp(-nslPow((dist/s),2)/2) ;
          }
}
```

ConnectW Module
The excitatory connection module **ConnectW** is defined as follows

```
nslModule ConnectW (int x1, int y1, int x2, int y2) {

    public NslDinFloat4 d(x1, y1, x1, y1);  // from a
    public NslDinFloat4 p(x2, y2, x2, y2);  // from q
    public NslDoutFloat4 e(x1, x2, y1, y2); // to q

    private NslFloat4 w(x1, x2, y1, y2);

    private NslFloat0 maxinitval(); // max weight val
    private NslFloat0 seed(); // random seed

    private NslFloat0 alpha();// get weights out from zero
    private NslFloat0 beta();// integration parameter for act
    private NslFloat0 gamma();// cubic decay term for w
}
```

Parameters *x1*, *y1*, *x2* and *y2* are assigned to local attributes so they can later be used by local methods cycling on every array element. Weights are initialized by a random function

```
public void initWeights(float randa)
{
    int   i, j, k, l;          // loops

    for (i = 0; i < _x1; i++)
      for (j = 0; j < _x2; j++)
        for (k = 0; k < _y1; k++)
          for (l = 0; l < _y2; l++)
            w[j][i][l][k] = maxinitval*randa;
}
```

Function *nslNormRand*() is shown as follows

```
private int nslNormRand(NslFloat0 seed)
{
    // calculation of the random maximum value
    int j, max_rand = 0;
    for (int i = 0; i < 1000; i++) { // max number of iterations ?
      j = nslRand();
      if (j > max_rand)
        max_rand = j;
    }
    // random seed
    nslRand(seed);

    return nslRand()/max_rand; // normalization to 1
}
```

The **initRun** method simply initializes the weights by a normalized random function

```
public void initRun()
{
    int randa = nslNormRand(seed);
    initWeights(randa);
}
```

Function *convGauss*() is shown as follows

```
private void convGauss()
{
    int              i, j, k, l, m, n, o, p;          /* loops */
    float            sum, sum2;

    /* convolutions gaussian 1 w pp (from L2) */
    for (i = 0; i < x1; i++)
      for (j = 0; j < y1; j++)
        for (k = 0; k < x2; k++)
          for (l = 0; l < y2; l++) {
            sum = 0;
          for (m = 0; m < x1; m++)
            for (n = 0; n < y1; n++) {
          sum2 = 0;
          for (o = 0; o < x2; o++)
          for (p = 0; p < y2; p++)
          sum2=sum2+w[o][m][p][n]*pp[o][p][k][l];
            sum = sum + d[i][j][m][n] * sum2;
            }
            e[k][i][l][j] = sum;
          }
}
```

Function *modifyWeights*() is shown as follows

```
private void modifyWeights()
{
    int              i, j, k, l, m, n, o, p;          // loops
    float            sum, sum2;

    // weight modification

    for (i = 0; i < x1; i++)
      for (j = 0; j < y1; j++)
        for (k = 0; k < x2; k++)
          for (l = 0; l < y2; l++) {
            sum = 0;
          for (m = 0; m < x1; m++)
            for (n = 0; n < y1; n++)
          sum = sum + d[m][n][i][j] * e[k][m][l][n];
            w[k][i][l][j] = alpha + w[k][i][l][j] *
          (1 + beta*(sum - gamma * w[k][i][l][j]
          * w[k][i][l][j]));
          if (w[k][i][l][j] < 0)
            nslPrint("no");
          }
}
```

The **simRun** method processes the differential equation defining the weight activity

```
public void simRun()
{
    // convGauss()
    e = d * (w * p);
    // modifyWeights()
    nslDiff(w,1.0,alpha + beta*w(d*e - gamma*(w^w)); // eq
        (11.9)
}
```

LayerB Module

LayerB module defines only diffused activation *db* with the help of a gaussian distribution function,

```
nslModule LayerB (int x2, int y2)
{
    public NslDoutFloat4 d(x2, y2, x2, y2); // (db) to Q
    private NslFloat0 s();  // gaussian spread (sb)
    private NslFloat0 h();   // gaussian height (hb)
}
```

The **initRun** method computes *d* value. Note that a user defined external function is applied,

```
public void initRun()
{
    nslGaussian(d,delta,sp);
}
```

ConnectQ Module

The inhibitory connection module **ConnectQ** is defined as follows

```
nslModule LayerB (int x1, int y1, int x2, int y2)
{
    public NslDinFloat4 e(x1, x2, y1, y2);  // from w
    public NslDinFloat4 d(x2, y2, x2, y2);  // from b (db)
    public NslDoutFloat4 p(x2, y2, x2, y2); // to w

    private NslFloat4 q(x1, y1, x2, y2);//x2*y2,x2*y2 inhib(q)
    private NslFloat0 alpha(); // get weights out from zero
    private NslFloat0 beta();// integration parameter for act
    private NslFloat0 gamma();  // cubic decay term for w
}
```

The **initRun** method simply initializes the weights to zero

```
public void initRun()
{
    q = 0;
}
```

Function *convGauss*() is shown as follows

```
private void convGauss()
{
    int             i, j, k, l, m, n, o, p;        // loops
    float           sum, sum2;

    // convolutions q gaussian 2

    for (i = 0; i < x2; i++)
      for (j = 0; j < y2; j++)
        for (k = 0; k < x2; k++)
          for (l = 0; l < y2; l++) {
        sum = 0;
        for (m = 0; m < x2; m++)
            for (n = 0; n < y2; n++)
    sum = sum + d[i][j][m][n] * q[m][n][k][l];
        p[i][j][k][l] = d[i][j][k][l] - sum;
          }
}
```

Function *modifyWeights*() is shown as follows

```
private void modifyWeights()
{
    int             i, j, k, l, m, n, o, p;        // loops
    float           sum, sum2;

    // weight modification

    for (i = 0; i < x2; i++)
      for (j = 0; j < y2; j++)
        for (k = 0; k < x2; k++)
          for (l = 0; l < y2; l++) {
        sum = 0;
        for (m = 0; m < x1; m++)
            for (n = 0; n < y1; n++)
        sum = sum + e[i][m][j][n] * e[k][m][l][n];
        w[i][j][k][l] = alpha + w[i][j][k][l] * (1 + beta *
            (sum - gamma*q[i][j][k][l] * q[i][j][k][l]));
        if (q[i][j][k][l] < 0)
            nslPrint("no");
          }
}
```

The **simRun** method processes the differential equation defining the weight activity

```
public void simRun()
{
    // convGauss()
    p = d - (d * q);
    // modifyWeights()
    nslDiff(q,1.0,alpha + beta*q(e*e - ga*(q^q)); // eq (11.9)
}
```

11.4 Simulation and Results[1]

The simulation control file contains parameter value assignment. Note how we can assign common values to different module parameters (*alpha*, *beta* and *gamma*)

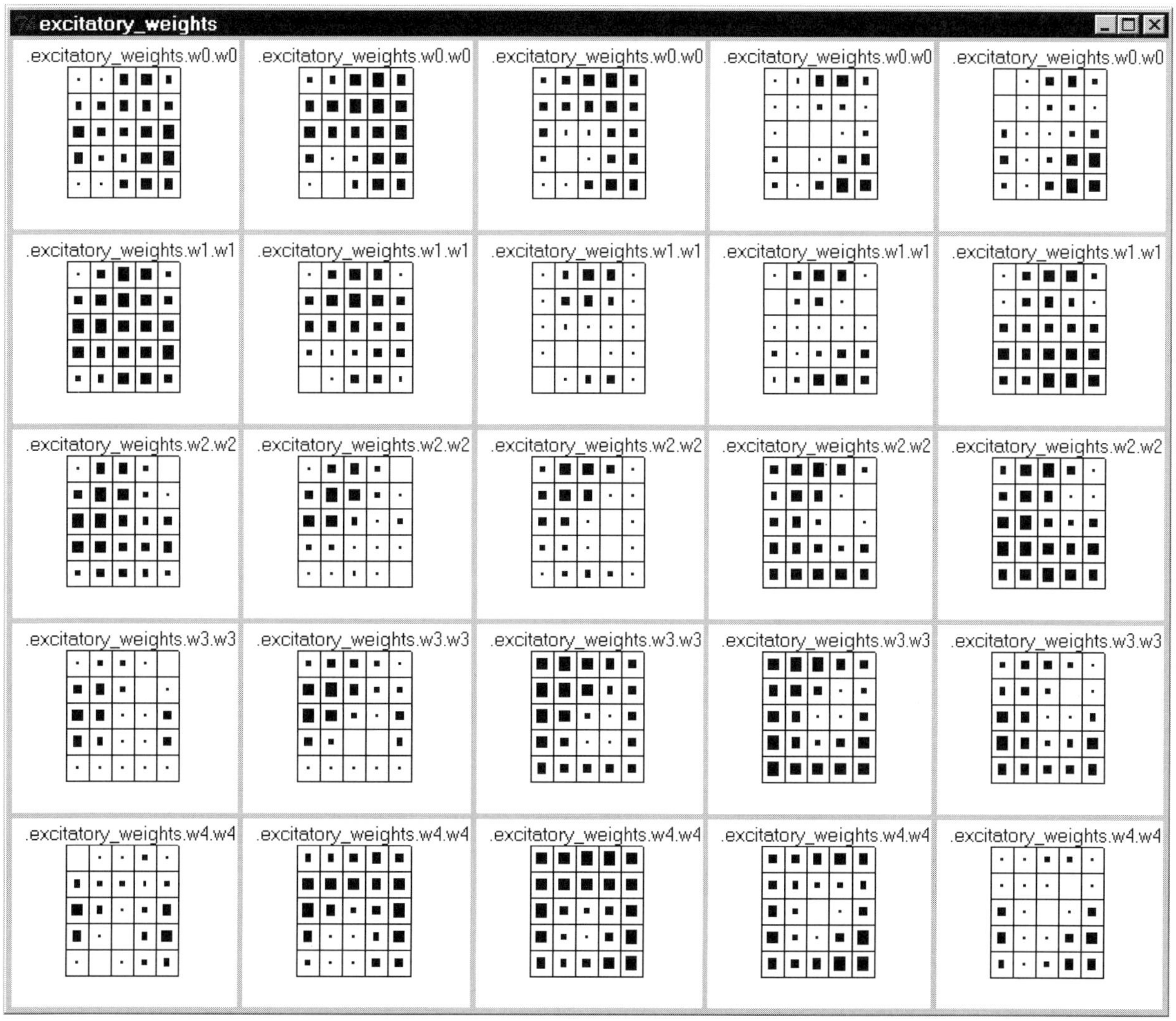

Figure 11.3
Excitatory connection weight *w* in **ConnectW** module.

```
nsl set system.simDelta 0.1
nsl set system.simEndTime 50

set alpha 0.00005
set beta 0.001
set gamma 1e4

nsl set recfield.w.alpha $alpha
nsl set recfield.w.beta $beta
nsl set recfield.w.gamma $gamma

nsl set recfield.q.alpha $alpha
nsl set recfield.q.beta $beta
nsl set recfield.q.gamma $gamma

nsl set recfield.a.seed 77
nsl set recfield.a.maxinitval 0.001
nsl set recfield.a.sp 1
nsl set recfield.a.delta 4

nsl set recfield.b.sp 1
nsl set recfield.b.delta 4
```

To simulate the model load "recfield.nsl" and then run it. Three display frames are created containing a display canvas each, for w, q and e respectively. The connection matrices w and q and the resulting matrix e are shown in the figures 11.3 to 11.5. Matrix e represents the excitatory/inhibition effect produced on each output layer neuron when the input layer neuron is activated and the signal is transmitted through the network. Therefore, it represents the set of receptive fields corresponding to the cortex neurons.

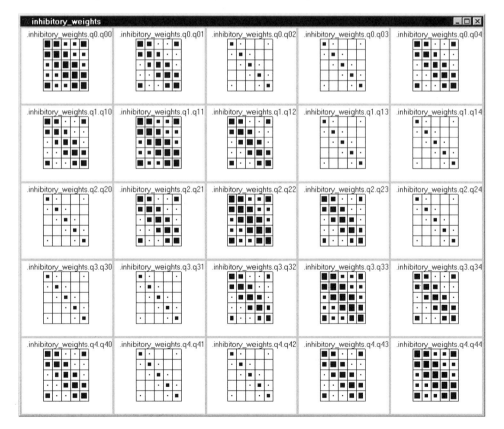

Figure 11.4
Inhibitory connection weight q in **ConnectQ** module.

In figure 11.3, the variations in geometry of the receptive fields can be noted, while in figure 11.4 the inhibitory weights show a more homogeneous shape, that is, each neuron is connected to its neighbors in a circular manner. These differences are more relevant if larger number of neurons are used (i.e., a layer of 8x8 neurons presents neurons with highly different oriented receptive fields)

The result of the joint action of the two weight matrices and the intra-layer lateral diffusion of signal become apparent in the receptive field values showed in figure 11.5. Thus, different receptive fields consist of a compact activation area placed in different positions, and the form of this area is also variable, showing oriented symmetries and different orientations. The size of the receptive fields is variable, too. When observed in detail, there is a spatial continuity between the receptive fields. So, closer neurons tend to coincide in the situation of its positive-area and to have similar geometry, either in orientations or sizes.

11.5 Summary

Through the simulation of this model, the essential characteristics of self-organization have been demonstrated. The kind of resulting connectivity let us to explain how the nervous system in general, and the visual system in particular, can obtain their specific connectivity through self-organizing process based in the system activity and a reduced number of local rules, easily justifiable from a physiological point of view.

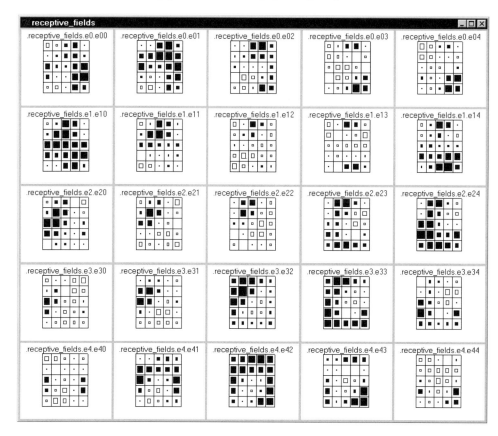

Figure 11.5 Receptive field *e* in ConnectW module.

Notes

1. This work has been supported in part by grants from the DGICYT, MEC, Spain (project no. PB92-0456) and from the CICYT, Spain. (project no. BIO96-0895). This work is part of the Doctoral Thesis of M.A.A. developed under a fellowship from the MEC, Spain. We thank Prof. Ch. von der Malsburg for his support and suggestions.

2. The Receptive Fields model was implemented and tested under NSLC.

12 The Associative Search Network: Landmark Learning and Hill Climbing

M. Bota and A. Guazzelli

12.1 Introduction

In 1981, Barto and Sutton showed how a simple network could be used to model landmark learning. Their work was based on a previous paper by Barto et al. (1981) which defined the associative search problem and presented the associative search network theory. The associative network described by Barto and Sutton (1981) controls locomotion in a spatial environment composed of distinct olfactory gradients, which are produced by landmarks. In this chapter, we show how this simple network and associated task can be easily implemented in NSL. Further discussion of this example is provided in Barto and Sutton (1981).

Figure 12.1 shows a NSL window, which was used to depict the network and its environment. For didactic reasons, from now on, we assume that a simple robot, which contains an associative search network is actually the agent in the environment. The robot's only task it to move from its current position to a tree located at the center. Four additional landmarks, located at the cardinal points exist in this rather simple and imaginary world.

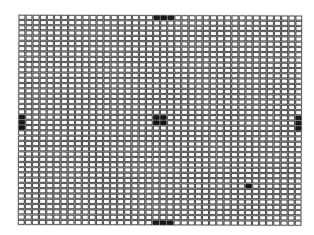

Figure 12.1
A window representing the robot's environment (40 x 40 small rectangles). Three consecutive filled rectangles located at the cardinal points represent the four landmarks: North, South, West, and East. The one filled rectangle on the Southeast quadrant represents the initial position of the robot. The four filled rectangles in the middle represent the tree.

Not only the tree, but also the landmarks emit each a distinctive odor, whose strengths decay with distance. However, only the odor emitted by the tree is attractive to the robot. The odors emitted by the landmarks can only be used as a cue to location in space.

12.2 Model Description

It can be shown that by using a hill-climbing algorithm, the robot can find its way towards the tree, even without an associative network or landmarks. If we imagine that the tree is located on the top of a hill, we can use a measure, a payoff function z, that tells the robot how high up in the hill it is each time it moves one step. Since the goal is to get to the tree, the higher the robot climbs, the closer it will get to its goal. In this case, the payoff function reaches its maximum at the goal, i.e. the top of the hill, and decreases smoothly with increasing distance from the tree. Note that the robot itself does not know how far it is from the goal. Its only concern is to maximize the value of the payoff function. In formal terms, at time t the robot takes one step in direction $d(t)$, moving from a position with payoff $z(t)$ to a new position with payoff $z(t+1)$. If $z(t+1) > z(t)$, then the robot will continue to move in the same direction, $d(t+1) = d(t)$, with a high probability. However, if $z(t+1) < z(t)$, then $d(t+1)$ is chosen randomly. This is like a goal-seeking strategy used by simple organisms, like *the bacterial chemotaxis* strategy used by several types of bacteria.

While this hill-climbing strategy alone can give the robot the capacity of eventually getting to the top of the hill, its trajectory, as we can imagine, will look rather clumsy and inefficient. Nevertheless, we can improve the robot's goal-seeking behavior by using Barto and Sutton's associative search network (figure 12.2). The network is composed of four input and four output units. Each input unit i, where $i = North, South, East,$ and *West*, receives an input $x_i(t)$ from their respective landmark. Moreover, each input unit is fully connected with all four output units j, where $j = North, South, East,$ and *West*. This allows each input unit to adapt four connection weights $w_{ji}(t)$ in the connection matrix. Each weight encodes a degree of confidence that, when the robot is near landmark i, it should proceed in direction j to get closer to the tree. An extra input unit (depicted in figure 12.2 as a triangle), represents the specialized payoff pathway z, which has no associated weights. The payoff function can also be seen as a reinforcement signal.

Landmarks (inputs)

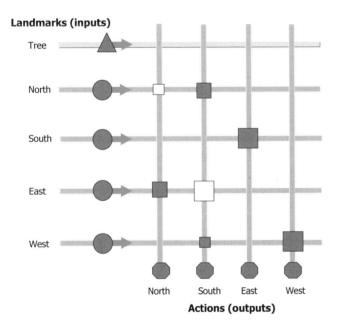

Actions (outputs)

Figure 12.2
The associative search network. The tree and the four additional landmarks are labeled vertically on the left. Each landmark releases an odor. The five distinct odors give rise to five different input pathways (input units are depicted as filled circles and as a triangle). At the bottom of the network, four distinct actions (representing the direction to be taken at the next step) give rise to four output pathways (output units are depicted as filled hexagons). Adaptable weights are depicted as rectangles: bigger weights are represented as bigger rectangles (negative weights are depicted as hollow rectangles; positive weights as filled rectangles). See text for more details.

When the robot is at a particular location in its environment, it is able to sense its distance from each of the landmarks. The degree of confidence $s_j(t)$ for a move in direction j is determined by the sum of the products of the current weights and the current signals received from the four landmarks:

$$s_j(t) = w_{0j}(t) + \Sigma_i \, w_{ji}(t) \, x_i(t) \qquad (12.1)$$

where $w_{0j}(t)$ can be seen as a bias term to be further described below. If we assume that the connection matrix contains appropriate weights, we can also assume that the chosen direction j is also appropriate. If, for example, our robot is close to the *Northern* landmark, the output unit *South* will be activated and the robot's next step will be towards *South*. Moreover, if the robot is in the *Southwest* quadrant, output units *North* and *East* will be activated and the robot's next step will be towards *Northeast*.

However, since it is still too early for us to assume that the network contains suitable weights, a noise term is added to $s_j(t)$, setting the output of unit j at time t to be

$$y_j(t) = 1 \text{ if } s_j(t) + \text{NOISE}_j(t) > 0, \text{ else } 0 \qquad (12.2)$$

where each $\text{NOISE}_j(t)$ is a normally distributed random variable with zero mean. If $s_j(t)$ is bigger than 0 when noise is added, the robot's next step will be towards direction j. If, on the other hand, $s_j(t)$ is smaller than 0, a random direction is chosen.

At this point, however, the biggest challenge for the robot is to learn appropriate weights. For this reason, a learning rule has to be implemented. This follows the following equation:

$$w_{ji}(t+1) = w_{ji}(t) + c[z(t) - z(t-1)] \, y_j(t-1) \, x_i(t-1) \qquad (12.3)$$

where c is a positive constant determining the learning rate. In the simulations depicted below, $c = 0.25$. According to this rule, a connection weight w_{ji} will only change if a movement towards direction j is performed ($y_j(t-1) > 0$) and if the robot is near an i-landmark ($x_i(t-1) > 0$). If we return to the view of $z(t)$ as height on a hill, we can see that w_{ji} will increase if z increases, which implies that direction j moves the robot uphill. In this situation, a j-movement will be more likely to happen again. If, on the other hand, w_{ji} decreases, z decreases, which implies the robot is moving downhill. In this case, a j-movement will be less likely to occur.

12.3 Model Implementation

In NSL, this learning rule is implemented by the following code:

```
NslDouble2 W(4,4);    // weight matrix
NslDouble1 Y(4);      // output vector
NslDouble1 X(4);      // input vector
double      tmp;
double      z;
double      z1;

...
tmp = 0.25 * (z1 - z);
W=W+tmp*Y*X;
for (i = 0; i < 4; i++){
  for (j = 0; j < 4; j++) {
      if ((W[i][j] >= (0.5))
          W[i][j] = 0.5;
      if (W[i][j]<= (-0.5))
          W[i][j] = -0.5;
  }
}
```

where $z1 = z(t)$ and $z = z(t-1)$. As it can be seen above, in the computations we performed, the weights are bounded inside the interval $[-0.5, 0.5]$.

The weights w_{0j} (formerly described as biases) are updated as follows:

$$w_{0j}(t+1) = f[w_{0j}(t) + c_0[z(t) - z(t-1)] \, y_j(t-1)], \qquad (12.4)$$

where $f(x) = \text{BOUND}$ if $x > \text{BOUND}$, 0 if $x < 0$, x otherwise (this will bound each w_{0j} to the interval $[0, \text{BOUND}]$), $c_0 = 0.5$, and $\text{BOUND} = 0.005$. Moreover, this learning rule is necessary only to permit the robot to climb the hill in the absence of landmark input information x_i.

12.4 Simulation and Results

By providing our robot with an associative search network and the appropriate values for its connection weights, we are giving the robot the chance of conducting hill climbing in weight space, instead of physical space. The simulations below try to show this newly acquired capacity. Figure 12.3a shows a NSL window containing the histogram of places occupied by the robot in its first attempt to get to the goal (training phase). Figure 12.3b shows the histogram of the robot's second attempt to get to the tree (testing phase), this time starting from a different position. If we compare (a) and (b), we can clearly see that there is a major improvement in the trajectory taken by the robot, since in 3b, it is using its long-term store acquired during the training phase. Both histograms are depicted over the environment as shown in figure 12.1.

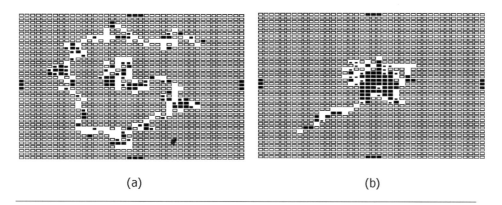

(a)   (b)

Figure 12.3

Two NSL windows containing the histogram of places occupied by the robot while in search of the tree during (a) the training phase and (b) the testing phase. In the test phase, the robot starts its trajectory from a different position than the one used for the training phase. Empty rectangles with a bold contour mean that the robot did not entered at that position. Empty rectangles with a light contour mean that the robot entered at that position at most one time. Each window displays a total of 400 steps for each phase.

This landmark-guided hill-climbing example illustrates how the results of explicit searches can be transferred to an associative long-term store so that in future encounters with similar (but not identical) situations the system need only access the store to find out what to do. As pointed out by Arbib (1989), the associative search network shows how all of this can be accomplished without centralized control. It is thus an improvement over a non-learning search method, and it also has the important property that the optimal responses need not be known a priori by the environment, the system, or the system's designer.

The NSL environment built to illustrate the robot's search for the tree is also composed by additional windows than the ones showed above. Figure 12.4 depicts a typical run. The main window is composed of six small windows. From left to right and top to bottom, the first window (x) shows the distance on the horizontal plane from the robot to the tree during the training phase. The second window (y) shows the distance on the vertical plane during the training phase. One can see that during the search, both distances are converging to 0. This is reflected in the third window (D), which shows the computed Euclidean distance between the robot and the tree during the training phase. The fourth window (Dtest) shows the computed Euclidean distance during the testing phase. The fifth window (Weight) shows the connection weights in the same way as shown in figure 12.2. The magnitude of the rectangles reflect the weights obtained at the end of the training phase. The next two windows (histtrain and histtest) show the histograms for the training and testing phases as in figure 12.3. In the present case, however, the robot started its trajectory from the same position in both phases. The last two windows (pathtest and pathtrain) show the trajectories of the robot on its path from the initial position to the goal. Each window displays a total of 400 steps.

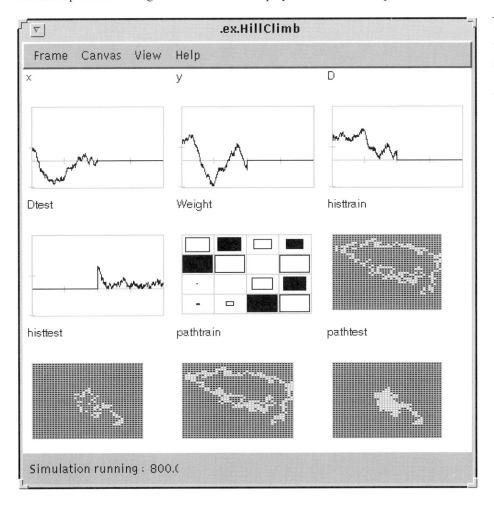

Figure 12.4
The NSL interface window used to simulate Barto & Sutton's (1981) landmark learning task. See text for details.

12.5 Summary

With this model we have shown how the hill-climbing strategy can give a robot the capability of getting to the top of a hill. However, we have also shown how to make the algorithm more efficient by improving the robot's goal-seeking behavior by using Barto and Sutton's associative search network (figure 12.2). Also, by using the NSL 3.0 simulation system we were able to easily encapsulated some of our more complex mathematical computation, and we were able to easily debug the model. We also used the NSL "Train and Run" feature to separate out the learning phase from the execution phase of the model. Finally, we were able to use NSL dynamic plot capability to plot the variables we were interested in and print the results for this book.

Notes

1. The Associative Search Network model was implemented and tested under NSLJ.

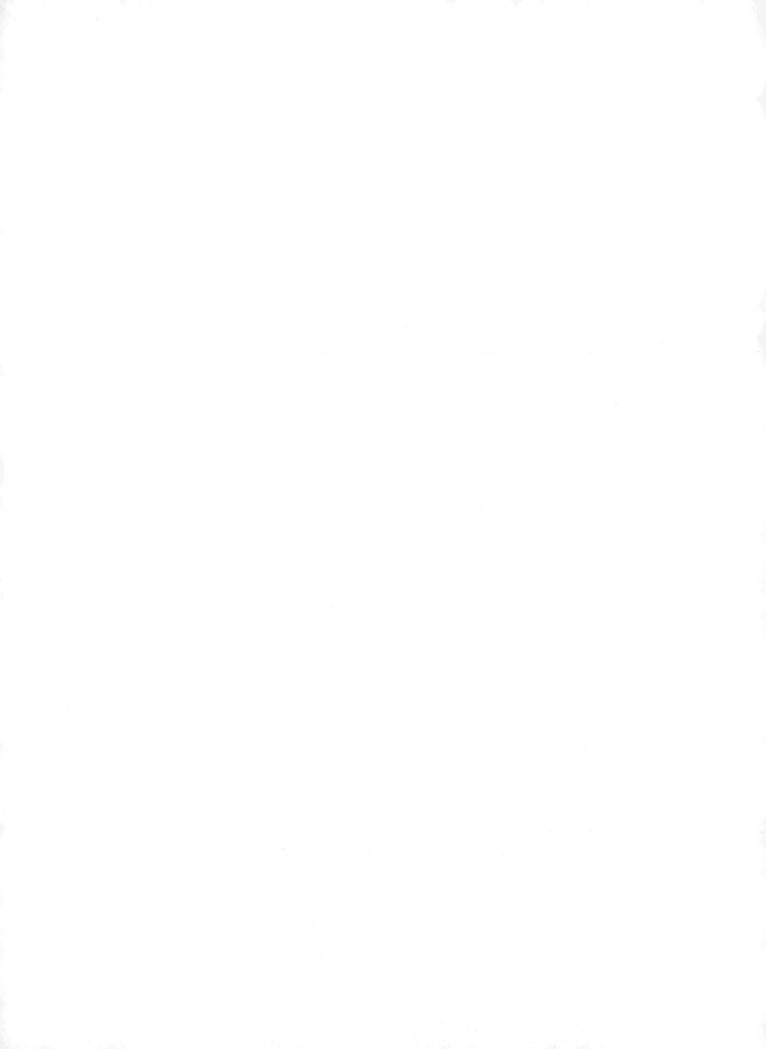

13 A Model of Primate Visual-Motor Conditional Learning[1]

A. H. Fagg and A. Weitzenfeld[2]

13.1 Introduction

Mitz, Godshalk and Wise (Mitz, Godshalk, and Wise, 1991) examine learning-dependent activity in the premotor cortex of two rhesus monkeys required to move a lever in a particular direction in response to a specific visual stimulus. Figure 13.1 shows the protocol and expected response for one such trial. The monkey is initially given a ready signal, which is followed by a visual stimulus (instruction stimulus, IS). The monkey is then expected to wait for a flash in the visual stimulus (trigger stimulus, TS), and then produce the appropriate motor response. The four possible motor responses are: move the handle left, right, down, or no movement. When a correct response is produced, the subject is rewarded with a squirt of juice and a stimulus is picked randomly for the next trial. On the other hand, when an incorrect response is produced, no reward is given and the same stimulus is kept for the next trial.

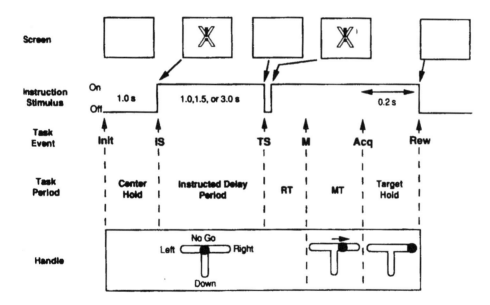

Figure 13.1
Top row: visual stimulus as seen on the video screen. Second row: temporal trace of the visual stimulus. Third and fourth rows: Primary events and periods of the experimental trial. Fifth row: expected motor response. (From Mitz et al., Figure 1; reprinted by permission of the Journal of Neuroscience.)

During the initial training phase, the two subjects were trained to perform the task with a fixed set of visual stimuli. This phase taught the protocol to the subjects, including the four appropriate motor responses. Through the second phase of learning, which we model here, the subjects were presented with novel stimuli and were expected to produce one of the four previously-learned motor responses. It was during this phase that single-unit recordings were taken from neurons in the primary- and pre-motor cortices.

Figure 13.2 demonstrates the results of a typical set of second-phase experiments. The left-hand column shows the correct response, and each row of the right-hand column shows the monkey's response over time. Two features of this figure are particularly interesting. First, there are a number of cases in which the monkey exhibits an incorrect response, and even though it does not receive the positive feedback, it will continue to output the same response for several additional trials. In most of these cases, the no-go response is given, which appears to be the "default" response. The second interesting feature, demonstrated in almost half of these response traces, is that once the monkey exhibits the correct response, it may give one or more improper responses before producing the correct response consistently.

Correct response	Trial number														
	1	2	3	4	5	6	7	8	9	10	11	12	13	14	15
Down (D)	L	+	+	+	+	+	+								
	R	L	L	+	R	+	+	+	+	+	+	+	+	+	
	R	+	R	L	+	+	+	+	+	+	+	+	+	+	+
	+	+	+	+	+	+	+	+							
	N	R	+	+	R	+	+	+							
	N	L	N	R	+	+	+	+	+	+	+	+	+	+	+
Right (R)	N	L	N	D	L	+	+	+							
	N	+	+	+	+										
	N	N	N	L	+	N	N	N	+	+	+				
	N	N	N	N	N	+	+	+	+						
	N	N	L	+	+	N	+	+	+						
Left (L)	R	D	+	N	+	+	+	+	+	+	+	+	+	+	+
	+	+	+	+	+	+	+	+	+	+	+	+	+	+	
	N	D	+	+	+	+	+	+	+	+	+	+	+	+	+
	N	D	+	+	+	+	+	+	+	+	+	+	+	+	+
	N	N	D	R	+	+	+	+	+	+	+	+			
	N	R	D	+	R	D	+	R	+	R	+	+	+		
No-go (N)	R	+	+	+	+	+	+	+	+	+	+	+	+	+	+
	+	+	+	+	+	+	+	+	+	+	+	+	+	+	+
	+	+	+	+	+	+	+	+	+	+	+	+	+	+	+
	L	L	R	D	L	+	L	+	+	+	+	+	+	+	+
	+	+	+	+	+	+	+	+	+	+	+	+	+	+	+
	D	R	D	+	D	L	R	+	L	D	R	D	+	+	+

Figure 13.2
Samples of responses to novel stimuli given example specific expected motor responses. Each row represents only those trials from an experiment that corresponds to a specific desired motor response. Correct answers are indicated with a '+'. (From Mitz et al., table 1; reprinted by permission of the Journal of Neuroscience.)

This behavior may be captured at a high level by considering a separate *decision box* for each stimulus (A more formal treatment of these computing elements (stochasitic learning automata) may be found in Bush (1958) and Williams (1988)). A box maintains a measure of confidence that each motor output is correct, given its particular input stimulus. When the system is presented with a stimulus, the appropriate box is chosen, and a motor output is selected based upon the confidence vector. When the monkey exhibits an incorrect response, positive reinforcement is not given. Therefore, the likelihood of the last response should be reduced slightly, while the probability of picking one of the other motor responses increases. When a correct response is given, the confidence value for the exhibited response is rewarded by a slight increase. Our challenge is to construct a neural implementation that is both distributed in nature and is capable of identifying novel stimuli as they are presented. The following data gives some hint as to how the implementation might look.

Mitz et al. recorded primarily from cells in the premotor cortex. A variety of cell types were identified. *Anticipatory* cells tend to fire between the ready signal and the IS. *Signal* cells respond to the presentation of a relevant stimulus, whereas *set-related* cells fire after the IS, in preparation for a particular motor response. *Movement-related* cells respond to the presentation of the TS and in some cases stay on for the duration of the movement. Most cells exhibit multiple response properties (e.g., combined set- and movement-related responses). Signal-, set-, and movement-related cells typically fired in correlation with a particular motor response. Thus, for any particular visual stimulus, only a small subset of cells fired significantly during the execution of the corresponding motor program. As learning progressed, some cells were seen to increase in their response activity towards a stimulus, while others decreased in their response.

Figure 13.3 shows normalized activity and performance curves for one experiment plotted against the trial number. The normalized activity is computed for a particular stimulus by looking at the activity of the ensemble of units that show an increase in activity over the course of learning. The performance curve is computed as a sliding window over a set range of trials. It is important to note that the performance curve precedes the activity curve in its sudden increase.

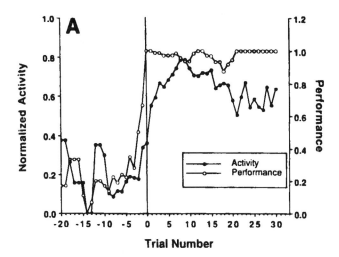

Figure 13.3
Normalized activity and performance curve plotted as a function of trial for the presentation of a novel stimulus. The rise in overall performance precedes that of cellular activity by about 3 trials. (From Mitz, figure 3; reprinted by permission of the Journal of Neuroscience.)

Mitz et al. (1991) identified a number of key features of learning-dependent activity in these experiments:

a.   The increase in cell activity (for those cells that increased their activity over the learning period) was closely correlated with, but was preceded by, the improvement in performance. Similar relations were seen in signal-, set-, and movement-related units.

b.   Activity of a particular unit for correct responses was, in most cases, higher than that during incorrect responses in the same movement direction.

c.   Activity for correct responses during times of good performance exceeded that at times of poor performance.

d.   When multiple sets of novel stimuli were presented to the monkey, similar learning-dependent responses of the signal-, set-, and movement-related cells were observed for stimuli that yielded the same motor response.

e.   The activity pattern resulting from a familiar stimulus closely correlated with the activity due to novel stimuli (after learning), although this correlation was not a perfect one. This and previous point (d) demonstrate that a similar set of premotor neurons are involved in responding to all stimuli mapping to the same motor output. From this, we can conclude that the pattern discrimination is probably not happening within the premotor cortex. If this were the case, one would expect separate groups of cells to respond to different stimuli, even if these stimuli mapped to the same motor output.

This set of experimental results presents a set of modeling challenges. We here list both those that we meet in the present model, and those that pose challenges for future research.

1.   Our neural model is capable of learning the stimulus/motor response mapping, producing qualitatively similar response traces to those of figure 13.2:

   a.   The appropriate number of trials that are required to learn the mapping.

   b.   Incorrect responses are sometimes given on several repeated trials.

   c.   Correct responses are sometimes followed by a block of incorrect responses.

The model can generate the variety of response traces, with the network starting conditions determining the actual behavior.

2. The model produces realistic normalized activity/performance curves (figure 13.3). The performance curve leads the activity curve by a number of learning trials.

3. A complete model will also reproduce the temporal activity of various neurons in the premotor cortex, including: anticipatory units, signal-related units, set-related units, and movement-related units.

13.2 Model Description

Much of neural network research has concentrated upon supervised learning techniques, such as the generalized delta rule or backpropagation (Rumelhart, Hinton and Williams, 1986). In our modeling efforts, we have chosen to explore other algorithms within an architecture that can be related (at least at a high level) to the biological architecture, while perhaps also offering greater computational capability.

Backpropagation with sigmoidal units suffers from the problem of global representation—in general, every unit in the network, and thus every weight, participates in a single input-output mapping. As a result, the gradient in weight space due to a single pattern will contain a component for almost every weight, and therefore learning can become rather slow. A related problem is that, in order to maintain an older memory for at least some amount of time, the learning of a new memory cannot alter the older memory to all but a very small degree. This is difficult to accomplish if all units are participating in every mapping and all weights are altered as a result of learning a single pattern.

With these problems in mind, we have sought *distributed representations* in which a single pattern (or task) is coded by a small subset of the units in the network. Although different subsets of units are allowed to overlap to a certain degree, interference between two patterns is minimized by the non-overlapping components. Inspired by the cell activities observed by Mitz et al., we see a unit that has not learned to participate in a motor program as being able to respond to a wide range of different inputs. As learning progresses for this unit, its response increases significantly for some stimuli, while it decreases for the remainder.

Network Dynamics

The primary computational unit in the proposed model is the *motor selection column*, each consisting of two neurons: the *feature detector unit* and the *voting unit* (figure 13.4). The overall network is composed of a large number of these columns, each performing a small portion of the stimulus-to-motor program mapping.

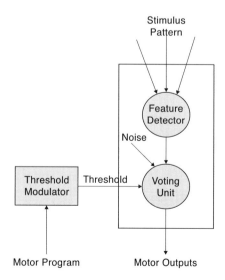

Figure 13.4
The motor selection column model. The feature detector detects specific events from the sensory input. The voting unit produces a vote for an appropriate set of motor programs. This unit, along with the noise and the threshold modulator, implements a search mechanism.

The feature detector recognizes small patterns (microfeatures) in the input stimulus. Due to the distributed construction of the circuit, a particular signal unit is not restricted to recognize patterns from a single stimulus, but may be excited by multiple patterns, even if these patterns code for different responses. A particular signal unit is physically connected to only a small subset of the input units. This enforces the constraint that only a small subset of the columns will participate in the recognition of a particular pattern. As will be discussed later, this reduces the interference between patterns during learning.

The state of the feature detector units are described by the equations:

$$\tau_f \frac{dFeature_{mem}}{dt} = -Feature_{mem} - Threshold_f + W_{in.feature} * Inputs \tag{13.1}$$

$$Feature = ramp(Feature_{mem})$$

where:

- τ_f is the time constant (scalar) of membrane potential change.
- $Threshold_f$ is the internal threshold of the feature detector units (a scalar).
- $Feature_{mem}$ is a vector of membrane potentials for the set of feature detector units. The initial condition (at the beginning of a trial) is $Feature_{mem} = - Threshold_f$ for all elements of the vector.
- $W_{in.feature}$ is the weight matrix between the input stimulus and the feature detector units. These weights are updated by learning.
- $Inputs$ is the vector of stimulus inputs.
- $Feature$ is the vector of firing rates of the feature detector units.

The voting unit receives input from its corresponding feature detector, as well as from a noise process and the threshold modulator. Based upon the resulting activity, the voting unit instantiates its *votes* for one or more motor programs. The strength of this vote depends upon the firing rate of this neuron and the strength of the connection between the voting unit and the motor program selector units.

The behavior of the voting units is governed by the equations:

$$\tau \frac{dVoting_{mem}}{dt} = -Voting_{mem} - Threshold_v(t) + Feature + Noise \tag{13.2}$$

$$Voting = saturation(Voting_{mem})$$

where :

- τ_v is the time constant of the voting units.
- $Voting_{mem}$ is the membrane potential of the voting units (vector). The initial conditions are $Voting_{mem} = -Threshold_v(t)$ for all units.
- $Threshold_v(t)$ is the time-dependent threshold determined by the threshold modulator (a scalar).
- $Feature$ is the vector of firing rates. Each voting unit receives input **only** from its corresponding feature unit.
- $Noise$ is a low-amplitude noise process that changes slowly relative to τ_v (vector).
- $Voting$ is the firing rate vector.

As shown in figure 13.5, the votes from each column are collected by the *motor program selection units*, labeled "Left", "Right", "Down", and "No-Go". The final activity of these units determines whether or not a particular motor program is activated, and thus executed.

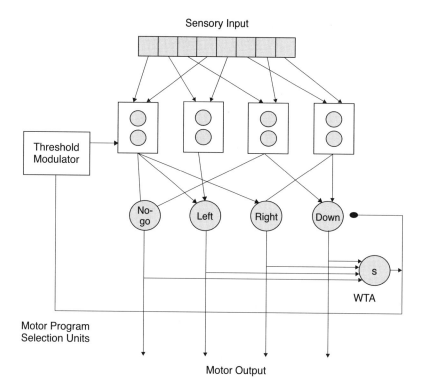

Sensory Input

Threshold Modulator

No-go Left Right Down

S

WTA

Motor Program Selection Units

Motor Output

Figure 13.5
The motor program selection units label corresponds to the four action circles (no-go, left, right, down). A set of motor selection columns votes for the motor responses. The votes are collected by units representing the activity of the schemas for each of the legal motor responses. The winner-take-all circuit ensures that only one motor program is selected.

Depending upon the state of the voting units, the motor program selection units/winner-take-all circuit attempts to choose a single motor program to activate. This selection process is governed by the following equations:

$$\tau_m \frac{dMotor_{mem}}{dt} = -Motor_{mem} - Threshold_m + W_{vote,motor} * Voting - S + Motor + Motor\_Noise$$ (13.3)

where :

- τ_m is the motor selection unit time constant.
- $Motor_{mem}$ is the membrane potential of the motor selection units (a vector). The initial conditions are $Motor_{mem} = -Threshold_m$ for all elements in the vector.
- $Threshold_m$ is the scalar threshold of the motor selection units.
- $W_{vote,motor}$ is the weight matrix representing the projection from the voting units to the motor selection units.
- S is the firing rate of the inhibitory neuron. The initial condition of this neuron is $S = 0$.
- $Motor$ is the firing rate vector. Initially, Motor = 0 for all elements.
- $Motor\_noise$ is a low-amplitude noise process, that changes slowly relative to τ_m (a vector).
- The winner-take-all circuit (Didday 1976) ensures that at most one motor program will be activated at any one time. This is accomplished through the inhibitory neuron (S).

$$\tau_S \frac{dS_{mem}}{dt} = -S_{mem} - Threshold_S + \sum_{i=1}^{N} Motor[i]$$ (13.4)

$$S = ramp(S_{mem})$$

- S_{mem} is the membrane potential of the inhibitory neuron (a scalar, since there is only one). The initial condition for this neuron is $S_{mem} = -Threshold_s$. $Threshold_s$ is the threshold of the inhibitory neuron.

When more than one motor program selection unit becomes active, this unit sends an inhibitory signal to the array of motor program selection units. The result is that all of the units will begin turning off, until only one is left (the unit receiving the largest total of votes from the motor columns; Amari and Arbib 1977). At this point, the one active unit will cue the execution of its motor program.

The reception of the trigger stimulus (TS) causes the execution of the selected motor program. Although only a single motor program selection unit will typically be active when the TS is received, two other cases are possible: none active, and more than one active. In both cases, the No-Go response is executed, irrespective of the state of the No-Go motor program selection unit. Thus, the No-Go response may be issued for one of two reasons: explicit selection of the response, or when the system is unsure as to an appropriate response by the time the TS is received.

The global threshold modulator and the local noise processes play an important role in the search for the appropriate motor program to activate. When a new visual stimulus is presented to the system, the feature detector units will often not respond significantly enough to bring the voting units above threshold. As a result, no voting information is passed on to the motor program selection units. The threshold modulator responds to this situation by slowly lowering the threshold of all of the voting units. Given time (before the TS), at least a few voting units are activated to contribute some votes to the motor program units. In this case, a response is forced, even though the system is very unsure as to what that response should be.

Noise processes have been used as an active element of several neural models. Noise is used in Boltzmann machines as a device for escaping local minima and as a way of breaking symmetry between two possible solution paths (Hinton & Sejnowski, 1986). Although the problem of local minima is not a concern in this work, the problem of choosing between two equally desirable solutions is a considerable one. By injecting a small amount of noise into the network, we randomly bias solutions so that a choice is forced within the winner-take-all (WTA) circuit. There are some cases in which two motor program selection units receive almost the same amount of activity. Due to the implementation of the winner-take-all circuit, this situation may send the system into oscillations, where it is not able to make a decision. The added noise coming into the voting units helps to bias one of the motor programs, to the point where a decision can be made quickly. Moreover, rather than always selecting the motor program that has the highest incoming feature support, the system is enabled by the noise to choose other possibilities. This keeps the system from prematurely committing to an incorrect solution, maintaining diversity during the search process (Barto, Sutton, & Anderson, 1983). Thus, the amount of time dedicated to the search process can be significantly decreased.

Learning Dynamics

Learning in this model is reinforcement-based, and is implemented by modifying two sets of synapses: the sensory input to feature detector mapping and the voting unit to motor program selection unit mapping, i.e., the weight matrices $W_{in,feature}$ and $W_{vote,motor}$ corresponding to the fan-in and fan-out of figure 13.4, respectively. Only those columns that participate in the current computation adjust their weights. In the experimental setup, positive reinforcement is given when the monkey exhibits a correct response, but not otherwise. Similarly, in the model, a scalar quantity called *reinforcement* is set by the teacher to +1 if the selected motor program is correct, and to -1 otherwise.

However, a special case occurs when the system is unable to make a decision within the allotted time (causing the "No-Go" response to be selected). Two possible situations have occurred: no motor program selection units are active, or more than one are active. In the first case, the reinforcement term is set to +1 by the system itself, regardless of the teacher feedback. Therefore, the currently active columns are rewarded, ensuring that the next time the pattern is presented, these columns will yield a greater response. Thus, they will have a greater chance of activating one of the motor program selection units. Without this additional term, negative reinforcement from the teacher is disastrous. The negative reinforcement further decreases the response of the already poorly responding columns, further decreasing their response. The result is a self-reinforcing situation that can never discover the correct response.

In the second situation, where more than one motor program selection unit becomes active at one time, the reinforcement term is set by the system to -1. This decreases the response of all columns involved, adjusting the input to the two (or more) motor program selection units until one is able to achieve threshold significantly before the other(s). It is at this point that the symmetry between the two is broken.

When positive reinforcement is given, the weights leading into the feature detector units are adjusted such that the feature detector better recognizes the current sensory input. In the case of negative reinforcement, the weights are adjusted in the opposite direction, such that the current input is recognized by the feature detector unit to an even lesser degree. Note that this reinforcement depends on whether or not the overall system response was correct, not on the output of any individual motor selection column. We thus have:

$$lgain = \begin{cases} negative\_factor\_f & if\, reinforcement < 0 \\ 1 & otherwise \end{cases}$$

$$\Delta W_{in,feature} = reinforcement * lgain * lrate_f * \left(\left(Input \cdot Voting^T\right) \wedge W\_in\_feature\_mask\right) \quad (13.5)$$

where:

- $lrate_f$ is the learning rate coefficient for the stimulus-to-feature mapping
- $Input \cdot Voting^T$ is the outer product of the Input and Movement vectors.
- $lgain$ scales the effect of negative reinforcement relative to positive reinforcement.
- $\wedge$ is a point/wise multiplication operator.
- $W\_in\_feature\_mask$ is a binary matrix indicating the existence of a synapse.

In this case, the effect of negative reinforcement on the weights is intended to be less than that of positive reinforcement. This is done because negative reinforcement can be very devastating to columns that are just beginning to learn an appropriate mapping.

To simultaneously weaken those weights that are not strengthened by reinforcement, we then set:

$$W_{in,feature} = Normalize\left(W_{in,feature} + \Delta W_{in,feature}\right) \quad (13.6)$$

where:

- $Normalize()$ is a function that L1-normalizes the vector of weights leading into each feature detector unit to length 1, given by

$$Y_i = \frac{X_i}{\sum_j |X_j|} \quad (13.7)$$

- $W\_in\_feature\_mask$ is a matrix of ones and zeros that determines the existence of a weight between the corresponding voting and motor program selection units. The elements of this matrix are point-wise multiplied with those of $\Delta W_{in,feature}$ to mask out weight deltas for weights that do not exist.

Equation (13.2) produces a competition between the weights associated with a particular unit. Thus, the weights are self-regulating, forcing unneeded or undesirable weights to a value near zero. If a column continues to receive negative reinforcement (as a result of being involved in an incorrect response), then it becomes insensitive to the current stimulus, and is reallocated to recognize other stimuli.

The voting unit to motor selection mapping is adjusted similarly. Positive reinforcement increases the weight of the synapse to the correct motor program. When negative reinforcement is given, the synapse is weakened, allowing the other synapses from the voting unit to strengthen slightly through normalization. Thus, more voting power is allocated to the other alternatives:

$$\Delta W_{vote,motor} = reinforcement * lrate_v * \left(\left(Voting \cdot Motor^T\right) \wedge W\_vote\_motor\_mask\right) \quad (13.8)$$

$$W_{vote,motor} = Normalize\left(W_{vote,motor} + \Delta W_{vote,motor}\right) \quad (13.9)$$

where:

- $lrate_v$ is the learning rate coefficient for the voting-to-motor response mapping.

- $W\_vote\_motor\_mask$ is a weight matrix mask similar to the mask that appears in (13.2).

A similar type of reinforcement learning is utilized in Barto et al. (1983, see later discussion).

$W_{in,feature}$ and $W_{vote,motor}$ are initially selected at random. When a response is generated, learning is applied to each of the columns that are currently participating in the computation. The learning objective of an individual column is to recognize particular patterns (or subpatterns) and to identify which of the possible motor programs deserve its votes given its view of the sensory input. Equation (13.1) attempts to create feature detectors that are specific to the incoming patterns. As these feature detectors begin to better recognize the correct patterns, the activity of the signal units will grow, thus giving the column a larger voting power. The feature detecting algorithm is related to the competitive learning of von der Malsburg (1973) and Grossberg (1976) (discussed further in Rumelhart and Zipser 1986). Individual columns learn to become feature detectors for specific subpatterns of the visual stimulus. However, a column does not recognize a pattern to the exclusion of other patterns. Instead, several columns participate in the recognition at once. In addition, a column is responsible for directly generating an appropriate motor output. Therefore, the update of the feature detector weights not only depends upon recognition of the pattern (as in competitive learning), but also upon whether or not the network generates the correct motor output. In the case of a correct response, the feature detector weights become better tuned towards the incoming stimulus, as in the von der Malsburg formulation. For an incorrect response, the weights are adjusted in the opposite direction, such that recognition is lessened for the current input.

Note that in this scheme, all of the columns that participate in the voting are punished or rewarded as a whole, depending upon the strength of their activity. Thus, a column that votes for an incorrect choice may still be rewarded as long as the entire set of votes chose the correct motor program. This method works, in general, because this "incorrect column" will always be active in conjunction with several other columns that do vote appropriately and are always able to overrule its vote. This scheme is similar to that used by Barto et al. (1983) in that one or more elements may correct for errors made by another element. In their case, however, the correction is made sequentially through time, rather than in parallel.

It should be noted that there is a tradeoff in this algorithm between the speed of learning and the sensitivity to noise. Because this protocol always gives the correct feedback and the possible motor outputs are finite and discrete, this tradeoff is not quite as evident. Imagine the case where learning is very fast and the reinforcement function occasionally makes a mistake (as can easily be imagined in real-world situations). If the system has discovered the correct response, but is then given no positive reinforcement for the correct response, extremely rapid learning would cause this response to lose favor completely. Likewise, if an incorrect behavioral response is positively rewarded, a high learning rate would cause the incorrect response to rise quickly above the alternatives.

13.3 Model Implementation

The model is implemented by three top level models, **CondLearn** module, **TrainFile** module and **CondLearnModel** as shown in figure 13.6.

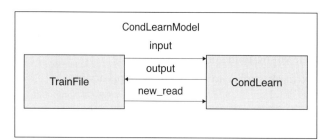

Figure 13.6
Conditional Learning model modules. CondLearn module where dynamics are described, TrainFile module where training data are read, and CondLearnModel which instantiates and connects the modules.

Model

The complete model is described in **CondLearnModel**. It is responsible for instantiating two modules, the **CondLearn** and **TrainFile** modules.

```
nslModel CondLearnModel ()
{
    private TrainFile tf();
    private CondLearn cl();
}
```

The **initModule** methods perform model initialization by reading training data and instantiating the number of layer elements dynamically specified.

```
public void initModule()
{
tf.readFile();
    NslInt0 inSize = tf.getValue("inSize");
    cl.memAlloc(inSize.getValue(),
    num_columns.getValue(),num_choices.getValue());
}
```

Note in this instantiation how we obtain the number of patterns from the **TrainFile** module as it reads this value from the training data file, and only then do we pass it to the **CondLearn** module to be used to instantiate data arrays. While the number of columns and number of choices are directly specified by the user, the input size is read from the training file. These sizes are then used to call all **memAlloc** methods in the model.

Train Module

The **TrainFile** module contains input and output ports for interconnections with the **CondLearn** module. It stores training data in memory similar to the **BackProp Train** module.

```
nslModule TrainFile()
{
public NslDinInt0 new_read();
    public NslDoutInt1 input();
    public NslDoutInt0 output();

    private NslFloat2 pInput();
    private NslFloat1 pOutput();
}
```

The **readFile** method reads the training data while the **intTrain** picks a new random pattern during each new epoch

```
public void initTrain()
{
    int pat = nslIntRand(numPats);
    input = pInput[pat];
    output = pOutput[pat];
}
```

CondLearn Module

The **CondLearn** module contains a number of submodules, **Feature**, **Vote**, **Motor**, **Threshold** and **WTA** (winner take all) modules, as shown in figure 13.7.

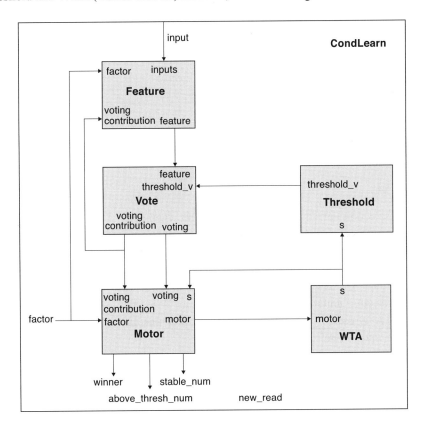

Figure 13.7
CondLearn module

The neural computational model for these modules are implemented using the leaky-integrator model (e.g., Arbib 1989), in which each neuron is represented by a membrane potential and a firing frequency. In the following set of equations, neural states are represented as vectors. Two vectors are connected through a set of weights through either a one-to-one connection scheme, or a fully-connected scheme (all neurons of the input layer are connected to each of the neurons of the output layer). The first case is represented by a vector addition, while the second case is represented by multiplying the vector *I* with a "mask" of synaptic weights *W* to yield *W@I*. The network is initialized by randomizing the input-to-feature and voting-to-motor projections and prepares the model to begin execution.

```
nslModule CondLearn()
{
    private Feature feature();
    private Threshold threshold();
    private Vote vote();
    private Motor motor();
    private WTA wta();
    public NslDinInt1 input();
    public NslDinInt0 output();
    public NslDoutInt0 new_read();
    public NslDoutInt0 factor();
    public NslDinInt0 above_thresh_num();
    public NslDinInt0 stable_num();
    public NslDinInt0 winner();
}
```

The **simTrain** method detects four termination conditions, computes the appropriate reinforcement, updates the weight matrices and prepares the network for the next trial.

```
public void simTrain()
{
    if(above_thresh_num.getData() == 1 && (stable_num.getData()
        == _num_choices || first_pole_mode.getData() != 0.0))
    {
    timer_flag = 1;
        punish_reward_func(winner.getData());
        system.breakCycles();
    }
}
```

The state of the motor program selection units is checked to determine whether or not the system is itself ready to generate an output. The model is ready to output a motor response in one of two cases, depending upon the state of the **first_pole_mode** flag. When this flag is FALSE, this indicates that the standard WTA is being used as the competition mechanism. This mechanism requires that exactly one motor program be selected and that all motor program selection units have reached equilibrium. When the flag is TRUE, first-past-the-pole WTA is used, which relaxes the constraint that the motor program selection units be in an equilibrium state.

```
public void endTrain()  // Timeout: NO-GO case
{
if (timer_flag == 1)
    return;

    if(above_thresh_num.getData() == 0)
        timer_flag = -1;
    else
    timer_flag = 1;

    punish_reward_func(NO_GO_CASE);
}
```

The trial is terminated and **timer_flag** is set to 1. Termination of the current trial may also be forced if the go signal has arrived. As stated earlier, two cases are possible: no motor program selection units active or more than one active. In either case, the trial is terminated and the weight matrices are updated. The reinforcement is set to 1 if the **timer_flag** = -1, meaning no winner has been found yet. Reward and punishment are the reinforcement signals used to update the weight matrices if there is at least one winner. Weights are modified in the **feature** and **vote** modules, respectively.

The **punish_reward_func()** routine selects a new input pattern to present to the system in preparation for the next trial.

```
public void punish_reward_func(int win)
 {
factor = 1;

if(output.getData() == win)
        new_read = 1;
    else
    {
        new_read = 0;
        if (timer_flag != -1)
            factor = -1;
    }
}
```

Feature Module

The **Feature** module computes the membrane potential **feature_mem**, the firing rate **feature** of the feature detector units and the feature detector weights, most important ones are **w_in_feature**, **w_in_feature_mask**, and **dw_in_feature**. It receives input **pInput** and the **voting_contribution** for learning, while its output is **feature**

```
nslModule Feature ()
{
    public NslDinFloat1 inputs();
    public NslDinFloat1 voting_contribution();
    public NslDinFloat0 threshold_v();
    public NslDinInt0 factor();

    public NslDoutFloat1 feature();

    private NslFloat1 feature_mem();

    private NslFloat2 w_in_feature();
    private NslFloat2 dw_in_feature();
    private NslFloat2 w_in_feature_mask();
    private NslFloat0 negative_factor_f();
}
```

The **initModule** method initializes the feature detector weights. Initially, the module configures the input-to-feature weight matrix **w_in_feature**.

```
public void initModule()
{
    nslRandom(w_in_feature);
    select_random(w_in_feature_mask,w_in_feature_probability.
        getData());
    w_in_feature = (w_in_feature/2.0 + 0.5 + input_weight_bias)

        ^ W_in_feature_mask;
    normal_col(w_in_feature);
}
```

A random value is selected for each of the individual weights (uniform distribution in the interval [0,1]). Then existing physically connections are found. The call to **select_random()** initializes **w_in_feature_mask** with a set of 0's and 1's (0 = no connection; 1 = connection). The probability that each element is set to 1 is determined by **w_in_feature_probability**. The **w_in_feature_mask** weight mask is applied to **w_in_feature**, after a linear transformation is applied to the weights. After this operation, **w_in_feature** will consist of elements that are either 0 (when no connection exists), or selected from the distribution [0.5+**input_weight_bias**, 1.0+**input_weight_bias**]. The linear transform of the weight elements guarantees that those that exist take on significant initial values. The random trimming out of connections from the weight matrix is important for giving us a wide diversity of feature detectors to begin with. This will play an important role both in the initial behavior of the network, as well as in limiting the interference during learning.

A normalization is applied to **w_in_feature** weight matrix. The call to **normal_col()** L1-normalizes the columns of **w_in_Feature**. This ensures that the total output weight from any single input unit is 1 (presynaptic normalization). As these weights change during learning, this condition will continue to hold, thus implementing a form of competition between the connections leading from the input unit.

The **simTrain** method processes the dynamics of the feature detector,

```
public void simTrain()
{
    nslDiff(feature_mem, u_feature, -feature_mem - threshold_f
        + w_in_feature * inputs);

    if (LIMITED_ACTIVITY_FLAG == true)
        feature = nslSat(feature_mem, 0, 1, 0, 1);
    else
        feature = nslRamp(feature_mem);
}
```

where **feature_mem** depends upon the **threshold_f**, and the matrix product of weight matrix **w_in_feature** by column vector **pInput**, this returns a vector containing the net input to the feature detector units.

The firing rate of the feature detector unit is limited to the range [0..1].

The **endTrain()** routine is responsible for the internal modulation of the reinforcement signal and the update of the weight matrices. As discussed earlier, if the system was unable to make a decision in the allotted time and no motor program selection units were active, then the reinforcement signal is set to 1. This will cause all of the currently active feature detector units to become a little more active the next time the same input is presented, improving the chances that a motor program selection unit will be activated. Note for the other degenerate case, where more than one motor program selection unit is active at the completion of the trial, **factor** has already been set to -1 (passed in to **endTrain()**).

```
public void endTrain()
{
    float f_factor;

    if(factor.getData() < 0.0)
        f_factor = factor.getData() * negative_factor_f.
            getData();
    else
        f_factor = factor.getData();

    dw_in_feature = f_factor * lrate_f *
        vec_mult_vec_trans(voting_contribution,inputs) ^
    w_in_feature_mask);

    w_in_feature = nslRamp(w_in_feature + dw_in_feature);

    normal_col(w_in_feature,L1_norm_mode.getData());
}
```

In the feature detector, the information content of a negative reinforcement is much less than that of positive reinforcement. This is the case because positive reinforcement indicates the exact answer that is expected, whereas negative reinforcement only tells the system that the selected action was not the correct one. Because this is the case, the connection strength adjustment due to negative reinforcement should be smaller than in the positive reinforcement case. This is implemented here by discounting the negative reinforcement signal, and leaving the positive reinforcement signal intact

voting_contribution identifies those columns that are currently participating in the computation and the degree to which they are participating. Only those connections which carry signals into or out of the active columns will change in strength. The update to the input-to-feature mapping is computed in. The call to **vec_mult_vec_trans**() computes the outer product of the two vectors, returning a matrix of elements which indicate coactivity of input unit and column pairs (Hebbian component). **W_in_feature_mask** filters out all elements of the resulting matrix except for those pairs between which a connection exists. **lrate_f** is the learning rate, and **f_factor** modulates the update based upon the incoming reinforcement signal. This update matrix is then combined into the weight matrix (the call to **nslRamp**() ensures that all connection strengths are always positive), and the weights are normalized.

The call to **normal_col**() L1-normalizes the columns of the weight matrix. This continues to maintain the constraint that the total output weight from any single input unit is 1 (presynaptic normalization). In other words, each input unit has a fixed amount of support that it can distribute between the feature detector units. When positive reinforcement is received, more of this support is allocated to the currently active columns at the expense of those columns that are not active. Likewise, when negative reinforcement is received, the support for the active columns is reduced, to the benefit of the remaining columns (driving the search for a more appropriate group of columns).

Noise Module

The **Noise** module computes the next noise signals that are to be injected into the voting units and the motor selection units. What is implemented here are noise processes that change value on occasional time-steps. This slow change of injected noise is important for the behavior of the network. As will be seen in the next two modules, the voting units and the motor selection units are also implemented as leaky-integrator neurons, which implement a low-pass filter on the inputs coming into them. If the injected noise changed drastically on every time-step, this high-frequency noise would for the most part be filtered out. By forcing the noise process to change more slowly, the neurons are given an opportunity to respond in a significant manner.

```
nslModule Noise ()
{
    private Noise noise();
}
```

Noise initialization.

```
public void initExec()
{
    randomize(noise);

    noise = noise_gain * noise;
}
```

In the **noise** vector is initialized.

Noise is modified if necessary in the **simExec** method

```
public void simExec()
{
    if(random_value2() < noise_change_probability.getData())

    {
        randomize(noise);
    noise = noise_gain * noise;
    }
}
```

In the frequency at which a new noise vector (**noise**) is selected is determined by the parameter **noise_change_probability**.

If it is time to update the noise vector, a completely new vector is generated, and then scaled by the **noise_gain** parameter.

Vote Module

The **Vote** module computes the state of the voting units.

```
nslModule Vote ()
{
    private Noise noise();
public NslDinFloat0 threshold_v();
public NslDinFloat1 feature();
public NslDoutFloat1 voting();
public NslDoutFloat1 voting_contribution();

    private NslFloat1 voting_mem();
    private NslFloat0 voting_contribution_mode();
    private NslFloat0 voting_contribution_scale();
    private NslFloat1 voting_participation();
}
```

The **simTrain** method specifies local processing

```
public void simTrain()
{
    noise.simExec();
nslDiff(voting_mem, u_voting, -voting_mem - threshold_v +
    feature + noise.noise);

if (LIMITED_VOTING_ACTIVITY_FLAG == true)
        voting = nslSat(voting_mem, 0, 1, 0, 1);
    else
voting = nslRamp(voting_mem);

    voting_participation = nslStep(voting);

    if (voting_contribution_mode.getData() == LINEAR)
        voting_contribution = voting;
    else if (voting_contribution_mode.getData() == BINARY)
        voting_contribution = voting_participation;
    else if (voting_contribution_mode.getData() ==
        COMPRESSED_LINEAR)
      voting_contribution = nslSat(voting,0.0,
           voting_contribution_scale.getData(),0.0, 1.0);
    else if (voting_contribution_mode.getData() == JUMP_LINEAR)
        voting_contribution = nslSat(
         nslRamp(voting, 0.0,
0.0,voting_contribution_scale.getData()));
    else
        nslPrintln("Unknown voting_contribution_mode:",
        voting_contribution_scale.getData());
}
```

The membrane potential of these units (**voting_mem**) is determined by the firing rate of the corresponding feature detector units, a noise signal, and the signal from the threshold modulator. When a visual stimulus is initially presented, the inhibitory signal from the threshold modulator is at a high level. If the stimulus is relatively unfamiliar, the input from the feature detector unit will typically not be above this threshold. As a result, no decision will be immediately made. However, the threshold modulator will begin to slowly drop this threshold, ultimately forcing several voting units to fire, causing a decision to be made at the motor selection unit level.

The noise process plays an important role in the search for the correct input/output mapping. At this level, the noise causes different columns to participate in the mapping from trial to trial. Over time, this allows the system to consider many combinations of sets of columns until an appropriate set can be found.

The firing rate of the voting units requires a membrane potential above some threshold.

The vector **voting_participation** is used to display to the user which columns are participating within any particular computation.

Threshold Module
The **Threshold** module implements the dynamics of the threshold modulator.

```
nslModule Threshold ()
{
    public NslDinFloat0 s();
    public NslDoutFloat0 threshold_v();
}
```

The **simTrain** method updates the threshold

```
public void simTrain()
{
    if(s <= 0.0)
        nslDiff(threshold_v,u_threshold_v, -threshold_v);
}
```

The threshold level, **threshold**, is initially set at the beginning of the trial to the parameter **init_threshold**. This value then decays exponentially. However, this decay only happens as long as no motor selection units have begun to fire (as measured by the activity level of the inhibitory unit). In order for this event to occur, several voting units must have begun to fire giving the system the ability to make some sort of decision.

Motor Module

The motor selection unit dynamics are described within the **Motor** module.

```
nslModule Motor ()
{
    private Noise noise();
    public NslDinFloat1 voting();
    public NslDinFloat1 voting_contribution();
    public NslDinFloat0 s();
    public NslDinInt0 factor();

    public NslDoutFloat1 motor();

    public NslDoutInt0 above_thresh_num();
    public NslDoutInt0 stable_num();
    public NslDoutInt0 winner();

    private NslFloat1 dmotor_mem();
    private NslFloat1 motor_mem();
    private NslFloat1 motor_inputs();

    private NslFloat2 w_vote_motor();
    private NslFloat2 dw_vote_motor();
    private NslFloat2 w_vote_motor_mask();
    private NslFloat0 voting_weight_bias();
    private NslFloat0 w_vote_motor_probability();
    private NslFloat0 voting_factor();

    private NslFloat0 normalize_input_mode();
    private NslFloat0 stable_detect_threshold();
}
```

The **initModule** method initializes the voting weights

```
public void initModule()
{
   noise.initExec();
   winner = 0;

      randomize(w_vote_motor);
   select_random(w_vote_motor_mask, w_vote_motor_probability.
      getData());
   w_vote_motor = (w_vote_motor/2.0 + 0.5 +
      voting_weight_bias) ^
   w_vote_motor_mask;

   if (normalize_input_mode.elem() == 1.0)
      normal_col(w_vote_motor,L1_norm_mode.getData());
   else
      normal_row(w_vote_motor,L1_norm_mode.getData());
}
```

The vote-to-motor weights **w_vote_motor** are initialized in a similar manner. However, normalization may be done one of two ways, depending upon the flag **normalize_input_mode**. Presynaptic normalization (**normalize_input_mode** = 1) is as above, maintaining the condition that the weights leading from the voting unit sum to 1. For postsynaptic normalization (**normalize_input_mode** = 0), the sum of the weights leading to the motor selection units would sum to 1. For the simulations results reported in this chapter, **normalize_input_mode** = 1 (presynaptic normalization).

The motor selection unit dynamics are determined within the **simTrain** method.

```
public void simTrain()
{
   noise.simExec();
   motor_inputs = mat_mult_col_vec(w_vote_motor,
      voting)/_num_columns;
   dmotor_mem = -motor_mem - threshold_m +
      voting_factor * motor_inputs - s + motor + noise.noise;
   nslDiff(motor_mem, u_motor,dmotor_mem);
   motor = nslStep(motor_mem);

   above_thresh_num = 0;
   stable_num = 0;

   for (int i = 0; i < _num_choices; ++i)
   {
      if (motor(i) > 0.0)      // Above threshold
      {
         above_thresh_num = above_thresh_num + 1;
         winner = i;
      }
      if(fabs(dmotor_mem[i]) <
         stable_detect_threshold.getData())
         stable_num = stable_num + 1;
   }
}
```

The membrane potential of these units is a function of the votes from the feature detector units (**motor_inputs**), the inhibitory signal from the WTA (Winner-Take-All) inhibitory unit **s**, and an injected noise signal (**motor_noise**). The inhibitory unit ensures that when the system has reached an equilibrium point, at most one motor program has become selected. This style of distributed Winner-Take-All computation is due to Amari & Arbib (1977).

The noise signal is important at this point for providing a diversity in the search for the correct mapping. In addition, it helps to prevent the system from becoming stuck onto a saddle point, where it cannot decide between one of two equally-active motor selection units.

The motor selection cells fire maximally whenever the membrane potential exceeds the cell's threshold. We consider that a selection has been made only when one motor program selection unit is firing.

The **endTrain()** routine is responsible for the internal modulation of the reinforcement signal and the update of the weight matrices. As discussed earlier, if the system was unable to make a decision in the allotted time and no motor program selection units were active, then the reinforcement signal is set to 1. This will cause all of the currently active feature detector units to become a little more active the next time the same input is presented, improving the chances that a motor program selection unit will be activated. Note for the other degenerate case, where more than one motor program selection unit is active at the completion of the trial, **factor** has already been set to -1 (passed in to **endTrain()**).

```
public void endTrain()
{
    dw_vote_motor = factor * lrate_v *
    (vec_mult_vec_trans(motor, voting_contribution) ^
        w_vote_motor_mask);

    w_vote_motor = nslRamp(w_vote_motor + dw_vote_motor);

    if(normalize_input_mode.getData() == 1.0)
        normal_col(w_vote_motor,L1_norm_mode.getData());
    else
        normal_row(w_vote_motor,L1_norm_mode.getData());
}
```

A similar learning rule to that of the input-to-feature mapping is applied to the voting-to-motor mapping. The change in weights is a function of the co-activity of voting columns and the motor program selection units, modulated by the learning rate (**lrate_v**) and the reinforcement signal. These delta values are then added into the weight matrix, and normalized. For this mapping, the type of normalization is selectable as either presynaptic or postsynaptic. For the results reported in this chapter, presynaptic normalization is used, implementing a competition between the different motor program selection units for support from the columns.

WTA Module
The **WTA** module implements the dynamics of the winner-take-all inhibitory unit.

```
nslModule WTA ()
{
    public NslDinFloat1 motor();
    public NslDoutFloat0 s();
    private NslFloat0 s_mem();
}
```

The **simTrain** method executes the wta dynamics

```
public void simTrain()
{
    nslDiff(s_mem, u_s, - s_mem - threshold_s + nslSum(motor));
    s = nslRamp(s_mem);
}
```

The membrane potential of this unit is driven to a level that is essentially proportional to the number of motor selection units that have become active (these units either have an activity level of 0 or 1). The firing rate of this unit also reflects the number of currently active motor selection units.

13.4 Simulation and Results[3]

Simulation

Parameters

The set of parameters used to produce the results presented in this paper are described next. Table 13.1 to 13.9 show the complete list of parameters and the values used in the simulation.

Network Parameters	Value	Description
num_columns	30	Number of columns in the middle layer.
num_inputs	14	Number of inputs into the columns.
num_choices	4	Number of motor program selection units (no-go, left, right, down)

Table 13.1

Network Parameters

Simulation Parameters	Value	Description
delta	0.01	Integration step

Table 13.2

Simulation Parameters

Weight Initialization	Value	Description
voting_weight_bias	4.0	
w_vote_motor_probability	1.0	
normalize_input_mode	1	Determines whether postsynaptic or presynaptic normalization is used for this set of weights (0 = postsynaptic; 1 = presynaptic).
input_weight_bias	1.0	Constant added to random weight value (see weight initialization)
w_in_feature_probability	0.3	Probability that a particular weight will exist.

Table 13.3

Weight Initialization
Parameters

Feature detector parameters	Value	Description
threshold_f	0.1	Threshold
u_feature	0.05	Time constant

Table 13.4
Feature Detector Parameters

Threshold Modulator	Value	Description
init_threshold_v	0.2	Initial threshold (threshold is determined by the threshold modulator).
u_threshold_v	4.0	Time constant of threshold modulator for voting units.

Table 13.5
Threshold Modulator
Parameters

Voting Unit	Value	Description
u_voting	0.05	Time constant
gain	0.045	Injected noise to voting units.
change_probability	0.01	Determines how often the injected noise term changes value.

Table 13.6
Voting Unit Parameters

Motor Program Selecion Unit	Value	Description
u_motor	2.0	Time constant
gain	0.05	Injected noise to motor units
change_probability	0.01	Determines how often the injected noise term changes value.
threshold_m	0.035	Motor program unit threshold.

Table 13.7
Motor Program Selection
Unit Parameters

Analysis Parameters	Value	Description
α	0.8	Used to compute average performance.

Table 13.8
Analysis Parameters

Simulation Parameters	Value	Description
display_participation_mode	0	1 indicates that the participation vector is printed to the screen at the end of each trial.
collect_mode	0	If 1, collecting statistics.
	1	If no MPSUs are active at time of punishment, then reward to get voting activity up.

Table 13.9
Simulation Parameters

A number of parameters play a crucial role in the behavior of the network. These are further discussed here:

w_in_feature_probability determines how likely that a connection exists between an input unit and a feature unit. For this work, it was important to keep this parameter at a low value (0.3). This serves to minimize the number of columns that will respond at all to an input stimulus, thus minimizing the interference between columns. If set too low, not enough columns will react to a particular input.

input_weight_bias determines the distribution of weight values for those weights that do exist. A high value forces the existing weights synapsing on a particular feature to be very similar. On the other hand, a low value causes the weights to be more randomly distributed. In the case of our simulation, this value is set to 1.0 (a low value), yielding a reasonable distribution that allows different columns to respond differently to an individual stimulus. Thus, the weight initialization procedure biases the symmetry breaking between stimuli that goes on during the learning process.

noise_gain determines the magnitude of noise injected into the voting units. It is important that this value is significantly less than **init_threshold_v**. Otherwise, the voting unit may fire spontaneously (without feature unit support) before the threshold is lowered.

noise_change_probability is set such that the noise value changes slowly relative to the time constant of the voting unit (**u_voting**). When the noise changes at this time scale, on average, the effects of the noise are allowed to propagate through the system before the noise value changes again. Thus, in the early stages of learning, different groups of voting units may fire given the same input stimulus, allowing the system to experiment with what the appropriate set of voting units might be. If the noise changes too quickly, then the average effect will be very little noise injected into the system. Therefore, all eligible columns will fire together, and not in different subsets.

WTA (Inhibitory Unit)	Value	Description
u_s	0.5	Time constant of membrane potential.
threshold_s	0.1	Unit threshold.

Table 13.10
WTA parameters.

Learning Parameters	Value	Description
lrate_v	0.035	Voting/motor program selection unit lrate
lrate_f	0.4	Input/feature detector unit lrate
negative_factor_f	0.25	Input/feature factor for negative reinforcement
L1_norm_mode	1	1 indicates L1-normalization is used (0 indicates L2-normalization).

Table 13.11
Learning parameters.

Protocol Parameters	Value	Description
first_pole_mode	1	1 indicates first-passed-the-pole mode is turned on.
repeat_mode	1	1 indicates stimuli are repeated when an incorrect response is generated by the system.
max_time_counter	200	Maximum number of time steps alotted to the system for making a decision.

Table 13.12
Protocol parameters.

The constraints on **motor.noise_gain** and **threshold_m** are similar.

lrate_f determines how much effect that one trial will have on the weight matrix that maps from the input units to the feature units (the value used in these simulations was 0.4). When set too low, the slope of the overall activity curve begins to decrease and the system will take longer before it achieves perfect performance. On the other hand, setting this parameter too high will amplify the interference between the various weights (this is critical during the early stages of learning). Thus, the learning of one pattern may erase (in one trial) the information associated with another pattern.

lrate_v is the learning constant for the vote-to-motor weight matrix (the value used was 0.035). Setting this constant too high will cause the system to very quickly commit columns to particular motor responses. The result is that the network is able to learn the mapping much quicker than in the cases discussed in this paper. Although it appears to be advantageous to use a higher parameter value, we would move away from the behavioral results seen in the Mitz experiments. In addition, the network may become more sensitive to interference, a problem that will show itself as the task difficulty is increased.

negative_factor_f scales the effect of negative reinforcement on the network. When this value approaches 1, the effect of a negative signal can be devastating to the network (see discussion of learning dynamics). In general, we found that too high of a value will decrease the slope of the overall activity curve (evident when the network begins to produce the correct answer, but then tries other responses).

Training Patterns

The patterns shown in table 13.13 were used to train the network for most of the above experiments. The right-hand column denotes the expected motor response. For this case, the input patterns are orthogonal. Other training sets that were used for the comparison with backpropagation included overlapping patterns. One such training set is shown in table 13.14.

Training Pattern	Expected Response
1 1 1 0 0 0 0 0 0 0 0 0 0 0	No-Go
0 0 0 0 0 0 0 0 0 1 1 1 0	Left
0 0 0 0 1 1 1 0 0 0 0 0 0	Right
0 0 0 1 0 0 0 1 0 1 0 0 0 0	Down

Table 13.13
Input patterns and expected motor responses.

Training Pattern	Expected Response
1 1 1 0 0 0 0 0 0 0 0 0 0 0	No-Go
1 0 0 0 0 0 1 0 0 1 0 0 0 0	Left
0 0 0 1 0 1 1 0 0 0 0 0 0 0	Right
0 0 0 1 0 0 0 1 0 1 0 0 0 0	Down

Table 13.14
Input patterns and expected motor responses (more difficult case). Each of the patterns overlaps at least one other pattern.

Simulation Results

Once NSL has been compiled for the model, the simulation is started by loading the *startup* script, which loads in the standard set of parameters (CondLearn.nsl) together with graphics (CondGraphics.nsl):

```
nsl% source startup.nsl
```

The system parameters involve 100 epochs of 200 training cycles each:

```
nsl set system.epochSteps 100
nsl set system.trainDelta 1
nsl set system.trainEndTime 200
```

The *seed* is used to configure the random number generator (useful for forcing the same conditions for multiple experiments):

```
nsl set condLearnModel.condLearn.seed 10
```

The *pattern file* contains a list of input patterns and the corresponding desired outputs.

```
nsl set condLearnModel.trainFile.pName a1.dat
```

For example, the "a1.dat" train file looks as follows:

```
4
1
24
1 1 1 0 0 0 0 0 0 0 0 0 0 0 0 0 0 0 0 0 0 0 0 0   0
0 0 0 1 1 1 0 0 0 0 0 0 0 0 0 0 0 0 0 0 0 0 0 0   1
0 0 0 0 0 0 1 1 1 0 0 0 0 0 0 0 0 0 0 0 0 0 0 0   2
0 0 0 0 0 0 0 0 0 1 1 1 0 0 0 0 0 0 0 0 0 0 0 0   3
```

The first line specifies the number of train patterns in the file, "4" in this example. The second line specifies the number of elements in the output pattern, while the third line specifies the number of elements in the input pattern, "1" and "24" respectively. Finally, each additional line specifies the actual train pattern consisting of the input pattern followed by its corresponding desired output.

Once configuration is complete, begin execution as follows:

```
nsl% nsl train
```

In this configuration, at the end of each trial the system reports if it is unable to make a decision by the time the trigger stimulus is received:

```
No-pick no-go!
```

On the following line, the number of time steps (equivalent to train steps) required to obtain a decision is printed (in this case, 200 is the maximum number of time steps).

```
200
```

On the next line, the system prints the current trial (followed by a ":"), presented pattern number ("p"), expected motor output ("s"), selected motor output ("w"), indication of correctness (+/-), and a measure of total activity of the voting units.

```
0 : p0 s0 w0 + 0.022166
```

Next the system prints the participation vector, which indicates those columns that were active at the end of the trial.

```
voting_participation
1 0 0 0 1 0 1 0 0 0 0 0 0 0 0 0 0 1 0 0 0 0 0 1 1 0 0 0 0
```

To perform an entire experiment, the simulation continues executing until the system has learned the mapping completely. A good indication of this is that all mapping have been learned, and all decisions are made in a very short amount of time (for the given parameters, 50 time steps should be sufficient).

```
32
50 : p3 s3 w3 + 0.123120
voting_participation
0 0 0 0 0 1 0 0 1 0 1 0 0 0 0 1 1 0 0 0 0 0 0 1 0 0 0 1 0 0

77
51 : p0 s0 w0 + 0.057379
voting_participation
1 0 0 0 0 0 0 0 0 0 0 0 0 0 0 0 0 0 0 1 0 0 0 0 0 0 1 0 0 0 0

55
52 : p1 s1 w1 + 0.094080
voting_participation
0 0 1 0 1 0 1 0 0 0 0 0 0 0 0 0 0 0 0 0 0 0 1 1 0 0 0 1 0 0 0
.
.
.
68
58 : p2 s2 w2 + 0.069137

nsl set voting_participation
0 0 0 1 1 0 0 0 0 0 0 0 0 0 0 0 0 0 0 0 1 1 0 0 0 1 0 0 0 1 0
```

In figure 13.8 we show a sample graphical display as the system has already learned.

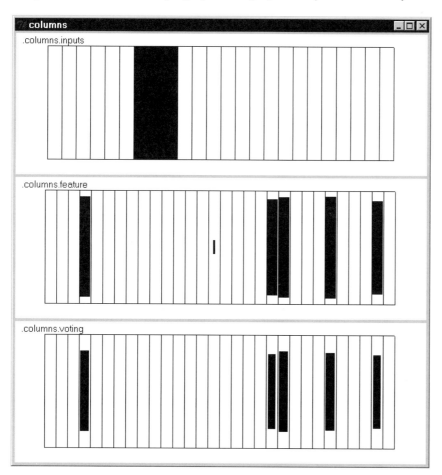

Figure 13.8
The top portion of the display, ".columns.input", represents the train pattern input, in this case corresponding to the third input pattern with corresponding desired output "2". The display in the middle represents the corresponding ".columns.feature" pattern while the bottom display represents the ".columns.voting" pattern. The more correspondence between the two bottom displays the better the learning.

Results

The following experiment utilized a variant of the winner-take-all (WTA) algorithm in the simulation, referred to as first-past-the-pole WTA. Rather than requiring that the network settle down into a stable state, the first unit that achieves a membrane potential above the threshold is declared the winner. In the case that more than one unit activated at the same instant, the standard winner-take-all circuit is used to squelch the activity of all but one. Using this particular algorithm allows for a faster simulation, since more time is required if the units must settle down to equilibrium.

During the testing/learning trials, a pattern is randomly presented to the system. The overall control system waits until a single selection is made (after the TS is presented), before moving on to the next trial. When the network produces an incorrect answer, the same pattern is presented on the next trial (as in the primate experiments). This protocol allows for much quicker learning, as opposed to a completely random sequence of stimulus/response pairs.

Primary Experiments

Next we show the behavioral traces resulting from a single experiment. In two of the three traces, the network produces a correct answer, and then attempts other choices (given the identical pattern). This happens due to the fact that the voting strengths are influenced by the noise process. Even though a correct answer has been given, there is still a probability that another answer will be output at a later time. Eventually, however, the learning biases the correct motor program to a level sufficiently above the noise. After this point, the correct motor program is always chosen. The behavioral responses of one experiment broken into sequences corresponding to a particular stimulus/motor output pair. +'s indicate correct responses, letters indicate an incorrect response of a particular type.

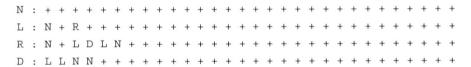

```
N : + + + + + + + + + + + + + + + + + + + + + + + + + + +
L : N + R + + + + + + + + + + + + + + + + + + + + + + + + +
R : N + L D L N + + + + + + + + + + + + + + + + + + + + + +
D : L L N N + + + + + + + + + + + + + + + + + + + + + + + +
```

For the same experiment, the pattern of activity for a particular motor response and the behavioral performance were compared to those of the monkey. The overall activity of the resulting voting unit response is measured by using the final voting unit activity pattern (i.e. after learning) as a reference. The overall activity is defined as the dot product between this reference and the voting unit activity pattern from every trial in the learning sequence. As in the results reported by Mitz et al., the normalized activity and performance curves for a single motor response are plotted together. The performance is computed by low-pass filtering the performance value (where 0 corresponds to an incorrect response and 1 corresponds to a correct response).

Figure 13.9 shows the resulting set of curves for one such experiment. The solid curve corresponds to the activity measure and the dotted line is the behavioral performance of the subject. These values are plotted over the number of trials. In this, as in several other experiments, the performance begins its steady increase 3 to 4 trials before the activity measure becomes significant.

(A)

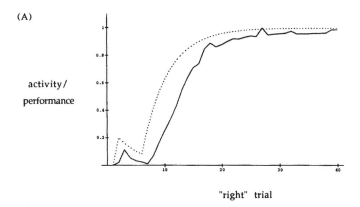

activity/
performance

"right" trial

(B)

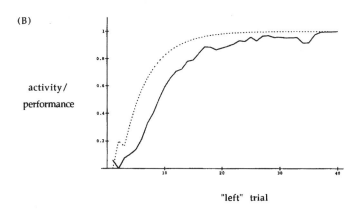

activity/
performance

"left" trial

Figure 13.9
Overall activity (solid) curve and performance (dotted) curve plotted against trial for the (A) "Right" and (B) "Left" responses. As in the experimental curves, the performance curve begins to increase prior to the increase in the activity curve. Note that the trial axis represents only those trials for which the "Right" and "Left" responses are expected, respectively.

When a naive network is first tested, the presentation of a pattern causes some random set of columns to be active, as determined by the initial weight values from the input units to the feature detector units. Based on the strength of the pattern match, the corresponding voting units may not immediately become active, but instead have to wait for the Threshold Modulator to lower the threshold to an appropriate level. Given time, this function forces the system to vote for some response, even though it is not very sure about what the correct response might be.

With respect to identifying the correct response, positive reinforcement gives the system more information than does negative reinforcement. For the case of positive reinforcement, we are telling the system what the correct response is (specific feedback), but negative reinforcement only tells the system that the correct response is one of three choices (nonspecific feedback).

Because the system is essentially guessing on these initial trials, the performance is very poor at first. Therefore, the system is primarily receiving negative reinforcement, keeping the overall response activity at a low level. An occasional correct response, in combination with the negative feedback for other choices, begins to bias the voting unit output towards the correct motor program selection unit. In turn, this effect begins to increase the probability of selecting the correct motor response.

Once the performance of a set of columns begins to increase, the positive feedback becomes significant enough to reward the correctly responding feature detector units on average, thus switching over from nonspecific to specific feedback information (in the weight update equations, the **reinforcement** term becomes +1 for the most cases). In figure 13.10, as in other experiments, the overall activity does not begin to rise significantly until the performance passes the 0.5 mark. This also appears to be the case in most of the graphs provided by Mitz et al. (1991). Once the performance is correct on average, the activity of the feature detector units belonging to the "correct" set of columns increases. This increase comes from the fine-tuning of the feature detector weights towards the incoming pattern.

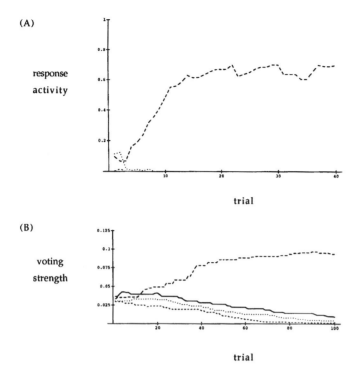

(A)

response activity

trial

(B)

voting strength

trial

Figure 13.10
(A) Activity of a single voting unit plotted against trial number. The four curves represent responses to each of the four input stimuli (solid = no-go, long dash = left, dotted = right, and short dash = down). Note that trial number *N* corresponds to the Nth occurrence of each of the four stimuli, and does not necessarily correspond to the same moment in time. (B) Evolution of the voting strength of the same unit. The four curves (designated as above) represent the voting strength to each of the four motor program selection units. Note that in this graph, the trial axis represents all trials.

As a result, we see an overall increase in activity in response to the learned stimulus, and, most importantly, we see this increase **after** the increase in performance.

In addition to looking at the overall activity of the network, it is also possible to examine an individual column's response to input stimuli as learning progresses. Figure 13.10A shows the response activity of one voting unit from the same experiment. In this particular case, the unit initially responds equally well to two different stimuli. As learning progresses, however, the response to one stimulus grows to a significant level. Ultimately, this unit becomes allocated to the recognition of the stimulus pattern that maps to the Left response.

Figure 13.10B represents the same unit's orientation towards a particular motor program, as measured by the weight from the unit to the motor program selection unit. Initially, the unit supports the four motor program selection units almost equally, but within 12 trials, the weight corresponding to the Leftward motor unit begins increase above the others possibilities. After learning has completed, this weight completely dominates the others.

Changes in Protocol

In initially examining the protocol described by Mitz et al. (1991), we found it interesting that when the monkey responded incorrectly to a particular stimulus, the same stimulus was presented for the next trial. This repetition was continued until the monkey produced the correct response. The question that came immediately to mind was why a totally random presentation sequence was not used. We presented this question to our model through a simple modification of the protocol. The results shown in figure 13.11 represent a typical behavioral trace under this new protocol. In this case, the system requires almost twice as many trials before it begins to perform the task perfectly. This is especially evident in the Rightward response.

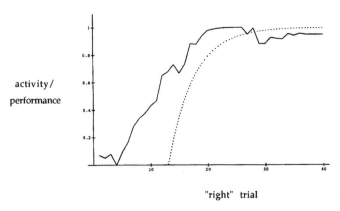

activity/
performance

"right" trial

Figure 13.11
The behavioral responses of one experiment with a completely random sequence of stimulus presentations. Under these conditions, the task requires more trials of learning.

This effect can best be explained by looking at the competition between the different stimuli. The degree of competition is determined by the amount of overlap between the sets of columns that are activated by each of the stimuli. In addition, certain stimuli may activate their set of columns more strongly than other stimuli, due to the initial random selection of weights. This activity difference can give the stronger stimulus a slight advantage in the learning process, since a weight update is related to the degree of activation of the voting unit. Therefore, given that a significant overlap exists between groups of columns, as well as an activity bias towards one or more stimuli, the learning induced by the stronger patterns can often cancel out any learning caused by the weaker stimulus. In the original protocol, this interference is not as much of a problem, since incorrectly mapped stimuli are allocated a larger number of consecutive trials. Within the new protocol, the probability of a favorable set of trials is relatively low.

Figure 13.11 shows the overall activity curve corresponding to the Right response in the above experiment. It is interesting to note that the activity curve increases prior to the performance curve. This can be explained by looking closer at the individual unit participation for the Rightward mapping. In this case, only a single column takes on the task of performing this particular mapping. During the early stages of learning, the network quickly learns the other three mappings. This particular column initially responds to both the Rightward and Downward stimuli (figure 13.12 A). When the Rightward stimulus is presented, the support to the columns is so weak that the system does not make a decision in the allotted time. Therefore, the input/feature weights are adjusted to maintain recognition of the Rightward stimulus. As shown in figure 13.12B, the system finally discovers the correct motor program to output at about trial 95. At this point, though, it still significantly supports the Downward response, but not enough to make incorrect decisions.

(A)

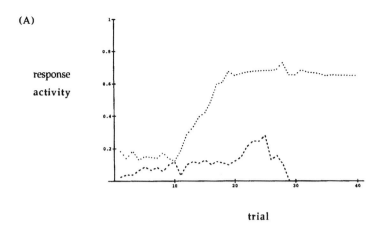

response activity

trial

(B)

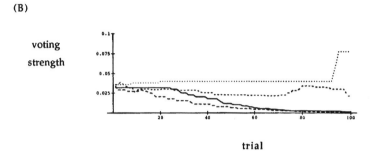

voting strength

trial

Figure 13.12
(A) Activity of the one voting unit that learned to perform the mapping plotted against trial number. Because this is the only unit that learns the mapping, it determines the curve of figure 13.10. (B) Evolution of the voting strength of the same unit. Only towards the end of the experiment (95th trial) does the unit discover the correct motor program selection unit.

Reversal Experiments

Another set of experiments performed on the model asked about the system's behavioral and neural responses after a reversal takes place. In this experiment the network is presented with the standard set of four novel stimuli. After a given number of trials, the teaching system switches the mapping of two responses. In this case, the stimulus that originally mapped to the No-Go motor response, now maps to the Down motor response, and vice versa. In looking at this experiment, we are interested in seeing how quickly the network is able to recover from the change in mapping and in understanding the underlying neural basis for this change. Next we show the behavioral results of one such experiment. After 26 trials, the visual/motor mapping had been learned perfectly for all cases. The first few responses that are generated after the reversal correspond to the original mapping. The system requires only a few trials of negative reinforcement to the Left and Right responses before the original mappings lose their dominance. At this point, the system continues its search as in the other experiments. Behavioral response during a reversal task. The break in the strings indicates the point at which the reversal (between the No-Go and Down responses) takes place.

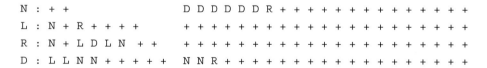

```
N : + +                    D D D D D D R + + + + + + + + + + + + + +
L : N + R + + + +            + + + + + + + + + + + + + + + + + + + + +
R : N + L D L N  + +         + + + + + + + + + + + + + + + + + + + + +
D : L L N N + + + + +      N N R + + + + + + + + + + + + + + + + + + +
```

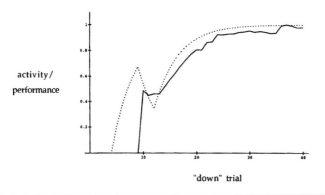

"down" trial

Figure 13.13.

Graph displays activity/performance curve for the reversal case ("Down" motor mapping). The solid (activity) curve corresponds to the overall activity in response to the stimulus that maps to the "Down" motor response, which switches between the 9th and 10th trials. The drastic change in overall activity after the reversal indicates that two separate sets of columns are being used to process the two different stimuli (recall that overall activity is measured by comparing the current activity pattern of the voting units to their activity pattern after learning is complete, in this case, trial 40). This also shows that the column continues responding to the same input before and after the reversal.

The activity/performance curve for the Left response is shown in figure 13.13. Recall that the activity curve is computed by taking the dot product between current activity of the voting unit vector and the same vector of activity after the learning is complete. The sudden jump in the activity curve indicates the point at which the reversal takes place. This jump happens because although the column continues to respond to the same stimulus, the stimulus is now supposed to map to the No-Go response (which has also been plotted). This and figure 13.14 A demonstrate that the column maintains its mapping to the specific stimulus. Figure 13.14 B (the output weights from the same column) demonstrates that it is these weights that are adjusted to deal with the new mapping. Note in this figure, the reversal takes place over just a few trials (both in the reduction of the Downward weight and the increase of the No-Go weight.

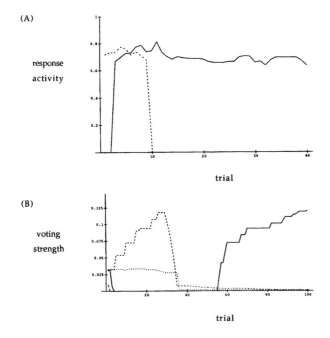

Figure 13.14

(A) A single unit's response to the various input stimuli over time. The solid curve represents the unit's response to the Nth occurrence of the stimulus that maps to the "No-Go" response. Likewise, the dashed curve represents the unit's response to the Nth occurrence of the stimulus that maps to the "Down" response. The drastic increase of the solid curve and decrease of the dashed curve indicate the point of reversal (after the 2nd occurrence of the stimulus that maps to "No-Go", and the 9th occurrence of the stimulus that maps to "Down, respectively). Note that the unit continues to respond to the same stimulus after the reversal, although the stimulus now maps to a different motor program.

13.5 Summary

Our model has primarily addressed the computational issues involved in learning appropriate stimulus/motor program mappings. However, we believe that the functional role of voting units within our network may be related to that of set units within the premotor cortex. The actual visual/motor mapping is considered to be taking place further upstream from premotor cortex (within the $W_{in,feature}$ weights in our model). We believe this to be the case, due to the fact the Mitz et al. (1991) observed similar set unit activity patterns in response to *different* visual stimuli that mapped to the same motor response.

The motor programs, themselves, are most likely stored in regions further downstream from premotor cortex, as is the circuitry that chooses a single motor program to execute (motor program selection units and the winner-take-all circuit of our model).

This model was successful in meeting a number of the challenges set forth earlier It produces a behavior similar to that which was seen in the monkey experiments (goals 1a–c), and also produces normalized activity/performance curves that are qualitatively similar to the experimental data. Although neither of these two challenges (goal 2) were explicitly designed into the neural algorithm, the two features resulted from the original formulation of the model. Finally, the model produces neuronal activity phenomena that are representative of those observed by Mitz et al. (Mitz challenges a–c).

The primary computation within the model was performed using distributed coding of the information, thus demonstrating that not all of the relevant information need be present at a single location to perform a complex task. Rather, a distributed set of computers, each acting with a limited set of information, is capable of producing a global decision through a voting mechanism. However, in this model, votes were cast in a more centralized manner than is appropriate for a more faithful model of the brain's circuitry.

The concept of the column served to bind together a minimal set of computational capabilities needed to perform the local computation. This structure was then replicated to solve the more global computation. The claim here is not that a cortical column in the neurophysiological sense consists strictly of feature detector and voting units, but that a local organization is sufficient to perform a significant part of the computation. Allowing all neurons to connect to all other neurons is not practical from a hardware standpoint, and may impede the learning process.

The learning algorithm was a local one. Except for the reinforcement signal, the update of a particular weight only used the information available locally (the activation of the presynaptic and postsynaptic neurons, and the surrounding weights that shared common dendritic tree). This feature adds to the biological plausibility of the process, and may also have important consequences such as easy implementation in VLSI. In addition, the learned function was stored in a local manner (any particular column was active for only a subset of the inputs). This type of representation can limit the amount of interference between different input patterns, and thus the learning may be faster and more effective in achieving its goal.

The model, however, does not attempt to account for the different types of units observed within the premotor cortex (goal 3). In particular, Mitz challenges d and e are not in general satisfied by the model (multiple stimulus patterns that map to the same motor response do not necessarily activate the same set of columns). This is due to the normalization operation that is performed on the input to the feature detector units. Again, in the premotor cortex of monkey, one would expect a set unit to continue participating in the same motor program after a reversal has taken place, rather than responding continually to the same input stimulus. This would be due in part to the fact that the monkey has already created and solidified its motor programs in memory (during the first stage of learning). Because the mapping from visual stimulus to motor program is transient, the synaptic changes are more likely taking place in regions upstream from premotor cortex.

Finally, the behavior of the model under different experimental conditions may yield some predictions as to the monkey's behavior under similar conditions. As discussed earlier, the use of a completely random sequence of stimuli (as opposed to repeating trials in which the incorrect response was given) significantly hindered the system's ability to learn the visual-motor mapping. From this observation, we would like to posit that the monkey would suffer a similar fate given the completely random trial presentation. This is not meant to say that the monkey would necessarily be unable to learn the task, but that the learning would at least be significantly more difficult. The degree to which this is true can ultimately feed back to future work on this model, since it would tell us something about the degree of interference between the different mappings.

Notes

1. This work was supported in part by a fellowship from the Graduate School, the School of Engineering, and the Computer Science Department of the University of Southern California, and in part by a grant from the Human Frontiers Science Program. We thank Steven Wise and Andy Mitz for correspondence that formed the basis for this project, and George Bekey for his help in the shaping of this document. In addition, we would like to thank Rob Redekopp for his aid in performing some of the backpropagation experiments.
2. A. Weitzenfeld developed the NSL3.0 version from the original NSL2.1 model implementation written by A.H. Fagg as well as contributed Section 13.3 to this chapter.
3. The Primate Visual-Motor Conditional Learning Model model was implemented and tested under NSLC.

14 The Modular Design of the Oculomotor System in Monkeys

P. Dominey, M. Arbib, and A. Alexander

14.1 Introduction

In this model we examine the modular design methodology as it applies to the design of both cortical and subcortical regions in the monkey. We will examine the topographic relations between the Posterior Parietal Cortex (PP), the Frontal-Eye Field (FEF), the Basal Ganglia (BG), the Superior Colliculus (SC), and the Mediodorsal thalamus (MD) as they work together to control the oculomotor regions of the brainstem (BS). We will also describe several experiments that can be performed on the model that demonstrate the modulation of eye movement "motor error maps", sustained potentiation (memory), and dynamic remapping of spatial targets within the "motor error maps". Although, the experiments were originally documented in Cerebral Cortex in 1992 (Dominey and Arbib), we have modified the model to make it easier to understand and to take advantage of the new features in NSL.

This work was initially motivated by data on the double saccade by Mays and Sparks, 1980 and 1983. In their testing, they found that monkeys could perform the double saccade task (as described below), though their accuracy was considerably affected by the delay between the retinal error input and the representation of eye position. Also, single unit recording studies of the Frontal-Eye Field, the Superior Colliculus, and the Lateral Inter Parietal (LIP) during visual and memory guided saccades indicate that cells in these regions code saccades in terms of direction and amplitude rather than head-centric spatial locations (Sparks 1986, Segraves and Goldberg 1987, Anderson et al. 1990, and Barash et al. 1991). We will attempt to duplicate their findings by examining two saccade paradigms in which retinotopic coding alone is inadequate to explain the spatial accuracy of the saccade. The five catagories of saccade experiments that we will be looking at are the simple saccade task, the double saccade task, the memory guided saccade task, the lesioning of FEF or SC, and the compensatory (or stimulated) saccade task.

14.2 Model Description

In the simple saccade task, a monkey is seated in a primate chair with its head fixed and eyes free to move. An illuminated point appears in the center of a grid of lights in front of him. We call this the fixation point. The fixation point disappears and a single light is illuminated. To get his reward, the monkey must saccade to this target. The timing diagram of these sequences and the resultant saccade are shown in figure 14.1.

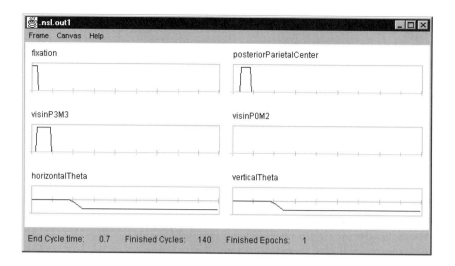

Figure 14.1
Timing Diagram for Simple Saccade Experiment. "visinP3M3" is the stimulus for the first target, "fixation" is the fixation timing, "verticalTheta" is the vertical eye movement response, and "horizontalTheta" is the horizontal eye movement response. Notice that the eyes do not move until the "posteriorParietalCenter" goes low.

After performing several simple saccade experiments, it became clear that the longer the saccade, the more likely the error in acquiring the target became.

In the double saccade task, an illuminated point appears in the center of a grid of lights in front of him (figure 14.2). The illumination point disappears and two different lights are illuminated in rapid succession. To get his reward, the monkey must saccade to the first target and then to the second. The total duration of the two targets presentation is less than the time it takes to saccade to the first target. Because there are two targets, the representation of the second target, visinM3P3, in the motor error map would move as visinM3P3 itself would move across the retina during the saccade to the first target, visinM3P0.

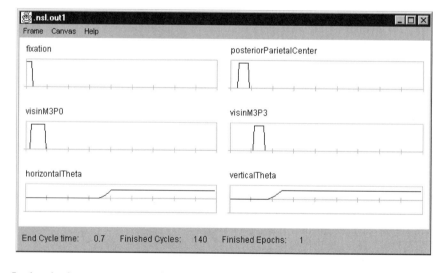

Figure 14.2
Timing Diagram for the Double Saccade Experiment I. "visinM3P0" is the stimulus for the first target and "visinM3P3" is the stimulus for the second target. "fixation" is the fixation timing., "verticalThet" is the vertical eye movement response, and "horizontalTheta" is the horizontal eye movement response.

In the single, memory saccade task, an illuminated fixation point appears, then a target is while the fixation point is still illuminated (figure 14.3.) Once the fixation point is un-illuminated, the monkey is free to move his eye to the target. Thus, he has to remember where this target was to saccade to it.

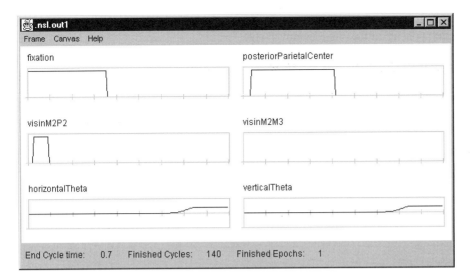

Figure 14.3
Timing Diagram for Single, Memory Saccade Experiment. "visinM2P2" is the stimulus for the first target "fixation" is the fixation timing, "verticalTheta" is the vertical eye movement response, and "horizontalTheta" is the horizontal eye movement response.

In the lesioning experiments we simply disable the output of the FEF (actually the fefsac variable) when we lesion FEF, and when we lesion SC we disable the output of the SC (actually the "supcol" variable). The lesioning experiments we describe here are different than the lesioning experiments we will talk about later where we combine the lesioning with stimulation. In these experiments the Long Lead Burst Neurons (LLBN) are strengthened due to the lesioning; however, it is not the case when we combine lesioning with the stimulation.

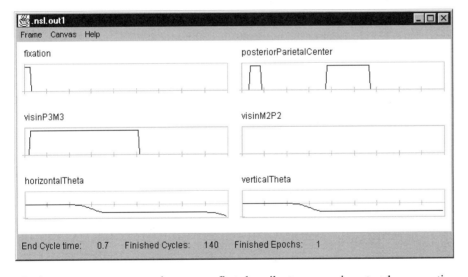

Figure 14.4
Timing Diagram for Lesioning of SC Experiment."sisinP3M3" is the stimulus for the first target , "fixation" is the fixation timing, "verticalTheta" is the vertical eye movement response, and "horizontalTheta" is the horizontal eye movement response.

In the compensatory experiments we first describe two experiments where we stimulate the SC, and then we describe two experiments where we stimulated the FEF. Finally we describe an experiment where we stimulate the SC but lesion the FEF, and then describe an experiment where we stimulate the FEF but lesion the SC. When performing the stimulate and lesion experiment (Schiller and Sandell, 1983; Keating and Gooley, 1988) a visual target is briefly presented and removed before a saccade can begin. Before the visual saccade can begin, an electrical stimulus is applied to either the FEF or SC. The monkey will first saccade to the stimulated location and then to the real target (Dassaonville, Schlag, Schlag-Rey, 1990) even though timewise the real target appeared first. This is due to the fact that the visual signal takes much longer to get from the retina to either the FEF or SC. After performing either of these experiments we will see that when either the FEF or SC is externally stimulated during an ongoing saccade that the brain compensates for different components of the ongoing movement.

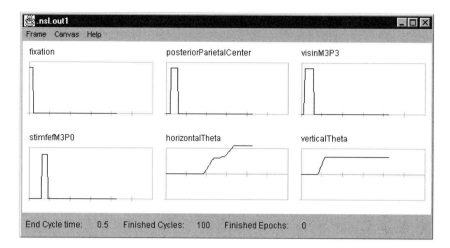

The simple saccade experiment allows us to study the topographic relations between sensory and motor areas, including inhibitory projections that manage motor field activities during the saccade. The double saccade experiment allows us to study the dynamic remapping of the target representation to compensate for intervening movement. The memory saccade experiment allows us to study the cortical and subcortical activity that sustains spatial memory. The lesioning experiments allow us to study the affects of lesioning. And the compensatory experiments allow us to study both the affects of stimulation to the FEF and of stimulation to the SC.

In the model, (figure 14.6) we have tried to localize the mechanisms that allow the monkey to accurately attain its target when an intervening saccade takes the eyes away from the location where the target was illuminated. The problem is that in many oculomotor structures, saccades are coded as a displacement from a given eye position, rather than as a final location. This means that the displacement code is only valid if it is updated almost continuously to account for the intervening changes in eye position, or if the saccade begins from the eye position at which the target was specified. Some experimental results indicate that the updating of the displacement code occurs before the signal reaches the FEF while other experiments indicate that this transformation occurs downstream from the FEF. In our model, we have chosen to represent this remapping in the lateral intra parietal (LIP) (part of the PP) before the signal reaches the FEF. Gnadt and Andersen (1988) found cells in the LIP that appear to code for future eye movement and show quasi-visual (QV) cell behavior. In a double saccade task they found cells that code for the second eye movement, though a visual target never falls in these cells' receptive fields. They proposed that PP might receive corollary feedback activity from saccades, suggesting that PP has access to eye position information that could be used to generate the QV shift. And since PP projects to both FEF and SC, it is likely that the PP is the origin of the QV activity seen in those two areas.

Looking at figure 14.6 we see that the dynamic re-mapping of spatial information contributes to the second saccade via multiple routes:

> LIP/PP to SC to the Brain Stem
> LIP/PP to FEF to the Brain Stem
> LIP/PP to FEF to SC to the Brain Stem

These multiple routes also contribute to the monkey's ability to saccade to the a target even though the SC or the FEF has been lesioned.

14.3 Model Implementation

The eye movement or saccade model as portrayed in figure 14.5 has been a useful system for studying how spatial information is transformed in the brain from a retinotopic coordinate system to the appropriate temporal discharge pattern of the motor plant. In this schematic we see the images transmitted to the Retina, and then to the Visual Cortex. From the Visual Cortex the image is transferred to the Posterior Parietal Cortex (PP) and specifically the Lateral Intra Parietal (LIP) within the PP. The Quasi Visual (QV) cells of the LIP/PP project to the intermediate layers of the SC (Lynch et al. 1985) and to the FEF (Petrides and Pandya 1984). Lesion studies have demonstrated that either the frontal eye field (FEF) or the superior colliculus (SC) is sufficient for commanding the execution of saccades. (Schiller and Sandell 1983; Keating and Gooley 1988). Also in figure 14.5, we see the basic mechanisms for calculating spatial accuracy. Mechanism A performs a dynamic memory remapping that updates motor error via an efferent velocity signal that is approximated by the damped change in eye position (DCEP).

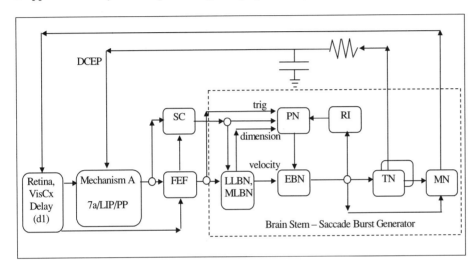

Figure 14.6

Spacial Accuracy within the Saccade Model. DCEP-Damped Change in Eye Position, 7a/LIP-Oculomotor Region of Posterior Parietal Cortex, FEF-Frontal Eye Field,SCd-Deep, Motor Layer in Superior Colliculus, LLBN-Long Lead Burst Neurons, MLBN-Medium Lead Burst Neurons, EBN-Excitatory Burst Neurons,PN-Omni-Pause Neurons, RI-Resettable Integrator, TN-Tonic Neurons, MN-Oculomotor Neurons

Also in figure 14.6 we see the Saccade Burst Generator. The saccade burst generator (SBG) performs the spatiotemporal transformation from the motor error maps of the SC and FEF to generate eye movements as a function of activity in tonic position cells and excitatory burst neurons (Robinson 1970, 1972).

The two neural areas we do not see in the figure 14.6 but which are included in our model in figure 14.7 are the mediodorsal thalamus (THAL) and the basal ganglia (BG). The thalamus with the FEF provides a reciprocal connection that implements the spatial memory loop. The basal ganglia (BG), on the other hand, provides a mechanism for the initiation of cortico-thalamic interactions via the removal of inhibition from the basal ganglia's substantia nigra pars reticulata (Snr) on the mediodorsal thalamus. The BG also plays a role in the disinhibition of SC and THAL for saccades requiring spatial memory (Fuster and Alexander 1973; Hikosaka and Wurtz 1983; Ilinsky et al 1985; Goldman-Rakic 1987).

The computer model emulates the above system as closely as possible. In figure 14.7 below, we see the exact schematic that is used to generate the code for the top level of the model, DomineyTop. DomineyTop contains many of the same components as in figure 14.6 above; however, we have encapsulated the Burst Saccade Generator (BSG) as part of the brainstem into one module. We have also changed the names of the neural areas to conform to the NSLM naming conventions (names begin with lower case letters for instances of objects).

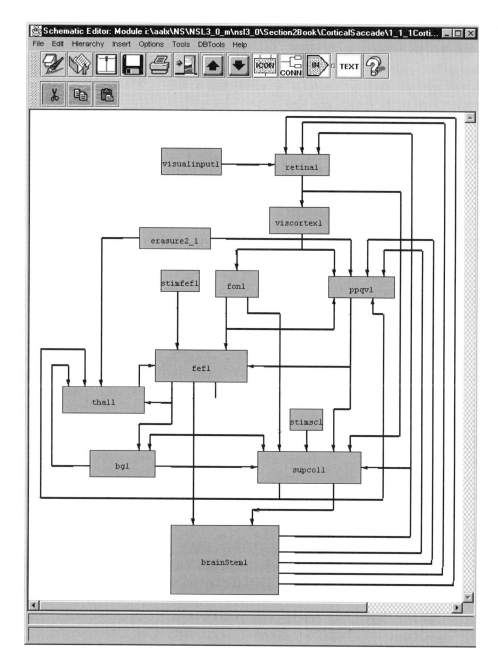

Figure 14.7
DomineyModel or
CorticalSaccade Schematic

In figure 14.7, we see the complete Dominey Model for all of the saccade experiments we will be performing. The external world is represented by a 27 by 27 neural element array, called visualinput. The fixation point and targets are specified on this array via the user interface or by using the default parameters. The visual input is remapped on to the retina, in retinotopic coordinates and then the visual image travels through the Visual Cortex (viscortex) to the Posterior Parietal. At this point, we connect the PP to both the FEF and to the Lateral Inter Parietal within the Posterior Parietal (ppqv1). In PPQV, we have implemented a variation of the Dynamic Memory algorithm by Droulez and Berthoz, 1991, for shifting targets on a motor error map, (what we called Mechanism A in figure 14.6.) This algorithm for the dynamic shifting of targets is called from PPQV but located in a library class we call DomineyLib. By providing special functions in library classes instead of buried in the model, we make it easier for other modelers to reuse these functions. This library is also used in the case of the Superior Colliculus, SC, which uses the "WinnerTakeAll" algrorithm to compute the tonic quasi-visual property seen in the superior colliculus (Mays and Sparks 1980). We call the variable that represents these cells scqv. SC also contains cells that receive direct input from the retinal ganglion cells, and are active in generating reflexive saccades to visual targets. We call these cells scsup. If a fixation target is not present, then these cells will drive SC, generating short latency saccades (Braun and Breitmeyer 1988) via the transcollicular pathway (Sparks 1986). Note that since scsup cells are connected to both the retinal input and the fovea on cells, FOn, these cells will not fire until the FOn turns off. Also SC contains cells that generate presaccadic bursts before voluntary saccades. We call these cells scsac. Experimental data indicates that SC receives an excitatory topographic projection from presaccadic cells in FEF (Segraves and Goldberg 1987). This is accomplished via fefsac in our model.

The FEF module has three classes of saccadic cells. Visual cells (fefvis) respond to all visual stimulus (Bruce and Goldberg 1984). We have grouped these with our Quasi-visual like cells. Coding for the second saccade in the double saccade, these QV cells demonstrate the *right movement field* and the *wrong receptive field* responses, characteristic of QV cells, and are referred to as right-MF/wrong-RF cells (Goldberg and Bruce 1990) or fefvis within our model. Memory cells (fefmem) sustain activity during the delay period in memory experiments (Funahashi et all 1989) while movement cells, fefsac, discharge before all voluntary saccades corresponding to the cell's preferred dimensions (Segraves and Goldberg 1987).

In figure 14.7 , we see the FON module which contains cells distinguished in the FEF that have an on or off response to visual stimulation in the fovea. These foveal cells are not localized to a particular location of the topographic map of FEF, and they project to a wide range of locations within the SC (Seagraves and Goldberg 1987). We model the Foveal On cells, FOn, projecting the center element of the PP layer (the fovea) to a standard size array, that is used to provide inhibition to the elements of the caudate (CD in BG). In each of the following experiments we note that the removal of the illumination of the fixation point signals the monkey that he is free to move his eyes; thus, when FOn is off, the monkey is free to perform the saccades.

Also in figure 14.7 we see several darkened modules. These are the input modules where the user can change the defaults. The visual input module is used for specifying the targets and fixation point. The stimulation modules are used to provide stimulus to the FEF or SC in the compensatory saccade cases. The user is also free to dynamically change these NSL type variables at run-time using the NSLS scripting language. (However, note that variables must be writable to change them from the scripting language. Currently we have declared the variables "visualinput1/visualinput", "stimfef1/stimFEF", "stimsc1/stimSC", "brainstem1/llbn1/llbnPot_k1", "brainstem1-/llbn1/llbnPot_k3", "fef1/fefmemPot_k2", "fef1/fefsac", "supcol1/supcol", "supcol1/supcol_k3", and "ppqv1/qvMask_k1" as writable variables since their values change depending on the protocol used.)

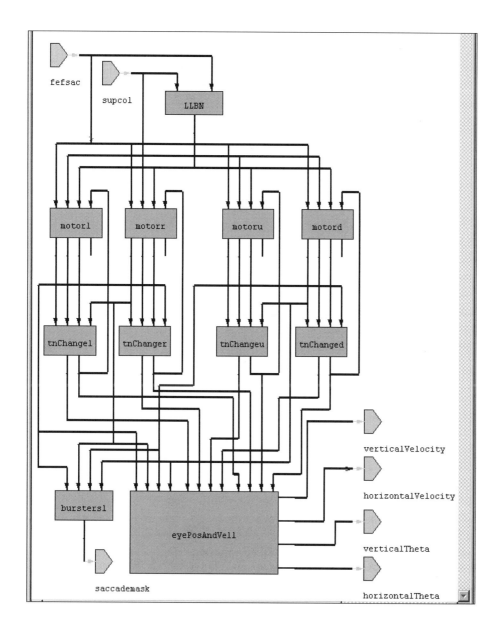

Figure 14.8
Saccade Burst Generator or
BrainStem Schematic

As stated in the earlier, the saccade burst generator (SBG) or the BrainStem Saccade Burst Generator (figure 14.8) performs the spatiotemporal transformations from the motor error maps of the SC and FEF (Robinson 1970, 1972). This SBG is based on one by Scudder (1988). Two of the properties of this model are that it will yield a saccade with the topographically coded metrics in response to either FEF or SC stimulation or both, and it accurately emulates the FEF and SC in that increased firing at a given point will increase the velocity and decrease the latency without changing the metrics of the saccade.

Also in figure 14.8 we see the Tonic Neuron modules. The tonic neurons (TN) provide corollary discharge signals lefttn, righttn, uptn, downtn, which, together with a delayed version of these signals, provide the input used by our model of the PP for the dynamic remapping function which underlies successful completion of the double saccade task (Mechanism A).

The main module in the BrainStem is the Motor Schema shown and described in figure 14.9.

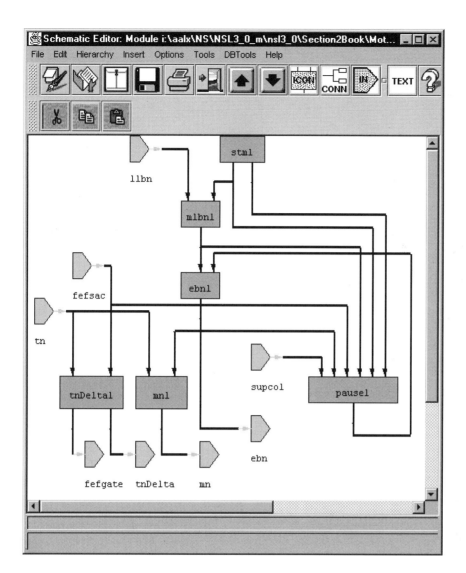

Figure 14.9
The Motor Module's
Schematic

In figure 14.9 we see the Motor Schema. This schematic represents the bulk of the Saccade Burst Generator (SBG). We can compare this to the schematic given by Dominey and Arbib 1992 describing the shared and cooperating spatial accuracy mechanisms. (See figure 14.6.) The Medium Lead Burst Neurons (mlbn) provide input to the Excitatory Burst Neurons (ebn). And the ebn neurons provide inputs to the tonic neurons, the resetable integrator within the Pause module, and the motor neurons, MN. The Pause module contains the resetable integrator, trigger cells, and the Omni-Pause Neurons. The TNDelta module gates the tonic neuron response. The oculer motor neurons (MN) move the eyes, and the STM module calculates spatio temporal transformations.

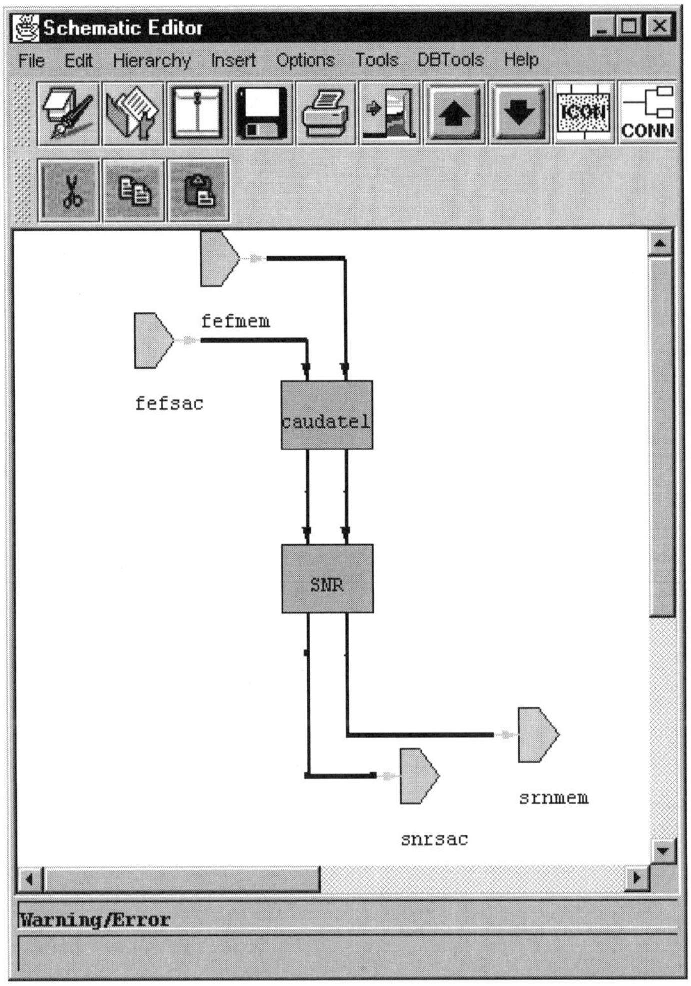

Figure 14.10
Basal Ganglia Schematic

In figure 14.10, we see two inhibitory nuclei of the basal ganglia (BG), caudate (CD) and substantia nigra pars reticulata (SNr). They provide an additional, indirect link between FEF and SC (Chevalier et al 1985). This link allows FEF to selectively modulate the tonic inhibition of the SNr on the SC and the thalamus (Deniau and Chevalier, 1985; Alexander et al. 1986) through the caudate nucleus.

Originally this model was written in NSL2.1 as a series of functions which were executed sequentially. We have re-written the model to make it more object-oriented and modular. The first thing we did was to stop representing neural areas as functions and start representing them as classes. This allowed us the ability to set the initialization parameters in each class/neural area as well as provide other functionality that was local to the neural area.

Next, we instantiated those classes where practical in the model. For instance, in the Saccade Burst Generator (figure 14.5) we instantiate the Motor Schema module four times: once for each direction (left, right, up, down). This of course reduced the amount of code we needed to write for the saccade burst generator in the brain stem: we only had to write MLBN, EBN, Pause, TNDelta, and MN once, instead of four times: one for each direction of right, left, up, and down.

We also made the model hierarchical, grouping together neural areas by schema. Thus the MLBN, EBN, Pause, RI, TN, and MN are all part of Motor which is part of the Brainstem which is part of the top level model. Other schemas include the Memory System, and the Vision System.

Once we had grouped the modules together, and added ports to connect the different modules, it was clear that we had created the same circuit as that documented in Dominey and Arbib (1992) (see figure 14.6). Since the model was now in the Schematic Capture System (SCS), we could automatically generates the structural part of the model code (see figure 14.7).

Another aspect of the new model, is ability to change the dimension of the internal layer sizes (arrays) by changing just one variable. In the original model, we needed to improve the spatial resolution and thus changed the model from using a visual input layer of 27 by 27 neurons to 57 by 57 neurons (Dominey 1991); which meant that the retina and the rest of the neural arrays were 19 by 19. Since there are over 80 of these structures, being able to change 80 structures by changing just one variable is a big improvement over the old model.

Some of the more interesting uses of the NSLM code appeared in the SC and FEF modules. In both modules we have called custom routines from the library we created called "DomineyLib". Code Segment 14.1 shows the code for the SC, and code segment 14.2 shows the code for the FEF.

```
public void simRun() {
    scsupPot=nslDiff(scsupPot,scsupPot_tm, - scsupPot -
        scsupPot_k1*fon + scsupPot_k2*retina);
    ppqv_winner = DomineyLib.winnerTakeAll
        (ppqv,nWTAThreshold.get(),stdsz);
    scqvPot=nslDiff(scqvPot,scqvPot_tm,-scqvPot + ppqv_winner);
    scsacPot=nslDiff(scsacPot,scsacPot_tm, -scsacPot
        +scsacPot_k1*fefsac -
        scsacPot_k2*snrsac);
    supcolPot=nslDiff(supcolPot,supcolPot_tm, -supcolPot +
        supcolPot_k2*scsac +
        supcolPot_k3*scqv -
        supcolPot_k4*fon +
        supcolPot_k6*scsup -
        supcolPot_k1*scDelay); // this is zero.
    supcolPot[center][center] = 0; // no saccades to where we
        already are!
    sc_winner = DomineyLib.winnerTakeAll(supcolPot,
    nWTAThreshold.get(),stdsz);
    scsup = nslSigmoid
        (scsupPot,scsup_x1,scsup_x2,scsup_y1,scsup_y2);
    scqv = (saccademask^scqvPot);
    scsac = nslSigmoid
        (scsacPot,scsac_x1,scsac_x2,scsac_y1,scsac_y2);
    //aa: from the 92 paper equation 15 is set to zero if
        lesioning SC
    if ((protocolNum==6)|| (protocolNum==13)) { // lesion SC
        supcol=0;
    } else {
        supcol = nslSigmoid(sc_winner,supcol_
            x1,supcol_x2,supcol_y1,supcol_y2);
        supcol = supcol + (supcol_k3*stimulation);
    }
    scDelay=nslDiff(scDelay,scDelay_tm, -scDelay + supcol);
}
```

Code Segment 14.1
Code Segment from SC

```
public void simRun() {
    fefvisPot=nslDiff(fefvisPot,fefvisPot_tm,
        (- fefvisPot + ppqv));
    fefmemPot=nslDiff(fefmemPot,fefmemPot_tm,(- fefmemPot +
        fefmemPot_k4*thmem + fefmemPot_k2*fefvis -
            fefmemPot_k1*fon));
    fefsacPot=nslDiff(fefsacPot,fefsacPot_tm,( - fefsacPot +
        fefsacPot_k1*fefvis +fefsacPot_k2*fefmem -
            fefsacPot_k3*fon));
    fefsacPot[center][center] = 0;
    fefvis = nslSigmoid
        (fefvisPot,fefvis_x1,fefvis_x2,fefvis_y1,fefvis_y2);
    fefmem = nslSigmoid
        (fefmemPot,fefmem_x1,fefmem_x2,fefmem_y1,fefmem_y2);
    fefsactmp = nslSigmoid(fefsacPot,
        fefsac_x1,fefsac_x2,fefsac_y1,fefsac_y2);
    fefsac = fefsactmp + (fefsac_k1*stimulation);
    if ((protocolNum==7)||(protocolNum==14)) {//lesion fef
        fefsac=0;
    }
}
```

14.4 Simulation Results[1]

We now report the simulation results. We note that the neural populations we model carry information in terms of their discharge frequencies, the durations of discharge, and the latencies both between stimulus and firing, and between neural events in connected regions. All of the experiments can be found on line at our website, at http://www-hbp.usc.edu/~nsl/unprotected. The World Wide Web applet for this model and these experiments can also be found at the same location, as well as, example experimental results. We will note here that the run delta was set to 0.005, or 5 milli seconds and the run end-time was set to 0.7 seconds for each of the following 15 experiments/protocols.

The Single Location Saccade Experiment

In the single saccade experiment a light illuminates the fixation point which for the monkey is in the center of a screen, but for us is in the center of an array called visualinput. After .02 seconds the light goes away and a target appears someplace on the screen. For the monkey to get his reward he must saccade to the target location.

> **Protocol 1: single saccade**
> Fixation 0-0.02 at [(i=center,j=center)]
> Target A 0.02-0.07 at [(i=center+3,j=(center-3)]

Figure 14.11 displays the system at time equal 0.16 seconds.

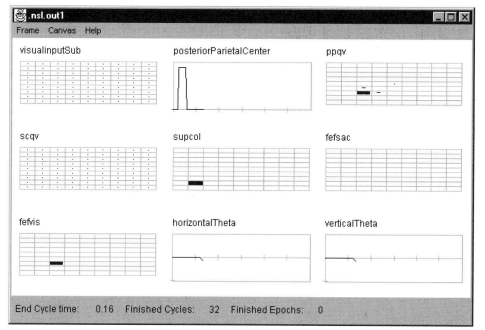

Figure 14.11
Single Saccade Protocol 1 at time t=0.16 seconds.

At 0.16 seconds the saccade is under way and we can see activity in several of the major brain areas. After the fixation has been removed and the target appears, the center of the Posterior Parietal (PP) is off, and the FOn signal is off, which releases the inhibition on the caudate. The caudate after receiving the fovea off signal and the target information from the FEF, then projects an inhibitory signal to the SNR which releases the inhibition on the SC which contains the information of where the target is. Target information contained in SC and FEF output drive the brainstem to reposition the eye such that the target is in the center of the fovea. If the target is still lit, then this causes the center element of the PP to be on. If the target is not still lit, then the center of PP will be off, as in figure 14.12.

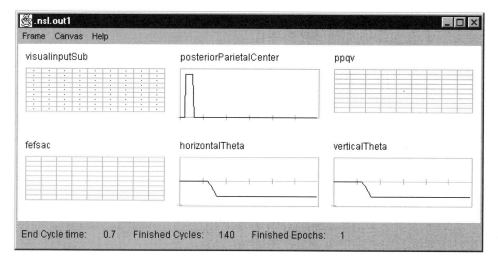

Figure 14.12
The final results of the simple saccade protocol at time=0.7.

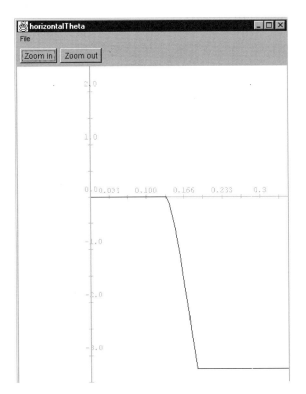

Figure 14.13
The final values for horizontalTheta for the simple saccade protocol at time=0.7.

The Single Location Saccade Experiments Using Memory

The memory saccade experiment requires the thalamus to store spatial locations in memories via a reciprocal excitatory connections with FEF. When the target disappears, it is held in FEF memory (fefmem) by the reciprocal excitatory connection between MD of the thalamus and FEF. The removal of the fixation point causes the FOn signal to be reduced which allows the fefsac to fire and removes a source of inhibition from the SC. The combination of these events allows the stored spatial memory to command a saccade. The effect of the spatial memory is to keep the target position in the FEF active after it is extinguished.

Protocol 2: memorySingleI saccade.

Fixation 0-0.28 at [(i=center),(center)]
Target A & fixation 0.02 - 0.07 at [(i=center-2),(j=center+2)]
Note: Fixation off at off at 0.28

Protocol 3: memorySingleI saccade.

Fixation 0-0.28 at [(i=center),(center)]
Target A & fixation 0.02 - 0.07 at [(i=center-2),(j=center-3)]
Note: Fixation off at off at 0.28

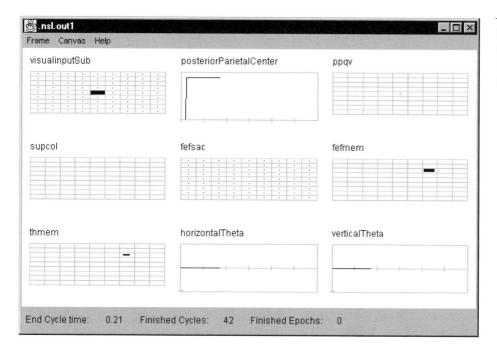

Figure 14.14
Single Memory I Saccade
Protocol 2 at time=0.2
seconds.

In figure 14.14, we see that at time equal 0.21 seconds no saccade has happened yet, but we can see that the location of the saccade is stored in the Thalmus (thmem) and the FEF (fefmem). As long as the fixation point remains on, the Thalamus and FEF will maintain the memory loop.

The Double Location Saccade Experiments

When performing the double saccade task, the motor error representation of the second target is dynamically remapped to com-pensate for the intervening movement. By using the ppqv layer as input to the fefvis layer, the FEF can contribute to the correct specification of both saccades in the double step task.

Protocol 4. doubleI saccade.
Fixation 0-0.02 at [(i=center),(j=center)]
Target A 0.02 - 0.07 at [(i=center-3),j=(center)]
Target B 0.09 - 0.13 at [(i=center-3),j=(center+3)]

Protocol 4. doubleII saccade.
Setup: delta = 0.005 = 5 msec; end-time 0.7 = .7 sec
Fixation 0-0.02 at [(i=center),(j=center)]
Target A 0.02 - 0.07 at [(i=center),j=(center-2)]
Target B 0.085 - 0.125 at [(i=center-3),j=(center)]

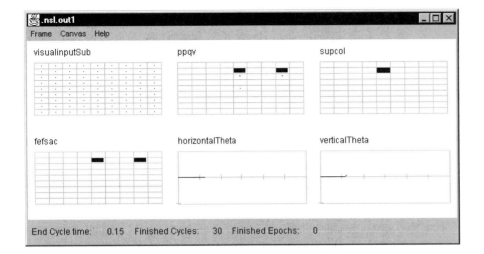

Figure 14.15
Double Saccade Experiment - Protocol 4 at time=.15 seconds.

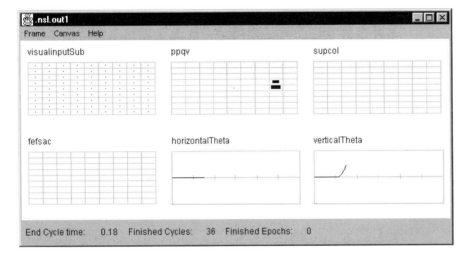

Figure 14.16
Double Saccade Experiment - Protocol 4 at time=.18 seconds

In figure 14.15 we see the activity in the ppqv before the dynamic remapping of the target takes place. The quasi-visual (QV) convolution mask (qvmask) is generated from the temporal offset of the horizontal and vertical eye position. When convolved with ppqv, the qvmask represents interactions thought to implement the quasi-visual shifting seen in the parietal cortex. The initial upward saccade along with the qvmask causes the cells on the upper part of ppqv to be excited, while the cells on the bottom part of ppqv are in inhibited, which causes the second target contained within ppqv to be shifted three cells down (the opposite direction). Or in otherwords, as the first target moves into the fovea or center of ppqv, the distance between the first and second target must be maintained, and thus it looks like the second target is moving away from its original location (see figure 14.16).

The Lesioning of SC or FEF Experiments

In the lesioning experiments either the SC or the FEF is lesioned. The protocol is the same as that for the simple saccade experiment except for the lesion.

> **Protocol 6 - lesionSC saccade.**
> Fixation 0-0.02 at [(i=center,j=center)]
> Target A 0.02-0.4 at [(i=center+3,j=(center-3)]
>
> **Protocol 7 - lesionFEF saccade.**
> Fixation 0-0.02 at [(i=center,j=center)]
> Target A 0.02-0.4 at [(i=center+3,j=(center-3)]

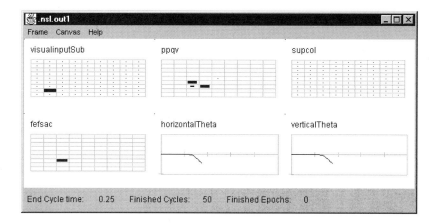

Figure 14.17
Lesion SC experiment -
Protocol 6 at time=0.25
seconds

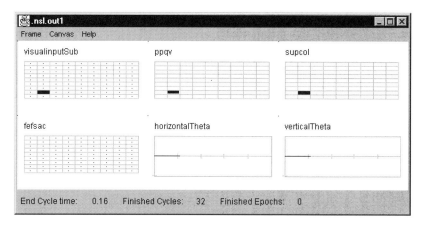

Figure 14.18
Lesion FEF experiment -
Protocol 7 at time=0.16

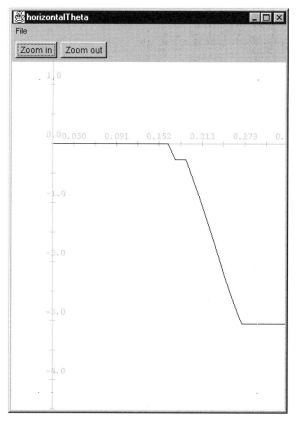

Figure 14.19
Lesion SC experiment -
Protocol 6 at time=0.4
seconds

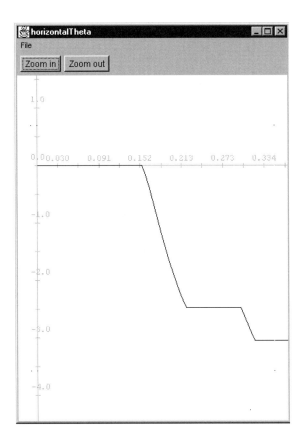

Figure 14.20
Lesion FEF experiment -
Protocol 7 at time=0.4

Note that in figure 14.17 we see that when we lesion the SC, there is no activity in "supcol". In figure 14.18 we see that when we lesion FEF, there is no activity in "fefsac". In figure 14.19 we see that lesioning the SC causes about a 0.34 second delay (.167-.133) and shortens the amplitude by a small amount when compared to the simple saccade of figure 14.12. In figure 14.20 we see that lesioning the FEF causes a 0.19 second delay in the saccade when compared to the simple saccade of figure 14.12. and shortens the amplitude by a small amount but then tries to correct for the mistake. When the amplitude of the saccade is reduced, the eyes do not move as far, and it can take several saccades to acquire the target in the center of the fovea.

The Double Location Memory Saccade Experiments

In the double location memory saccade experiments the quasi-visual field shifting is used to reposition the location of the second target in "ppqv" as the eyes moves to the first location. In addition, when the first target location goes on again, fixation re-occurs and the memory elements within the FEF and Thalamus are activated, causing the location of the second target to be stored until the fixation (or in this case the illumination of the first target) goes off. Thus this experiment combines attributes of the double saccade experiment with the memory saccade experiment. The timing on these types of experiments is very critical. If the second saccade happens too late it will not be shifted in ppqv. If the second saccade happens too early, the location will not get stored in the FEF and Thalamus memory loop.

Protocol 8 - memoryDouble saccade
Fixation 0-0.02 at [(i=center),(j=center)]
Target A 0.02 - 0.05 at [(i=center-3),(j=center)]
Target B 0.095 - 0.11 at [(i=center-3),(j=center+3)]
Target A 0.165 - 0.5 at [(i=center-3),(j=center)]

Protocol 15 - memoryDouble2 saccade

Fixation 0-0.02 at [(i=center),(j=center)]

Target A 0.02 - 0.07 at [(i=center),(j=center-2)]

Target B 0.09 - 0.105 at [(i=center-3),(j=center)]

Target A 0.17 - 0.5 at [(i=center),(j=center-2)]

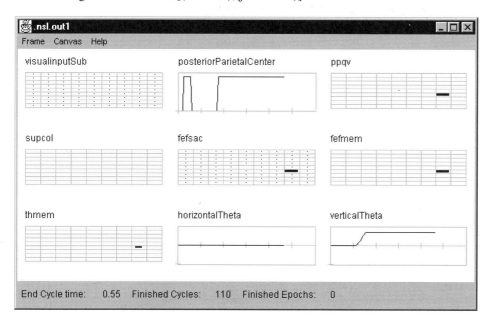

Figure 14.21
The First Memory Double Saccade Experiment - Protocol 8 at time =0.55

Just as in the single memory saccade we can see in figure 14.21 some activity in fefmem and thmem for storing memory. Also, we see that the remapped location of the second target is off by a couple of degrees. This is probably due to the fact that the saccade falls short of the target and thus retains some of the information needed to acquire the first target. However, the second double memory saccade experiment (protocol 15) does not have this problem since it acquires the first target without overshooting. Its first saccade is also a shorter saccade than protocol 8's first saccade.

The Compensatory Saccade Experiments

In the first four compensatory saccade experiments, no lesioning is involved. Only stimulation of the indicated areas.

Protocol 9 - stimulated SC CompensatoryI saccade.

Fixation 0-0.02 at [(i=center,center)]

Target A 0.02 - 0.07 at [(i=center-3),(j=center+3)]

Stimulation 0.07 - .11 at [(i=center-3),(j=center)]

Note: Reduced target error due to location - only going 1 direction

Protocol 10 - stimulated SC CompensatoryII saccade.

Fixation 0-0.02 at [(i=center,center)]

Target A 0.02 - 0.07 at [(i=center-3),(j=center)]

Stimulation 0.07 - 0.11 at [(i=center),(j=center-2)]

Note: Increased target error due to location - must go two directions

Protocol 11 - stimulated FEF CompensatoryI saccade.

Fixation 0-0.02 at [(i=center,center)]

Target A 0.02 - 0.07 at [(i=center-3),(j=center+3)]

Stimulation 0.07 - 0.11 at [(i=center-3),(j=center)]

Protocol 12. stimulated FEF Compensatory II saccade.
Fixation 0-0.02 at [(i=center,center)]
Target A 0.02 - 0.07 at [(i=center-3),(j=center)]
Stimulation 0.07 - 0.11 at [(i=center),(j=center-2)]

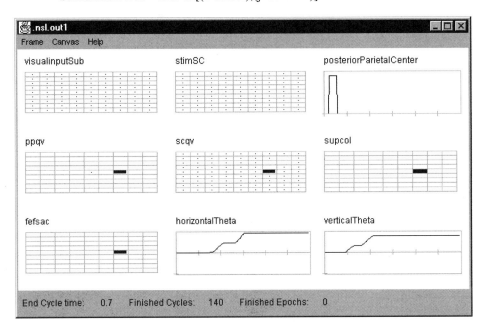

As can be seen in the figure 14.22, the activity within "ppqv" is very similar to that as shown for the double saccade experiment. However, we can also see that the stimulated target is acquired first even though the stimulus was applied after the visual input cue was illuminated. Again this is due to the long path between the retina and the SC.

In the compensatory saccade experiment with lesioning simulated the electrical stimulation of both FEF and SC (figure 14.6), as described in Schiller and Sandell (1983) in which one of the two neural area was lesioned and the other was stimulated. For FEF stimulation we set the k1 parameter to 1.58, and applied electrical stimulation at 175 Hz for 40ms to fefsac. For SC stimulation we set the k1 parameter to 2.9, and applied electrical stimulation at 175 Hz for 40 ms to various locations in SC. The timing and movement data for these trials are summarized below and the results for protocol 14 are shown in figure 14.21.

Protocol 13 - stimulated FEF LesionSC I saccade. - no SC
Setup: delta = 0.005 = 5 msec; end-time 0.7 = .7 sec
Fixation 0-0.02 at [(i=center,center)]
Target A 0.02 - 0.07 at [(i=center-3),(j=center+3)]
Stimulation 0.07 - 0.11 at [(i=center-3),(j=center)]

Protocol 14 - stimulated SC LesionFEF I saccade. no FEF
Setup: delta = 0.005 = 5 msec; end-time 0.7 = .7 sec
Fixation 0-0.02 at [(i=center,center)]
Target A 0.02 - 0.07 at [(i=center-3),(j=center+3)]
Stimulation 0.07 - 0.11 at [(i=center-3),(j=center)]

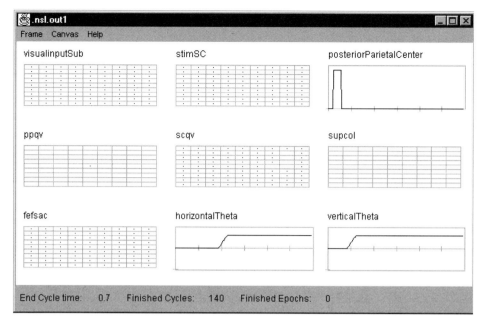

As can be seen in figure 14.23, the stimulation of the SC causes the second target to be acquired first; while the lesioning of FEF causes some delay in making the saccade. However, in this group of experiments we also increase the strength of the projections from either the SC or the FEF (which ever was not lesioned) to the long lead burst neurons. The changes corresponding to the postoperative adaptation of the system reported by Schiller and Sandell (1983).

14.5 Summary

We have discussed the basis of our computer model and how NSL 3.0 has made it easier to represent and understand. In 1992 Dominey compared his simulated results as far as timing and output amplitude with the corresponding literature and found that they compared well. The original model demonstrates that:

1. The inhibitory projection from BG to SC allows selective cortical control of remembered target locations.
2. The topographic position codes in motor error maps of future saccades can be dynamically updated to account for ongoing eye movement (ppqv).
3. Saccades can be driven by memory that is hosted in reciprocal connections between FEF and the Thalamus.
4. Either the projection from SCS to the LLBNs or the projection from FEF to the LLBNs can trigger a saccade but in degraded mode.

This new model demonstrates the same concepts but at the same time does it in a more user friendly fashion. We have demonstrated that with the new NSL 3.0, one can represent neural areas in a more natural fashion, treating neural areas as objects or classes incorporating all of the features of one neural area into one section of the code instead of strewn about the code. We have added the "protocol" interface which allows us to switch from one protocol to another without leaving the simulator or loading a nsl script file. We have also added the ability to see the temporal plots with their X and Y markings within the Zoom Window. We have also added the ability to add new plots dynamically at run time for debugging the model dynamically. Also, not shown here, but another plot feature that can be used is color for encapsulating more information in one plot. Finally, we would like to offer that the ability to see the structure of the model before performing an experimentis a very valuable tool since it allows the experimenter to better understand the model so that he/she does not waste time before performing possibly computer intensive and time consuming experiments with the model.

Notes

1. The Oculomotor model was implemented and tested under NSLJ.

15 Crowley-Arbib Saccade Model

M. Crowley, E. Oztop, and S. Mármol

15.1 Introduction

The visual system provides the primary sensory input to human brains. Nearly every activity we undertake first requires some information to be obtained from the visual system, whether it is identifying a face, or locating an object for manipulation. To obtain this information, the visual system must first move the eyes so that the region of interest falls upon the fovea, the most sensitive part of the eye. Additionally, moving objects must be tracked once they are foveated. These two aspects of "target" acquisition illustrate the two types of movements the oculomotor system are capable of producing. The former is called as saccades, which are quick eye movements to bring an object into the fovea. The latter is referred as smooth pursuit eye movements which are for tracking moving objects.

Crowley-Arbib model is a saccade model with an emphasis on the functional role of the Basal Ganglia (BG) in production of saccadic eye movements. It is based on the hypothesis that the BG has two primary roles the first being the inhibition of a planned voluntary saccade until a GO signal is established by the prefrontal cortex and the second being the provision a remapping signal to parietal and prefrontal cortex, through thalamic projections, that is a learned estimate of the future sensory state based upon the execution of the planned motor command.

The hypothesis that one of the basal ganglia roles is to inhibit a planned motor command prior to its execution was also used by Dominey and Arbib (1992) but is different than the action selection proposed by Dominey, Arbib, and Joseph and by Berns and Sejnowski (1995). However, both ideas require the involvement in the BG in motor preparatory activity. The issue is whether this preparatory activity assists cortical areas in selecting an action, or whether it instead is involved in "freezing" the execution of the motor command until the planning cortical areas, e.g., prefrontal cortex, execute a go signal. We suggest that nearly all motor planning occurs in cortical areas and that these areas use subcortical regions to provide specific information to aid in the motor planning.

15.2 Model Description

This model includes a number of cortical and subcortical areas known to be involved in saccadic eye movements: Lateral Intraparietal Cortex (LIP), Thalamus (Thal), Prefrontal Cortex (PFC), Superior Colliculus (SC), Frontal Eye Field (FEF), Basal Ganglia (BG), Brainstem (BS). For each of these areas we will arrange one or more modules depending on their individual functionality (i.e., for each of the two main roles of the BG described above we are going to create two different modules: Lateral Basal Ganglia (Lat) and Medial Basal Ganglia (Med)). In addition each module could be an assemblage of more submodules, creating with this a hierarchy where the leaves implement the details of the neurons involved. figure 1 shows the top level modules and how they are interconnected, as implemented by means of the Schematic Editor. We will discuss more about each module in the next paragraphs.

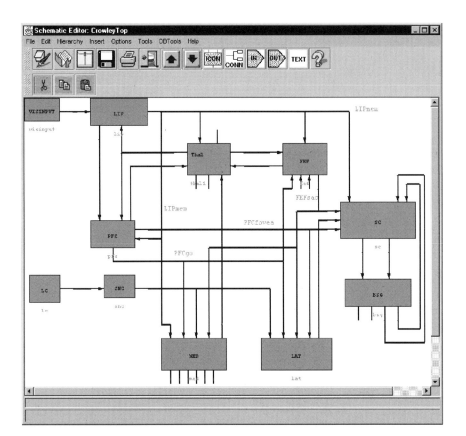

Figure 15.1
Top Level of the Crowley and
Arbib Model

Lateral Intraparietal Cortex (LIP)

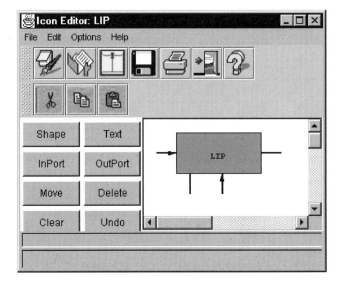

Figure 15.2
Lateral Inter Parietal Cortex I

LIP provides the retinotopic location of saccade targets through excitatory connections form its memory related neurons to SC, FEF and BG. It also exhibits the result of the remapping of saccade targets.

This module is modeled as composed of two types of cells due to the data from Gnadt and Andersen (1988). They found cells in area LIP that responded to a visual cue that did not last through the delay period in a delay saccade task. They also found sustained response cells whose firing was turned off by the eye movement. We will model the first class of neurons as visually responsive neurons (LIPvis) and the second class as memory-responsive neurons (LIPmem).

Visual Response Cells (LIPvis) only respond to visual stimuli. These neurons are modeled as receiving visual input from primary visual centers. In order to obtain saccade latencies that match experimental data we have included a chain of primary visual cortex regions that simply pass the visual signal to the next layer with a slight delay.

Memory Response Cells (LIPmem) fire continuously during the delay portion of a delay saccade task. These cells would fire even if the stimulus never entered their receptive field when second saccade was arranged so that it matched the cell's movement or receptive field. We propose that a memory loop is established between these cells in LIP and mediodorsal thalamus. The connection strength between LIP and thalamus were chosen so that the memory of saccade targets would remain without the target. Also the strength had to be not too strong to disable BG's power to eliminate memory traces.

Thalamus (Thal)

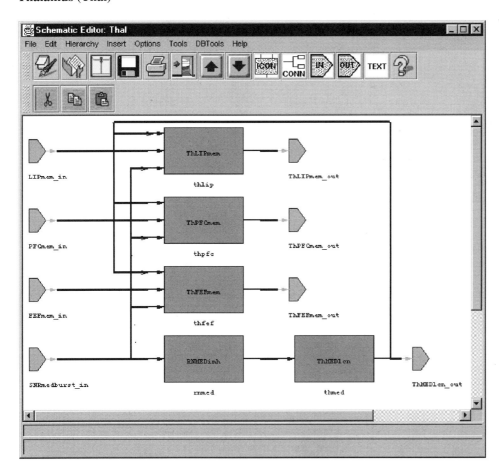

Figure 15.3
Thalamus

The thalamus relays sensory input to the primary sensory areas of the cerebral cortex, as well as information about motor behavior to the motor areas of the cortex. Based on the experimental data discussed below, we will consider only the mediodorsal nucleus and ventral anterior thalamic areas in our model. Additionally, these two areas will be implemented as a single layer within the model as the afferent and efferent connections are very similar between these two areas. In the model three types of cells in the thalamus and reticular nucleus are used as described next.

Thalamic Relay Cells (THrelay) have reciprocal connections with specific cortical areas. These are further divided into different sets for LIP, FEF, and PFC. These reciprocal loops maintain neuronal activity during delay periods of memory tasks essentially forming a memory loop.

Thalamic Local Circuit Cells (THlcn) fire continuously providing inhibition to the relay cells. But they are controlled by the inhibitory actions of the thalamic reticular nucleus (RNinh) neurons. When inhibition upon these LCN neurons drops below a threshold, their increased inhibition puts the thalamic relay neurons into a bursting mode until the corresponding cortical cells begin firing and inhibitory activity of the SNr returns to its normal levels.

Reticular Inhibitory Cells (RNinh) are tonically firing neurons receiving inhibition from SNr. They provide inhibition of the thalamic local circuit neurons.

Prefrontal Cortex (PFC)

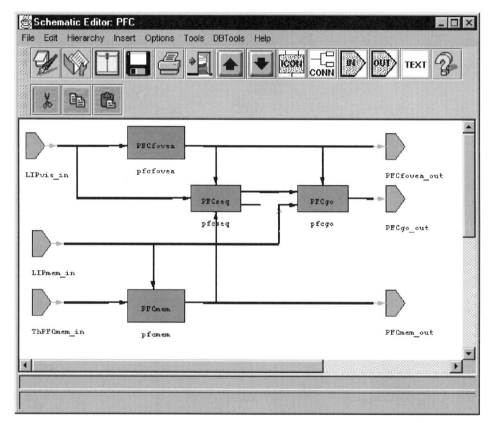

Figure 15.4
Prefrontal Cortex

It has been fairly well agreed that PFC is crucial for the process of working memory (Boussaoud and Wise 1993; Goldman-Rakic 1987; Kojima and Goldman-Rakic 1984; Sawaguchi and Goldman-Rakic 1994; Sawaguchi and Goldman-Rakic 1991). Lesions of this area render monkeys unable to perform spatial memory tasks even when the delay period is only a few seconds. We introduce the following layers in our model.

Visual Memory Cells (PFCmem) simulate the spatial working memory cells found in prefrontal cortex. These cells maintain a memory loop with the thalamus, as well FEF and LIP. We use the go signal (PFCgo) to inhibit the activation letting the remapped target information to be created. This mimics a memory state change from a current state to a future state. The connection strength was chosen to be strong enough to form target memory but not strong enough to disable BG from washing out the memory traces.

Go Cells (PFCgo) pass the trigger signal to FEF and the BG. This trigger will increase the receiving layers' activation for the selected target to cause the activation through to the superior colliculus to effect the saccade selected by prefrontal cortex. They receive visual memory information from LIP (LIPmem), the next saccade target location (PFCseq) and a cortical fixation signal (PFCfixation).

Fixation Cells (PFCfixation) provide a fixation signal as FEFfovea cells. The difference is that these cells have a large time constant. Thus it takes longer time to activate and deactivate the PFCfixation cells.This allows for the maintenance of fixation without a foveal signal.

Sequence Memory Cells (PFCseq) maintain a representation of the order in which the saccades are to be performed. The target locations are channeled via PFCmem.

Saccade Selector Cells (PFCsel) select the next saccade to be performed. We use refractory period to control when saccades can occur. This is a decaying value that must be overridden by the level of excitation in the visual memory calls (PFCmem). These cells select the target memory in PFCmem that has the highest activation and project this signal to the go cells (PFCgo) to assist in the activation of a saccade.

Superior Colliculus (SC)

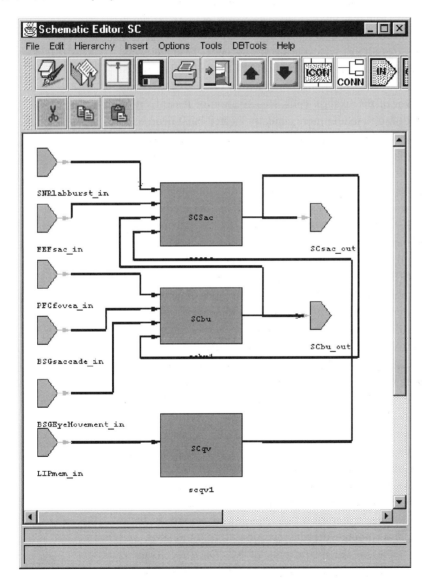

Figure 15.5
Superior Colliculus

The superior colliculus can be divided into two regions (Mason and Kandel 1991): the superficial layers and the intermediate and deep layers. The 3 superficial layers of SC receive both direct input from the retina and a projection from striate cortex for the entire contralateral visual hemifield. Neurons in the superficial SC have specific visual receptive fields: Half of the neurons have a higher frequency discharge in response to a visual stimulus when a monkey is going to make a saccade to that stimulus. If the monkey attends to the stimulus without making a saccade to it, for example by making a hand movement in response to a brightness change, these neurons do not give an enhanced response.

Cells in the two intermediate and deep layers are primarily related to the oculomotor system. These cells receive visual inputs from prestriate, middle temporal, and parietal cortices, and motor input from FEF. In addition, there is also representation of the body surface and of the locations of sound in space. All of these maps are in register with the visual maps. Among the various saccade generation and control by superior colliculus hypothesis we are using the relatively recent one due to (Munoz and Wurtz 1993; Optican 1994). This revised theory proposes that the activity of one class of saccade-related burst neurons (SRBN) declines sharply during saccades, but the spatial location of this activity remains fixed on the collicular motor map. The spatial activity profile in another class of saccade-related cells, called buildup neurons, expands as a forward progression in the location of its rostralmost edge during the saccade. Eventually the expanding activity reaches fixation neurons in the rostral pole of the colliculus, which become reactivated when the balance between the declining activity of the SRBNs and the fixation cells again tips in favor of the fixation cells. Reactivation of these fixation neurons, which have been hypothesized to inhibit more caudally located burst neurons in the rest of the colliculus in turn functions to terminate the saccade. Buildup neurons may also be located in the intermediate layers, but are more ventrally situated with respect to SRBNs.

Since the superficial SC layer does not project directly to the intermediate/deep layer, we will only model the intermediate/deep layer. We also will not use the FOn cells in FEF to directly inhibit the SC, instead we will use rostral SC as the inhibitory mechanism. Thus, saccades will be inhibited when there is fixation on the fovea and saccades will be terminated when the buildup neuron activity reaches the rostral pole of the SC. Target locations for the SRBNs will be mapped as quasi-visual cells receiving their input from LIP. The model implement SC as composed of four types of neurons.

Quasi-Visual Cells (SCqv) are visually responsive neurons and receive topographically organized output from the LIP (LIPvis). They project to saccade related burst neurons (SCsac), passing the visual information they have received from LIP.

Saccade Response Cells (SCsac) are the SRBN neurons responsible for the initiation of saccades by their projection to the long-lead burst neurons in the brainstem. These cells receive inhibitory afferents from the substantia nigra pars reticulata (SNr) and excitatory input from the SCqv cells, they also receive excitatory input from the FEF saccade-related neurons.

Buildup Cells (SCbu) are retinotopically organized, but the activity that arises at the beginning of a saccade acts as a moving hill towards the central element of this array which represents the fixation cells described below (SCfixation). Corollary feedback from the eye movement cells (BSGEyeMove) provide the information needed as to how far the eye is being moved. This controls the rate of progression of activity in these neurons towards the fixation cells, determining when the saccade is to be terminated.

Fixation Cells (SCfixation) represent the rostral pole of SC. Once the locus of activity in the buildup cells (SCbu) reaches the central element of this array, an inhibitory signal is propagated to the burst neurons (SCsac) in SC and the brainstem (BSGsac) to terminate the saccade.

Frontal Eye Field (FEF)

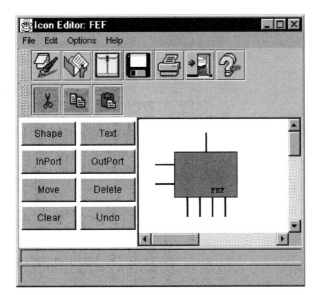

Figure 15.6
Frontal Eye Field

In FEF layer we model two types of saccade-related cells in FEF and a third type of cell relating to saccade inhibition (when a target is foveated)

Memory Response Cells (FEFmem) fire continuously during the delay portion of a delay saccade task. It has been found that there are neurons in FEF, in a double saccade task that would begin firing after the first saccade and continued firing until the second saccade (Goldberg and Bruce 1990). The cell would fire even if the stimulus never entered their receptive field when the second saccade was arranged so that it matched the cell's movement or receptive field. In the model a memory loop is established between these cells in FEF and mediodorsal thalamus (McEntee, Biber et al. 1976; Squire and Moore 1979; Fuster 1973). This memory loop is modulated by the inhibitory activity of BG upon the thalamus relay cells. The remapping of saccade targets performed by the BG is sent to thalamus. The connection strength between FEF and thalamus is chosen so that it is not strong enough to block BG from washing out the memory traces but strong enough to form a memory for the saccade targets.

Saccade Cells (FEFsac) are presaccadic movement neurons that respond to both visually and memory-guided saccades. These cells code for particular saccades.

Foveal Response Cells (FEFfovea) respond to visual stimuli falling on the fovea. They receive this input from LIP (LIPvis neurons) and project this information to BG and to the fixation neurons in SC (SCfixation neurons).

Basal Ganglia

The basal ganglia consist of five subcortical nuclei: the caudate nucleus (CD), putamen, globus pallidus, subthalamic nucleus, and substantia nigra. The neostriatum, or striatum, consists of both the caudate nucleus and putamen as they develop from the same telencephalic structure. The striatum receives nearly all of the input to the basal ganglia, receiving afferents from all four lobes of the cerebral cortex, including sensory, motor, association, and limbic areas. However, it only projects back to frontal cortex through the thalamus. This cortical input is topographically organized (Alexander, Crutcher et al. 1990; Alexander, R et al. 1986; Gerfen 1992; Parent, Mackey et al. 1983). There is also significant topographically organized input from the intralaminar nuclei of the thalamus (Cote and Crutcher 1991; Kitai, Kocsis et al. 1976; Sadikot, Parent et al. 1992; Wilson,

Chang et al. 1983): the centromedian nucleus projects to the putamen and the parafascicular nucleus projects to the caudate nucleus.

The model deals specifically with the saccadic oculomotor system within the brain. For this reason, the internal globus pallidus and the putamen in the model is not included in the model since they are more involved in motor control.

In terms of saccadic eye movement control the model proposes the purpose of the basal ganglia to be twofold:

- A lateral circuit that inhibits saccadic motor commands from execution until a trigger signal is received from higher motor centers, e.g., the prefrontal cortex.

- A medial circuit that estimates the next sensory state of the animal through an associative network for the execution of voluntary motor commands. This network receives as input the current sensory state, from LIP, and the currently planned motor command, from FEF, and outputs the next sensory state to limbic cortex and prefrontal cortex.

Lateral Basal Ganglia

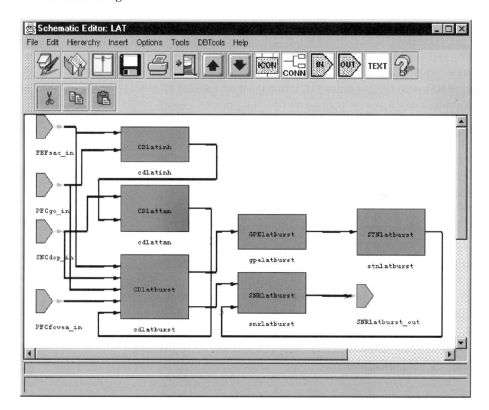

Figure 15.7
Lateral Basal Ganglia

The lateral basal ganglia circuit inhibits saccadic motor commands from execution until a trigger signal is received from higher motor centers, e.g., the prefrontal cortex. The lateral circuit is modeled as different set of cell groups. The following describes these cell groups.

Caudate Burst Cells (CDlatburst) are typically quiet and are tonically inhibited by the TAN interneurons. They receive excitatory input from cortex and the thalamus. These cells project to lateral SNr and GPe. They also receive afferents from the SNc dopaminergic cells.

Caudate Tonically Active Cells (CDlattan) are interneurons that fire continuously except when a go signal is received from prefrontal cortex. They are inhibited by the non-dopaminergic interneurons in the caudate. These cells also receive inhibitory input from the SNc dopaminergic neurons.

Caudate Non-dopaminergic Interneuron Cells (CDlatinh) are normally quiet. In the lateral circuit, these neurons receive the motor command from FEF and a go signal from PFC. When this input exceeds a certain threshold, these cells will fire and inhibit the tonically active interneurons (CDlattan).

GPe Burst Cells (GPElatburst) are tonically active and receive inhibition from the caudate burst cells. These cells project to the STN burst cells.

STN Burst Cells (STNlatburst) receive tonic inhibition from the GPe burst cells. These excitatory cells project to the SNr topographically, but with a wider projection area than that of the direct part from the striatum to SNr.

SNc Dopaminergic Cells (SNCdop) project to the burst cells and tonically active cells in the caudate. They receive excitatory afferents from limbic cortex about primary reward related events.

SNr Burst Cells (SNRlatburst) are tonically active and receive inhibition from the caudate burst cells and excitation from the STN burst cells. These cells project to the thalamus and SC and are responsible for inhibiting the execution of a saccade motor command until deactivated by a corticostriatal "go" signal.

Medial Basal Ganglia

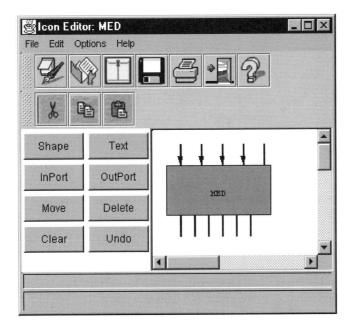

Figure 15.8
Medial Basal Ganglia

As in the lateral case the medial basal ganglia circuit is modeled as different set of cell groups. The following describes these cell groups that are modeled.

Caudate Burst Cells (CDmedburst) are typically quiet and are tonically inhibited by the TAN interneurons. They receive excitatory input from cortex and the thalamus. These cells project to medial SNr and GPe. They also receive afferents from the SNc dopaminergic cells.

Caudate Tonically Active Cells (CDmedtan) are interneurons that fire continuously except when a behaviorally significant, i.e., primary reward, signal is received from SNc through an increase in dopamine. They are inhibited by the non-dopaminergic interneurons in the caudate.

Caudate Non-dopaminergic Interneuron Cells (CDmedinh) are normally quiet. In the medial circuit, these neurons receive the motor command from FEF and the possible saccade targets from LIP. When this input exceeds a certain threshold, these cells will fire and inhibit the tonically active interneurons (CDmedtan).

GPe Burst Cells (GPEmedburst) are tonically active and receive inhibition from the caudate burst cells. These cells project to the STN burst cells.

STN Burst Cells (STNmedburst) are typically quiet and receive tonic inhibition from the GPe burst cells. These excitatory cells project to the SNr topographically, but with a wider projection area than that of the direct part from the striatum to SNr.

SNc Dopaminergic Cells (SNCdop) project to the burst cells and tonically active cells in the caudate. They receive excitatory afferents from limbic cortex about primary reward related events. These are the same cells as in the lateral circuit.

SNr Burst Cells (SNRmedburst) are tonically active and receive inhibition from the caudate burst cells and excitation from the STN burst cells. These cells project to the thalamus and thalamic reticular nucleus and are responsible for inhibiting the thalamic activity for the current sensory state and facilitating the growth of activation for the next sensory state.

Brain Stem Saccade Generator

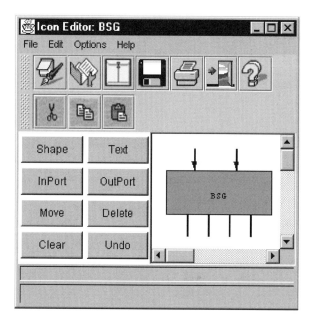

Figure 15.9
Brain Stem Saccade Generator I

Once the PFC issues a 'GO' signal the combination of increasing activity from PFC and decreased inhibition from BG allow activation to grow in the SC. This activation is projected to the brainstem where motor neurons are excited and cause the eye muscles to move the eyes to the new target location.

Brainstem Saccade Generator generates the saccade depending on the outputs of SC, where SCbu acts as inhibitory and SCsac excitatory. Once a saccade started SCbu neurons' activity start to grow and the activity of SCsac neurons start to decrease. Eventually the saccade ends (Note this is implemented in BSG). The BSG module is modeled as two types of cells:

BSG Saccade Generating Cells (BSGsac) are a composite of the burst, tonic and omnipause neurons in the brainstem. This layer receives the saccade command from SCsac and generates the saccade velocity and amplitude. They project to the BSGEyeMove layer. They also receive inhibitory feedback from SC buildup cells which inhibits saccades from occurring.

BSG Eye Movement Cells (BSGEyeMove) are equivalent to the brainstem motor neurons that actually drive the eye muscles. Corollary discharge from these neurons is received by SC buildup neurons (SCbu) to control the progression of their activity toward the rostral pole of SC. These neurons also receive activity from the SC buildup neurons (from the rostral pole only). This specific SC activity terminates an ongoing saccade.

15.3 Model Implementation

The complexity of this model in terms of the high number of brain areas and cell types involved, as well as the number of experiments implemented results in a wide use of the NSLM language functionality. Since the code is very long, we will focus on the special features that this model makes use of, like for example buffered ports to make processing order unimportant. The multiple experiments studied lead us to define new protocols and canvases. The protocols allow us to easily select and control the experiment to be simulated. The canvas offers an interactive way to collect and display experiment related information intuitively. Finally, we will explain how to extend NSLM to provide additional functionality not directly available in the language.

As always we need to define the top most module in the hierarchy, where we declare the model's constants, global variables, children modules, input and output modules and simulation methods such as initSys, initModule and makeConn. The top most module has to be defined with the reserved keyword nslModel. The children modules are those we previously saw in figure 1: Lateral Intraparietal Cortex (LIP), Thalamus (Thal), Basal Ganglia (Med, Lat, SNC), Prefrontal Cortex (PFC), Superior Colliculus (SC), Frontal Eye Field (FEF) and Brain Stem (BSG). To show the activity of the different cells we take advantage of the standard output interface (CrowleyOut). However, since we have different experiments we will extend the standard input interface with two canvases to collect the data for each of them (DoubleSaccadeInterface, GapSaccadeInterface).

At the instantiation of the model, the method initSys is called. Within this method we assign the values of the simulation parameters: simulation end time, step length and port buffering type. Once all the modules have been created, the scheduler executes the initModule method. Here we declare the protocols associated with each experiment using the method nslDeclareProtocol that adds new entries to the protocol menu (see figure 10). We will latter need to define which module will be part of which protocol. For that purpose we call the nslAddProtocolToAll function that add all modules to a particular protocol. Finally the method makeConn communicates the different modules by connecting their input and output ports. To connect siblings we use the nslConnect call, whereas nslRelabel allows a children module to inherit ports of their parents.

```
nslModelCrowleyTop()
{
    nslConst int CorticalArraySize = 9;
    nslConst int StriatalArraySize = 90;

    private int half_CorticalArraySize;
    public NslInt0 FOVEAX(half_CorticalArraySize);
    public NslInt0 FOVEAY(half_CorticalArraySize);

    // input modules that hold single output matrices
    VISINPUT visinput(CorticalArraySize);
    LC lc(CorticalArraySize);

    // LIP and Thalamus
    LIP lip(CorticalArraySize);
    Thal thal(CorticalArraySize);

    // Medial circuit
    Med med(CorticalArraySize, StriatalArraySize);

    // Lateral Circuit
    Lat lat(CorticalArraySize);
    SNC snc(CorticalArraySize);

    // Others
    PFC pfc(CorticalArraySize);
    SC  sc(CorticalArraySize);
    FEF fef(CorticalArraySize);
    BSG bsg(CorticalArraySize);

    // Graphic interfaces
    private   CrowleyOut
        crowout(CorticalArraySize,StriatalArraySize);
    private   DoubleSaccadeInterface doubleSaccade();
    private   GapSaccadeInterface gapSaccade();

    public void initSys(){
        system.setEndTime(0.55);
        system.nslSetRunDelta(0.001);
//all output ports will be double buffered
        system.nslSetBuffering(true);

        half_CorticalArraySize = CorticalArraySize / 2;
    }

    public void initModule(){
        nslDeclareProtocol("gap", "Gap Saccade");
        nslDeclareProtocol("double", "Double Saccade");

        system.addProtocolToAll("gap");
        system.addProtocolToAll("double");
    }

    public void makeConn() {
        // LIP inputs
        nslConnect(visinput.visinput_out , lip.SLIPvis_in);
        nslConnect(thal.ThLIPmem_out    , lip.ThLIPmem_in);
        ...
    }
}
```

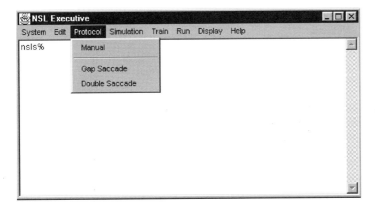

Figure 15.10
Standard executive interface
extended with new protocols.

As we mentioned before we utilize the standard output interface to graphically display the neural activity of the model. For that purpose we create a nslOutModule which includes all the functionality of a normal nslModule, but it incorporates a NslFrame, a window where graphs are displayed. Commonly this module contains the definition of input ports where the information will arrive. If we want this data to be displayed, we have to create a canvas and associate it with a particular input port. We do this with the nslAddCanvas methods family (e.g. nslAddAreaCanvas and nslAddSpatialCanvas).

```
nslOutModule CrowleyOut
    (int CorticalArraySize, int StriatalArraySize) {

    //input ports
    public NslDinFloat2
        visinput(CorticalArraySize, CorticalArraySize);
    public NslDinFloat2
        pfcGo(CorticalArraySize, CorticalArraySize);
    public NslDinFloat2
        lipMem(CorticalArraySize, CorticalArraySize);
    public NslDinFloat2
        thna(CorticalArraySize, CorticalArraySize);
    public NslDinFloat2
        fefsac(CorticalArraySize, CorticalArraySize);
    public NslDinFloat2
        scsac(CorticalArraySize, CorticalArraySize);
    public NslDinFloat2
        scbu(CorticalArraySize ,CorticalArraySize);

    public void initModule() {
        nslAddAreaCanvas(visinput,0,100);
        nslAddAreaCanvas(lipMem,0,100);
        nslAddAreaCanvas(thna,0,10);
        nslAddAreaCanvas(fefsac,0,100);
        nslAddAreaCanvas(scsac,0,100);
        nslAddSpatialCanvas(scbu,0,10);
    }
}
```

In order to build the new input user interface, two steps are required. The first one is the definition of a NslInModule. Within this module we associate an instance of the new canvas with an output port, where the information collected by the interface will be sent. For this purpose we use the nslAddUserCanvas method, which takes as parameters an outputPort and the name of the nslClass that implements the new canvas. In addition we call nslRemoveFromLocalProtocols function to remove this module and its window from the "manual" and "gap" protocols. This ensures that this interface will only be available when the "double" protocol is selected.

```
nslInModule DoubleSaccadeInterface() {

    NslDoutDouble1 params(8);

    public void initModule(){
        nslAddUserCanvas(params,"DoubleSaccade");
        nslRemoveFromLocalProtocols("manual");
        nslRemoveFromLocalProtocols("gap");
    }

}
```

In the second step is the implementation of nslClass that defines the new canvas. This has to be a subclass of NslInCanvas from which it inherits methods to handle input events and display graphics. As a NslInCanvas subclass it has to take two parameter, the first of them being the NslFrame where the canvas will be displayed and second a wrapping object that contains the port given by the parent NslInModule.

Every time the canvas has to be repainted, the nslRefresh method is called. Within this method we can draw lines, shapes, strings, change colors, etc. Every simulation step, the nslCollect function is executed, allowing input data to be gathered and sent to all the involved modules.

```
nslClass DoubleSaccade (NslFrame frame, NslVariableInfo vi)
    extends NslInCanvas(frame,vi) {
    public void nslInitCanvas() {
        nslClearDisplay();
    }

    public void nslRefresh() {
        drawSaccadeTargetLocations();
        drawSaccadeTargetDurations();
        ...
    }

    public void drawSaccadeTargetDurations() {
        int gx0, gx1, gy0, gy1, h, w;
        int x0, x1, y0, y1;

        float fix_start, fix_end;
        float t1_start, t1_end, t2_start, t2_end;

        NslString0 xTicks();

        int i;

        fix_start = (float) 0.;
            fix_end   = (float) 0.2;
        t1_start  = (float) 0.05;
        t1_end    = (float) 0.1;
        t2_start  = (float) 0.1;
        t2_end    = (float) 0.15;

        h = nslGetHeight();
        w = nslGetWidth();

        // Draw grid
        gx0 = w / 10;
```

```
gx1 = w - gx0;
gy0 = h / 5;
gy1 = h - gy0;
nslDrawLine(gx0,gy1,gx1,gy1,"black"); // X-axis
// X-ticks
y0 = gy1 - 5;
y1 = gy1 + 5;
for(i=0;i<=12;i++){
        x0 = x1 = gx0 + ((gx1 - gx0) * i)/12;
        nslDrawLine(x0,y0,x1,y1,"black");
        xTicks.set(i*5./100.);
        if(i%2 == 0)
            nslDrawString(xTicks.get(),x0-5,y1+15);
    }

// Draw time bars
y1 = gy0/2;
// Fixation
y0 = gy0;
x0 = gx0 + (int)((fix_start/.6)*(gx1-gx0));
x1 = (int) (((fix_end-fix_start)/.6)*(gx1-gx0));
if (x1<=0)
        x1 = 1;
nslFillRect(x0,y0,x1,y1,"red");

// T1
y0 = gy0*2;
x0 = gx0 + (int)((t1_start/.6)*(gx1-gx0));
x1 = (int)(((t1_end-t1_start)/.6)*(gx1-gx0));
if(x1<=0)
        x1 = 1;
nslFillRect(x0,y0,x1,y1,"green");

// T2
y0 = gy0*3;
x0 = gx0 + (int)((t2_start/.6)*(gx1-gx0));
x1 = (int)(((t2_end-t2_start)/.6)*(gx1-gx0));
if(x1<=0)
        x1 = 1;
nslFillRect(x0,y0,x1,y1,"blue");

}
public void nslCollect() {

    NslNumeric1 params = (NslNumeric1)vi.getNslVar();

params[0] = getXFixValue();
params[1] = getYFixValue();
...
}
...
}
```

To provide the continuous remmaping capability we utilized in the buildup neurons in the superior colliculus, we had to create a mechanism to keep track of the location of the centroid of the "moving hill", as we did not have enough neurons to allow the activity to propagate "naturally". We created a NSLM class called Target that had x and y coordinates as well as a variable to support a list of Target objects. We created a member function called Move that accepted a two-element vector of an x, y delta to be moved. This function applied the movement to the current location of the Target. A separate function applied to the new location of the buildup neuron targets onto the buildup neurons to simulate the continuous movement across the buildup cells.

```
nslClass Target() {
    // This class provides for a linked list of target objects
    // that all have the size of a single array element.
    // The contents of this class are the x,y coordinates
    // of the corner closest to array element 0,0, and a pointer
    // to the next Target in the list.  The x-coordinate is the
    // first sort.

    private double  xcor, ycor;
    private Target  next;

    initTarget() {
        xcor = 0; ycor = 0; next = nslNull;
    }

    ...

    void Move( NslDouble1 invec ){
    // This method applies the input movement vector to all of
        the
    // Targets in the linked list. The x,y-coordinates of each
    // Target have the input movement vector subtracted from
        their
    // corner coordinates as the motion of the Targets across
        the
    // visual space is in the opposite direction to the movement
    // of the eyes.
    Target cur;

    // Do the first target as it always exists

        xcor = xcor - invec[0];
        ycor = ycor - invec[1];

        cur = next;  //get pointer to next Target

        // The do-while will "move" the second and higher
        // Targets if they exist
        while ( cur != nslNull )      {
            cur.xcor = cur.xcor - invec[0];
            cur.ycor = cur.ycor - invec[1];
            cur = cur.next;
        }
    }

    ...

    double X() {return xcor;}
    double Y() {return ycor;}
    Target Next() {return next;}
}
```

Our most comprehensive extension to NSLM was the ability to map arbitrary neurons in one layer onto a larger layer. This was the basis of out remapping algorithm between the cortex and the basal ganglia. Specifically, we created a linked list mechanism for each element in the input layer (FEF, LIP and PFC) for our model that pointed to all neurons to which they project (striatum in or case). Thus, for any given input neuron, you only need to read the linked list out to determine its projections. We used the same mechanism to establish the remapping from striatum to SNr. In this case, however, there were multiple connections onto SNr from striatum, but the same principle applies. You can find out which striatal neurons talk to a specific SNr neuron by just indexing the linked list for that neuron. This "bi-directional" mapping made the teaching of the weights between cortex, striatum and SNr very simple, since we specified the cortical inputs and knew what SNr outputs we wanted. It was simple to match the linked lists that both pointed back to the striatum and then modify the weight matrix for the striatum. Summing the SNr inputs during runtime was also simplified as we accessed the linked list for each SNr neuron and summed the inputs for that neuron by reading the list only once per time step.

```
nslClass Element() {

    int x, y, xo, yo;
    Element next;

    nslConst int FOVEAX = 4;
    nslConst int FOVEAY = 4;
    ...
    public void initElement() {
        x = y = x0 = y0 = -1;
        next = nslNull;
    }
    ...
    public void Remap(int max, Element elem) {
        // This function "remaps" the calling Element and
            returns an
        // Element containing the remapped location.
        int xt, yt, xot, yot;

        xt = FOVEAX - x; yt = FOVEAY - y;
        xot = xt + xo;   yot = yt + yo;

        elem.x = FOVEAX; elem.y = FOVEAY;

        if ( ( xot > -1 ) && ( xot < max ) )
            elem.xo = xot;
        else
            elem.xo = -1;

        if ( ( yot > -1 ) && ( yot < max ) )
            elem.yo = yot;
        else
            elem.yo = -1;
    }
    public Element Next() { return next; }
    public int X() { return x; }
    public int Y() { return y; }
    public int XO() { return xo; }
    public int YO() { return yo; }
}

nslModule Med (int CorticalArraySize, int StriatalArraySize)
    extends Func (CorticalArraySize) {
    private nslConst int MaxConnections   = 50;
```

```
        private nslConst int NumberIterations = 10;
        // Output ports
        public NslDoutInt3
FEFxmap(CorticalArraySize,CorticalArraySize,MaxConnections);
        public NslDoutInt3
FEFymap(CorticalArraySize,CorticalArraySize,MaxConnections);
        public NslDoutInt3
LIPxmap(CorticalArraySize,CorticalArraySize,MaxConnections);
        public NslDoutInt3
LIPymap(CorticalArraySize,CorticalArraySize,MaxConnections);
        public NslDoutInt3
PFCxmap(CorticalArraySize,CorticalArraySize,MaxConnections);
        public NslDoutInt3
PFCymap(CorticalArraySize,CorticalArraySize,MaxConnections);

        // See MappingParameters
        private int FEFPatchCount;
        private int LIPPatchCount;
        private int PFCPatchCount;

        private Element LearnedElements();
        private Element UnlearnedElements();
        private Element Teacher();

        public void initRun () {
            MakeMapping();
            ...
            LearnNewElements();
        }
        ...
        public void MakeMapping() {
            int MapSize = StriatalArraySize/3;
            ...
            // Establish the direct path mapping from CD to SNr
            SNRMapping(FEFxmap, FEFymap, FEFPatchCount, MapSize);
            SNRMapping(LIPxmap, LIPymap, LIPPatchCount, MapSize);
            SNRMapping(PFCxmap, PFCymap, PFCPatchCount, MapSize);
            ...
        }
        public void learnNewElements() {
            LearnConnections(UnlearnedElements);
            LearnedElements.Merge(UnlearnedElements);
            UnlearnedElements.Remove();
        }
        public void LearnConnections(Element elem) {
            Element curelem(elem);
            while ( curelem != null ) {
            for (int ii=0; ii<NumberIterations; ii++ ) {
                //# of iterations
                // Set cortical excitation
                ...
                // Determine correct remappings for non-neural
                   Teacher
                curelem.Remap((int)CorticalArraySize, Teacher);
                MapToFovea(curelem.X(), curelem.Y());
                // Time to map the nonsaccade target as well
```

```
        ...
        // increment weights between active CD neurons
        // and remapped location
        MapToOffset(curelem.X(), curelem.Y(),
            curelem.XO(), curelem.YO());
        }
        curelem = curelem.Next();
    }
}
}

nslModule SNRmedburst (int CorticalArraySize,
        int StriatalArraySize) {
    public NslDinDouble3 SNRweights(CorticalArraySize,
        CorticalArraySize, CorticalArraySize);
    public NslDinInt3 SNRxmap(CorticalArraySize,
        CorticalArraySize, CorticalArraySize);
    public NslDinInt3 SNRymap(CorticalArraySize,
        CorticalArraySize, CorticalArraySize);
    public NslDinDouble2
        CDdirmedburst_in (StriatalArraySize, StriatalArraySize);

    private NslDouble2 SNRcdinput
        (CorticalArraySize, CorticalArraySize);
    ...
    public void SumCDtoSNR (NslDouble2 CD, NslDouble2 SNR) {
        // This function sums the activity in the medial CD
        // circuit onto the medial SNR circuit through
        // SNRweights, SNRxmap and SNRymap.

        int i, j, k, xmaploc, ymaploc;

        SNR = 0;  // Ensure new mapping only
        for (i = 0; i < CorticalArraySize; i ++) {
            for (j = 0; j < CorticalArraySize; j ++) {
                for (k = 0; k < SNRMapCount [i][j]; k ++) {
                    xmaploc = SNRxmap [i][j][k];
                    ymaploc = SNRymap [i][j][k];
                        SNR [i][j] = SNR[i][j]
                            + CD [xmaploc][ymaploc] *
                            SNRweights [i][j][k];
                }
            }
        }
    }
    ...
    public void simRun () {
        SumCDtoSNR (CDdirmedburst_in, SNRcdinput);
        ...
    }
}
```

15.4 Simulation and Results[1]

The Crowley model can be tailored to test various experimental saccade paradigms. The current version of the model has two built-in paradigms: gap saccade and double saccade. The latter is more subtle. So we are going to go over the double saccade paradigm and show how the model can reproduce real world experimental results.

The double saccade can be briefly described as the following. The subject is presented a fixation point which he must maintain a fixation until the stimuli is there. After some certain time delay first target is flashed somewhere in the visual field of the subject. It is followed by a second flash of target which may or may not overlap with the first stimuli. While the targets are being shown the subject must still maintain his fixation. Only after the fixation goes off the subject can make the saccades. The saccades he makes must follow the right temporal order. That is the first saccade to the first target and the second saccade to the second target.

In order to enable user to modify certain paradigm specific parameters in a convenient way a custom user interface is designed for Crowley Model. The user can bring either of the paradigms' user interface by using via experiment menu. The double saccade user interface gives user the convenience of setting up experiment parameters by dragging and clicking. Figure 15.11 shows how the double saccade interface looks like:

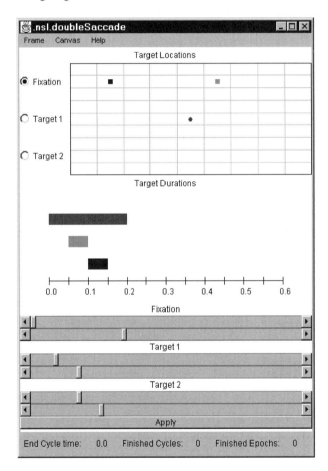

Figure 15.11
Double saccade experiment interface window

The upper part of the window is used to specify the location of the targets and the fixation point. The user needs simply to click on one of the buttons for fixation, target1 or target2 and point the position of the stimulus on the grid. Fixation point is denoted by blue, target 1 is by green and target 2 by red color. Once the user specifies the position of the stimuli then he/she has the opportunity to modify the timing of the stimuli by simply dragging the gauges on the lower level of the interface window. For example on the sample interface window the visual events that occur can be described as follows. At time 0.0 the fixation stimuli appears. At time 0.5 first target appears. At time 0.1 first target disappears and target two appears. At time 0.15 target two disappears. Finally the fixation stimulus goes away at time 0.2. Once the spatial and temporal characteristics of the double saccade paradigm is specified user has to click on Apply button to load the settings into the simulator. Then the double saccade experiment can be simulated by clicking the Start button. The simulator will, then, create the visual events defined by the user and simulate the model. NSL display window can be used to display the model variables as usual. The Crowley Model comes with a NSL display window with 8 graphic displays as shown in the below figure. The visual events specified occurs in the top left graph. Other graphs show the various model variables. For example the CrowleyTop.lip.LIPmem_out labeled graph shows the NSL variable LIPmem_out which is defined in lip module. In regard to model semantics this layers keeps the memory of the visual stimuli.

The activity of the buildup neurons in SC can be used to track the saccades that the model executes. The moving activity towards to center following by a decay at the center in SCbu1 layer corresponds to a saccade that the model executes. Thus a double saccade would mean two consecutive buildup neuron activity. The SCbu1 layer is retinotopically organized so the start of the activity corresponds to the target stimulus for the saccade. However the second target is remapped with anticipation of the first saccade. So the second saccade activity seen in buildup neurons are based on the remapped location.

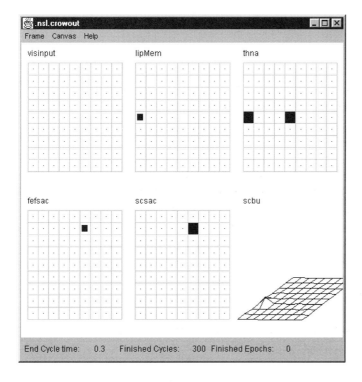

Figure 15.12
First saccade in progress

The buildup neuron activity is shown using a 3d graph (figures 15.12 and 15.13). The targets in this simulation run were horizontally aligned and above the fixation point. The first target were also aligned with the fixation point. The system was expected to make a vertical (upward) saccade then a horizontal (rightward) saccade to the second target. If there were no remapping the second saccade would not be horizontal but it would be an up-right one. The prediction for the buildup neuron activity was to have two perpen-dicular activities decaying at the center. The following two figures demonstrate the expected result. First figure shows the simulator display window during first saccade.

The second figure shows the expected second saccade (Note that the direction of the saccades are towards the center so they are perpendicular).

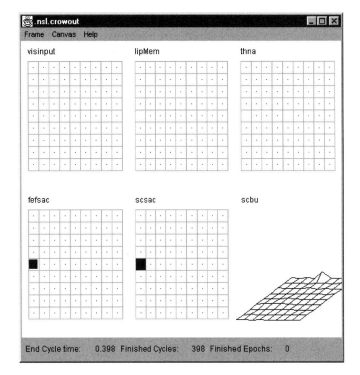

Figure 15.13
Second saccade in progress

15.5 Summary

We have developed a neural network model of the saccadic motor control system that includes a number of cortical and subcortical systems known to be involved in saccadic eye movements. One primary thesis of our model is that the basal ganglia has two primary roles in saccadic motor control: (1) inhibition of voluntary saccadic eye movements until cortical centers provide a go signal and (2) provide for the sensory remapping of potential saccade targets based upon an impeding saccade command. Additionally, we have implemented a mechanism simulating the effects of dopamine deficit in saccadic eye movements. Lastly, we have implemented a model that places the superior colliculus within a feedback control loop responsible for terminating saccades.

We have made use of the NSLM language functionality showing how buffered ports can be utilized to make the order in which modules are executed unimportant. We have explained the creation of standard and custom user interfaces. We reviewed how protocols are declared to simulate different experiments for the same model. We provided an example of how to extend NSLM to obtain additional functionality not directly available in the language. We ended showing how the NSL simulation environment can be used to run the implemented model for the double saccade experiment.

Notes

1. The Saccade model was implemented and tested under NSLJ.

16 A Cerebellar Model of Sensorimotor Adaptation

J. Spoelstra

16.1 Introduction

This chapter describes a neural network model of adaptation, based on the Martin *et al.* (1995) study of normal subjects and cerebellar patients throwing at a target after donning 30° prisms. The prisms caused subjects to miss the target by an angle corresponding to the prism deflection angle. With subsequent throws, however, normal subjects adjusted until they were once again throwing on target. After doffing the glasses the prism gaze-throw calibration remained and subjects made corresponding errors in the opposite direction. A cartoon sketch of the experiment is shown in figure 16.1.

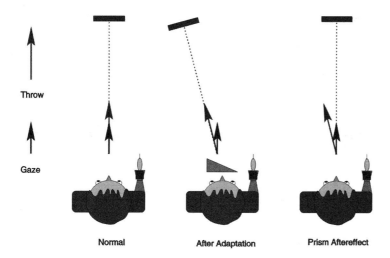

Figure 16.1
The experiment done by Martin et al. (1995). Subjects throw at a visual target while wearing prism glasses. Donning the glasses cause subjects to miss the target, but normal subjects adjust until they once again throw on target. After doffing the prism glasses, subjects make errors in the opposite direction and have to readjust their normal throwing.

From a modeling perspective, three results were particularly interesting:

- The calibration was throw-strategy specific: What was learned was not a general sensorimotor transformation; over- and under-hand throwing required independent adaptation.

- After a number of weeks of training subjects acquired the ability to throw accurately from the first throw, both with and without the prism glasses.

- Patients with lesions in the intermediate and medial cerebellum could not learn to throw accurately while wearing prisms, implicating the part of the cerebellum projecting "downstream" to the brainstem and spinal cord.

16.2 Model Description

Ito (1984) defined the basic building block of the cerebellar cortex and underlying nuclei as the microcomplex, shown in figure 16.2. Inputs arrive via mossy fibers (MF) to the granule cells (GC) whose axons bifurcate to form parallel fibers (PF) in the cerebellar cortex. Each Purkinje cell (PC) receives input from a large number of parallel fibers and one climbing fiber originating in the inferior olive (IO). Purkinje cells are the sole output from the cortex and inhibit the nuclear cells (NUC). Nuclear cell axons connect the cerebellum to the rest of the motor system, but have also been shown to produce an inhibitory effect on the same inferior olive cells that project to the overlying Purkinje cells to complete the loop. Learning occurs as long term depression (LTD) of parallel fiber-Purkinje dendrites after coactivation of parallel- and climbing fibers (Marr 1969; Albus 1971).

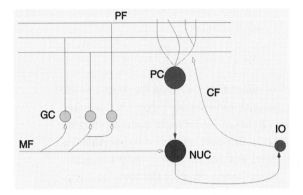

16.3 Model Implementation

Figure 16.3 shows the overall structure of the NSL implementation, including modules, submodules and input/output ports. The naming convention is that modules representing neuron populations are named xxx_layer, whereas high-level modules and other model systems "boxes" are named xxx_module.

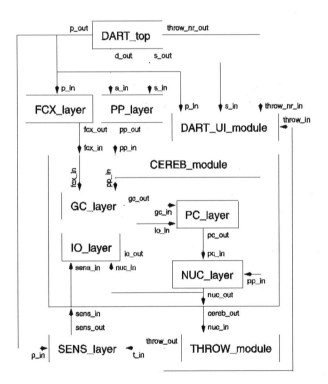

Neuron Populations

All neurons are modeled as having firing rate f computed from the membrane potential p using the sigmoid function:

$$f(p) = F_{max} \frac{1}{1 + \exp(-\alpha(p - \beta))} \qquad (16.1)$$

with F_{max} the maximum firing rate, α determining the slope and β the offset of the sigmoid. The membrane potential is simply the weighted sum of the inputs to the neuron

$$p = \sum_{j \in A} I_j \qquad (16.2)$$

with I_j the current synaptic input from neuron j and A denoting the set of projecting neurons.

PP_layer

The cerebellar granule cell layer receives input from two other layers, both containing a coarse coding of physical variables. The first input, putatively called posterior parietal (PP), is a 10x10 array with coordinates ranging from (0,0) to (9,9) and codes the arm configuration at the end of the throw. Because we are only interested in the horizontal throw direction, only the arm yaw angle relative to the head direction is represented. We also want to distinguish between over- and underhand throwing, so the PP layer arbitrarily codes both aiming angle (where the target appears visually) and throw strategy (over-/underhand).

A group of cells in a circular region with diameter of roughly 6 grid units were activated simultaneously, with activity maximal in the center and tapering off from there. As displayed by the NSL system, throw direction was coded on the Y-axis, with strategy on the X-axis. Using our coding convention, planning an overhand throw at a target centered in the visual field would cause a bump of activity centered at (3,4.5). If an underhand throw is planned the activity would be centered at (7,4.5).

The NSL code for generating this input is shown below. The parameter pp_sep determines the separation between the activity bumps for overarm and underarm throwing respectively, while pp_noise determines what portion of the signal will be generated by random to simulate noise. The inputs s_in and a_in represent throw strategy (0 for overarm, 1 for underarm) and aim direction respectively.

```
public void simRun(){
    int i,j;
    double mx, my;
    double dx,dy;

    if(s_in < .5)     // throw = over
        my = 4.5 - pp_sep/2.;
    else              // throw = under
        my = 4.5 + pp_sep/2.;
    mx = 4.5 + 4.5*a_in/30.; // Fit [-30:30] in [0:9]
    for(i=0;i<10;i++){
        dx = mx - i;
        for(j=0;j<10;j++){
            dy = my - j;
            pp_out[i][j] = pp_noise * nslRandom() +
                (1. - pp_noise) *
            nslExp(-1.*(dx*dx/sx2 + dy*dy/sy2));
        }
    }
}
```

FCX_layer

The second input layer contains a population code indicating an awareness of wearing prism glasses. Given enough time subjects could learn to throw accurately both with and without the prism glasses, indicating that the cerebellum received some information, possibly from the frontal cortex (FCX), telling it whether this was a prism-on or prism-off trial. In the model a 10x4 array was used with the Gaussian bump of activity centered around (2.5,2) normally, and at (2.5,7) when prism glasses were worn.

In the NSL code below p_in is the prism angle while the parameter fcx_noise determines the noise level as for the PP input.

```
public void simRun(){
    int i,j;
    double mx, my, dx, dy;

    mx = 1. + 9.*p_in/50.; // Fit [0:50] in [1:10]
    my = 1.5;
    for(i=0;i<10;i++){
        dx = mx-i;
        for(j=0;j<4;j++){
            dy = my - j;
            fcx_out[i][j] = fcx_noise*nslRandom() +
            (1.-fcx_noise)*nslExp(-1.*(dx*dx/sx2 +
                dy*dy/sy2));
        }
    }
}
```

GC_layer

Input arrives at the cerebellum via mossy fibers from the two input regions PP and FCX. Granule cells provide the input to the cerebellar cortex and are represented by a 30x30 array. In the real cerebellum each granule cell synapses with on average four mossy fibers—in the model four inputs were randomly selected with varying probability from the two input regions. The result is that the granule cell layer in a sense acts as the hidden layer in a multi-layer perceptron artificial neural network by providing nonlinear combinations of the raw inputs.

In order to produce this random mapping from the two input matrices onto the 30x30 GC grid, 5 arrays were set up in the initModule procedure: For each of the 3600 synapses (30x30x4) an input is selected randomly from the two input matrices. Vectors Xo and Yo record the coordinates on the input matrix; Xd and Yd record the coordinates on the GC matrix; and src records which of the two inputs was chosen.

During execution of the model the simRun method uses these vectors to map elements of the input matrices onto the GC inputs. The model is sensitive to GC parameters, so a number were made a available to the user for experimentation: The number of inputs each granule cell receives is determined by gc_nd; gc_dist determines the fraction of PP inputs versus FCX inputs chosen; gc_offset and gc_slope determine cell properties as described above.

```
public void initModule(){
    int gx,gy,i,x,y;
    double td;
    w = 1./((double)gc_nd);
    // Create mapping function
    NC = 0;
    for(gx=0;gx<30;gx++){
        for(gy=0;gy<30;gy++){
        for(i=0;i<gc_nd;i++){
            Xd[NC] = gx;
            Yd[NC] = gy;
            if(NslRandom() < gc_dist){ // PP input
                src[NC] = 0;
                td = (NslRandom()*5. + 3.);
                Xo[NC] = (int)td;
                td = (NslRandom()*10.);
                Yo[NC] = (int)td;
            } else { // FCX input
                    src[NC] = 1;
                    td = (NslRandom()*10.);
                    Xo[NC] = (int)td;
                    td = (NslRandom()*2. + 1);
                    Yo[NC] = (int)td;
            }
            NC++;
        }
        }
    }
}
```

```
public void simRun(){
    int i,j;
    int mx,my,ix,iy;

    // Map inputs onto 30x30 array using mapping function
    gc_mp = 0.;
    for(i=0;i<NC;i++){
        mx = Xd[i];
        my = Yd[i];
        ix = Xo[i];
        iy = Yo[i];
        if(src[i]==0)
            gc_mp[mx][my] = gc_mp[mx][my] + pp_in[ix][iy];
        else
            gc_mp[mx][my] = gc_mp[mx][my] + fcx_in[ix][iy];
    }

    gc_mp = w * gc_mp;
    for(i=0;i<30;i++){
        for(j=0;j<30;j++){
            gc_out[i][j] =
                f_max/(1.+nslExp(gc_slope*(gc_offset-
                    gc_mp[i][j])));
        }
    }
}
```

PC_layer

Granule cell axons bifurcate to give rise to the parallel fibers in the cortex that synapse with the Purkinje cell (PC) dendrites. The PCs are modeled as a 2x5 array. Parallel fibers run parallel to the X-direction and are modeled to span the entire width of the cerebellar patch modeled. Thus, if a PC receives input from one granule cell in a row, it receives input from all the granule cells in that row. The synaptic weights are excitatory and modifiable.

The section of NSL code below, taken from the simRun method shows how GC inputs are mapped onto the PC layer so that each PC receives input from a beam of GCs comprising one third of the total GC population. All the weights are stored in a single large vector.

```
// GC inputs
    pc_mp = 0.;
    wc = 0;
    for(px=0;px<2;px++){
        for(py=0;py<5;py++){
            beam_start = py*30/5;
            for(gx=0;gx<30;gx++){
                for(y=0;y<10;y++){
                    gy = (beam_start + y)%30;
                    pc_mp[px][py] = pc_mp[px][py]
                        + w[wc] * gc_in[gx][gy];
                    wc++;
                }
            }
        }
    }
```

We follow the current thinking that learning in the cerebellum occurs at the parallel fiber-Purkinje synapses and specifically that long term depression (LTD) of synaptic weights occur with simultaneous granule (pre synaptic), Purkinje (post synaptic) and climbing fiber activity. In order to prevent all weights systematically decreasing to zero, it is postulated that long term potentiation (LTP) will occur if pre- and post-synaptic activity is paired without climbing fiber activity.

Climbing fibers originate in the inferior olive (IO) and project topographically to the Purkinje layer: Each PC receives only one climbing fiber from the IO (Ito 1984). In this model we do not address the real-time role of climbing fiber activity on the firing rate of PCs; the inputs from the inferior olive (IO) are used solely as training signals.

The learning rule can be formalized as:

$$\Delta w = -\alpha F_g F_p \left(F_{io} - F_{io}^{back} \right) \tag{16.3}$$

with w the synaptic efficacy at one of the parallel fiber-Purkinje synapses, α some constant, F_g the firing rate of the granule cell, F_p the firing rate of the Purkinje cell, F_{io} the climbing fiber activity and F_{io}^{back} the tonic activity rate of the IO cells. IO activity below the tonic rate will result in LTP while any activity higher than the tonic rate will cause LTD.

In the NSL implementation below the same loop structure is used as above to make clear which PC, GC and IO cells are used when updating a specific weight. The test against getCurTime is made to ensure that all the inputs have filtered through the various stages of the process.

```
// Learning
if(system.getCurTime()>.055){ // give others time to settle
    (dart to fly)
    wc = 0;
    for(px=0;px<2;px++){
        for(py=0;py<5;py++){
            beam_start = py*30/5;
            for(gx=0;gx<30;gx++){
                for(y=0;y<10;y++){
                    gy = (beam_start + y)%30;
                    w[wc] = w[wc]
                        + alpha * (gc_in[gx][gy]*.01) *
                            (io_in[px] - 2.);
                    if(w[wc] < 0.)
                        w[wc] = 0.;
                    else if(w[wc] > 1.)
                        w[wc] = 1.;
                    wc++;
                }
            }
        }
    }
}
```

Purkinje cells inhibit nuclear cells which in turn inhibit IO cells, producing a stable system: Any activity (disturbance) in the IO higher than F_{io}^{back} will cause a decrease in the PC firing, leading to an increase in nuclear cell activity which inhibits the IO cell. Stability is reached when nuclear activity is such that inhibition has all IO cells firing at F_{io}^{back}. One could think of the nuclear cells providing an *expectation* of the disturbance.

NUC_layer

The PC layer projects topographically onto the 20x1 nuclear layer. Each nuclear cell synapses with all the PCs in its column. These synapses are fixed and inhibitory. Nuclear cells also receive topographical projections with fixed weights from PP. Each nuclear cell receives input from a column of PP cells (coding aim direction) so that without PC intervention (no adaptation) normal throws go in the aim direction. In order to facilitate nuclear cell activity through PC disinhibition, the offset and slope parameters for the nuclear cells are set so that the cells are tonically active at about 10% of their maximum firing rate.

```
public void simRun(){
    int i,j;
    int ix;
    double td;
    // Map PP and PC inputs onto 2x1 array
    nuc_mp = 0.;
    for(i=0;i<10;i++){
        ix = i/5;
        for(j=0;j<10;j++){
                nuc_mp[ix] = nuc_mp[ix]+ 2.*pp_in[i][j];
        }
    }
    for(i=0;i<2;i++){
        for(j=0;j<5;j++){
                nuc_mp[i] = nuc_mp[i] - .2 * pc_in[i][j];
        }
    }
    for(i=0;i<2;i++){
        nuc_out[i] = f_max/(1.+NslExp(slope*(offset-
            nuc_mp[i])));
    }
}
```

IO_layer

As discussed above, each IO cell receives inhibitory projections from the nuclear cells and an excitatory connection from a sensory layer that indicates an error in performance. An interesting aspect is that the IO cells receive inhibition not only from the corresponding nuclear cell (which closes the negative-feedback learning loop), but also from the other (opposing) nuclear cell. The reason for this is that the output of the nuclear cells drive the direction of the eventual throw in a push-pull manner. In such a system, if the slightest disparity exists between LTD and LTP, small random errors will eventually drive the system to saturate with all weights at either their maximum or minimum values. By adding inhibition from the opposing side, however, any coactivation suppresses IO activity (which would increase NUC activity by decreasing PC weights) and steers the system towards reciprocal nuclear cell activation.

```
public void simRun(){
    int i;
    double nuc_act;

    nuc_act = nuc_in[0] + nuc_in[1];
    io_mp = sens_in - .01*nuc_act;
    for(i=0;i<2;i++){
        io_out[i] = f_max/(1.+NslExp(slope*(offset-io_mp[i])));
    }
}
```

SENS_layer

We postulate that a system (also PP) codes the perceived error in the final arm configuration or dart flight direction. This system then projects onto the IO layer where it is combined with inhibition from the nuclear cells to generate the cerebellar training signal.

Each of two cells are proportionally receptive to either a leftward or rightward throw error. The module takes as input both the throw direction and the prism angle.

```
public void simRun(){
    double Derror;

    Derror = p_in - t_in;
    if(Derror < 0.){ /* go leftward */
        sens_out[0] = .1-Derror/10.;
        sens_out[1] = 0.1;
    } else { /* go right */
        sens_out[0] = 0.1;
        sens_out[1] = .1+Derror/10.;
    }
}
```

High-level modules

CEREB_module

This module is simply a convenient abstraction of the cell layers comprising the cerebellar part of the model. It does not do any processing, but simply instantiate its child modules and pass on inputs and outputs.

THROW_module

The output of the model is the yaw direction of the throw, derived from the activity of the two nuclear cells. Gilbert and Thach (1977) reported that cerebellar nuclear cells firing is related to arm yaw angle at the end of a trial. Following the hypothesis that cerebellar output influence brainstem motor pattern generators, it is assumed that each synergy cell will activate a combination of spring-like muscles to pull the final arm position to a side in a push-pull configuration. In a simplified model, the throw direction can be computed as the ratio of the activity of one cell to the total activity in both cells as shown below. The formula used gives a range of [-100:100] for the throw direction.

```
public void simRun(){
    throw_out = (.5 - (1.+nuc_in[0])/(2.+nuc_in[1] +
        nuc_in[0]))*100.;
}
```

DART_top

This module acts as a controller, automating the execution of specific experiments by executing a predetermined sequence of trials. A trial consists of setting up the inputs, then letting the simulation run for 6 steps at the end of which the throw direction is computed and the cerebellar weights adapted. An example of an experiment would be to execute a number of warm-up throws, followed by 20 throws while wearing prisms and 20 throws after doffing the prism glasses.

DART_UI_module

Although NSL provides an interface for displaying model variables and setting parameters, this module incorporates Java code for a model-specific user interface. It uses the standard NSL ports and facilities for hierarchical variables to communicate with the model, but is designed to present the experimenter with a more intuitive interface for displaying results and facilitate access to the model parameters.

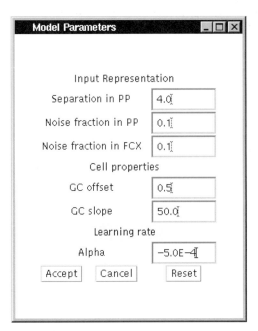

Figure 16.4
The custom user interface window for setting model parameters.

The custom interface window, shown in figure 16.5, pops up alongside the two NSL windows. The center panel indicates where consecutive throws hit the target, color-coded to indicate whether prisms were worn and differentiate between overarm and underarm throwing. From the menu bar users may select between three experiments or choose to set parameter values (shown in figure 16.4).

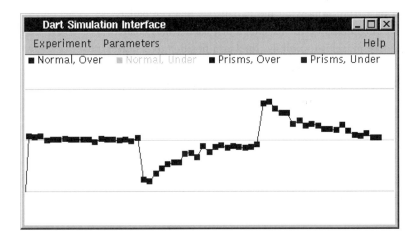

Figure 16.5
Simple adaptation experiment. 30° prism on at trial number 20, prism off at trial number 40

16.4 Simulation and Results[1]

There are three basic experiments: Simple adaptation to wearing prisms and readaptation to overcome the aftereffect; transfer between over- and underarm throwing; and the acquisition of two gaze-throw calibrations. To reproduce the data presented by Martin *et al.* (1995) and Kitazawa *et al.* (1995) it has to be shown that parameters exist to simultaneously satisfy 4 constraints:

1. Rate of adaptation: Approximately 30 throws are required to adapt to the prisms, slightly less to readapt. In both cases errors decrease exponentially, with readaptation occurring at a higher rate.

2. Magnitude of aftereffect: There is some variation, but the first throw after doffing the prisms usually misses by about 80% of the prism angle.

3. Transfer between over- and underarm throwing: Different levels of transfer should be possible.

4. Acquisition of two calibrations: This should take a large number of prism-on/prism-off adaptation trials. The initial error after donning or doffing the prisms should decrease exponentially.

After Effect of Prism Adaptation

Figure 16.5 depicts results of the basic experiment. A subject throws at a target, then dons 30° wedge prism glasses causing him to throw 30° off target. With repeated throws he improves until he once again throws on target. When the prisms are removed the subject misses by almost 30° on the opposite side and has to readjust his aim.

The activity of cells after adaptation to throwing with prisms as displayed by the NSL system is shown in figure 16.6. It can be seen how a depression in Purkinje cell activity (pc_out) leads to an increase in nuclear cell activity (nuc_out) that drives the direction of throwing.

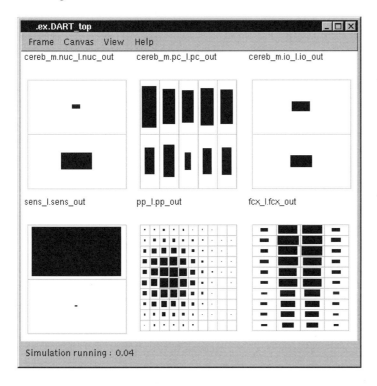

Figure 16.6
NSL output display of model variables after adaptation to prisms is complete. Note the depression in the activity of cells in the Purkinje layer and corresponding higher activity levels in the corresponding nuclear cells.

Transfer between Over- and Underhand Throwing

Martin reported that some patients showed no transfer, i.e., the first underhand throw without prisms after adapting overhand throwing with prisms was on target, while others showed partial transfer. He also noted that for patients that showed partial transfer, the first overhand throw after readjusting underhand throwing was closer to target by an amount roughly equal to the amount adjusted during underarm adaptation. In simulation we can replicated this phenomenon by adjusting the separation between over- and underhand in PP (parameter pp_sep). Due to the Gaussian shape of the activity bump in PP, a separation of 6.0 leads to almost no overlap, while a separation of 1.5 leads to substantial overlap in representation. The results shown in figure 16.7 were obtained with the default setting of 4.0 and produces only limited transfer.

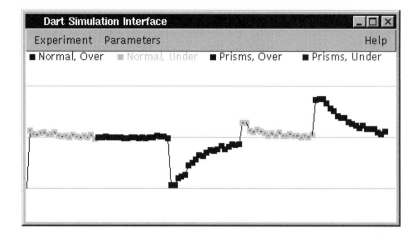

Figure 16.7
Transfer between over- and underhand throwing. At trial 20 30° prisms were donned while throwing overhand. At trial 40 the prisms were taken off but throwing was underhand. From trial 60 throwing is overhand again. In cases where the separation is large (solid line), the adaptation is independent—underhand throwing does not show the prism aftereffect. Where the separation is smaller, overhand adaptation affects underhand throwing and the overhand aftereffect is reduced proportional to the amount of adaptation that was required for underhand throwing.

Relating this result to human studies we would predict that the cortical representations for under- and overhand throwing could differ between subjects in terms of the amount of overlap. One interpretation could be that those who show partial overlap acquired underhand throwing as a variation of the overhand strategy, while those who showed no transfer learned two separate skills.

Relation to Other Models
The model shares many features with the AST model (Arbib, Schweighofer and Thach, 1994). In both models the cerebellar nuclear cells represent a population code of horizontal direction. However, in the AST model this direction is "added" as a rotation to the gaze angle in premotor cortex, whereas the current model does not need the complicated rotation computation and posits that the cerebellar nuclear neurons contain a direct code of the throw direction.

The AST model further required an artificial error detection system in register with the shoulder position that would activate an array of binary "leftward" and "rightward" cells in the inferior olive depending on where the throw went. While the current model does not yet offer a full explanation of the inferior olive, the error signal is generated in the IO through a combination of excitatory projections from PP and inhibitory projections from cerebellar nuclei to provide realistic IO firing rates and a stable learning system.

The learning circuitry based on inhibitory feedback from the cerebellar nuclear cells to the inferior olive has previously been suggested in models of cerebellar function in classical conditioning by Moore *et al.* [1989] and again by Bartha and Thompson (1995).

Martin et al. (1995) proposed a model where pairs of Purkinje cells, via disinhibition of nuclear cells, control eye, head and shoulder direction. The inputs are the current values of the controlled variables plus again the required "prism detector" input. However, no modeling results were published, so direct comparisons might not be appropriate.

16.5 Summary

The model described in this chapter shows how observed behavior could be generated in a cerebellar-like structure. In this context we offer explanations to the following questions:

What influences partial vs. zero transfer between over- and underhand throwing? The model can replicate the behavior by varying a single parameter that controls representations in (possibly) posterior parietal cortex.

What is the function of the known inhibitory projections from cerebellar nuclei to the inferior olive? The model demonstrates that when combined with a plausible cerebellar learning mechanism that incorporates both LTD and LTP, the loop results in a stable learning system that will adapt to provide the correct output and encourage reciprocal activation.

Notes

1. The Cerebellar model was implemented and tested under NSLJ.

17 Learning to Detour[1]

F. J. Corbacho and A. Weitzenfeld[2]

17.1 Introduction

Anurans (frogs and toads) show quite flexible behavior when confronted with stationary objects on their way to prey or when escaping from a threat. *Rana computatrix* (Arbib, 1987), an evolving computer model of anuran visuomotor coordination, models complex behaviors such as detouring around a stationary barrier to get to prey on the basis of an understanding of anuran prey and barrier recognition, depth perception, and appropriate motor pattern generation mechanisms based on sensory perception. This chapter presents a model of detour in *Rana computatrix* with an extension to learning of new schemas "How are schemas combined to form new schema assemblages acquired for the system to become more efficient?" We describe the construction mechanisms and interactions with the environment necessary to achieve higher levels of detour performance. This chapter describes a model that includes all these phenomena implemented in NSL. More details on some of the model components can be found in (Corbacho and Arbib, 1995) whereas Corbacho et al. (1996) present more behavioral data. This is a specific model in Schema-based Learning (SBL) but it serves to exemplify some of the general points and mechanisms included in the general framework of SBL. For the general framework we refer the reader to (Corbacho, 1998).

In this chapter we present a Schema-based model of learning to detour including different schemas implemented in some cases as functional units and in other cases as neural networks. The motivation for the study of Learning to Detour in frogs as our case study in Schema-based learning (SBL) is three-fold:

1. SBL is constrained by data on a neuro-ethologycally sound system -both the task, the environment and the agent.
2. The study of Rana Computatrix allows for horizontal integration (across many integrated functionalities) and not just vertical integration (action-perception within one central functionality, e.g., saccadic eye movements).
3. Learning to Detour has proved to be a very adaptive process relaying on important processes of learning (Corbacho et al., 1996).

Problem Background

Ingle (1983) and Collett (1983), to cite some examples, have observed that a frog/toad's approach to a prey or avoidance from a threat are also determined by the stationary objects in the animal's surround. A frog or toad, viewing a vertical paling fence barrier through which it can see a worm, may either approach directly to snap at the worm, or detour around the barrier. However, if no worm is visible, the animal does not move. Thus, it is the worm that triggers the animal's response but, when the barrier is present, the animal's trajectory to the worm changes in a way that reflects the relative spatial configuration of the worm and the barrier. Corbacho and Arbib (1995) modeled the different behavioral responses to different barrier configurations, as well as the learning involved in the behavioral transitions. The present section is based on behavioral studies of frogs, *Rana pipiens* (Corbacho et al., 1996). Here we sample a few of our observations of the main capabilities of frogs for detour behavior that set challenges for our learning model.

Experiment I: Barrier 10 cm Wide

Frogs that started from a long enough distance (15–25 cm) in front of a 10cm wide barrier (and with the worm 10 cm behind the barrier) showed (in 95% of the trials) reliable detour behaviors from the first interaction with the 10 cm barrier. They produced an immediate approach movement towards one of the edges of the barrier (see 17.1A). This experiment shows that an adult frog has the capability without training to perform detours when the barrier is narrow enough (10 cm long) and the frog is at a far enough distance (15-20 cm) from the barrier.

Experiment II: Barrier 20 cm wide

From now on we will refer to a frog which has not been exposed to the barrier paradigm as naive. If the chopsticks are placed the same distance apart, so that the gaps have the same width, and the barrier is 20 cm wide, then the naive frog tends to go for the gap in the direction of the prey (this was the case for 88% of the trials). The frog starts out approaching the fence trying to make its way through the gaps. During the first trials with the 20 cm barrier the frog goes straight towards the prey thus bumping into the barrier. When the frog is not able to go through a gap towards the prey it backs-up about 2 cm and then reorients towards one of the neighboring gaps (see figure 17.1B).

Observation: After 2 (43%) or 3 (57%) trials, the frog is already detouring around the barrier without bumping into the barrier (see figure 17.1C). The behavior involves a synergy of both forward and lateral body (sidestep) movements in a very smooth and continuous single movement.

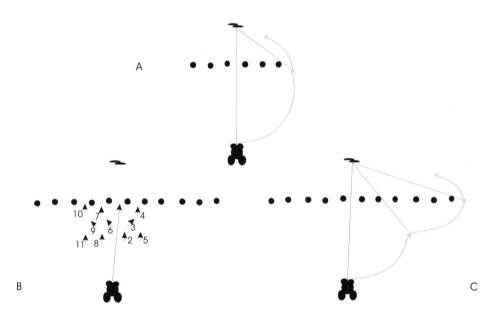

Figure 17.1
A. Approach to prey with single 10 cm barrier interposed. **B.** Approach to prey with single 20 cm barrier interposed: first trial with frog in front of 20 cm barrier (numbers indicate the succession of the movements). **C.** Approach to prey with single 20 cm barrier interposed: after 3 trials with frog in front of 20 cm barrier. Arrowheads indicate the position and orientation of the frog following a single continuous movement after which the frog pauses.

17.2 Model Description

We start by defining the environment and the agent (frog in this case). The environment provides the agent with an interaction space. Ultimately the behavior of any agent is very dependent on its environment so that the behavior can only be understood in relation to the synergy agent-environment. In order to define the structure of the agent we start by defining the spaces of interaction/communication with the environment and then follow with the functional units that constitute the agent.

Definition. An *Environment* is a space that includes a collection of entities and their relations (interactions). A particular instance configuration at time t will be denoted as

Environment(t). *Environment* is a 150x150 grid where different entities e.g., *frog*(x_f,y_f), *barrier*(x_b,y_b,*wh*,*g*). The simulation system contains simplified *Environment* functions designed to allow for an adequate interaction between the simulated agent and its environment, for instance the simulation system performs simple "shifts" of the agent's visual field as it moves in the environment and its coordinates change. The environmental functions will be described in more detail in the Model Architecture section.

Basically, the visual field of the agent corresponds to a sector of the *Environment*, and the coordinates of this sector are updated as the agent moves around. This 2D sector corresponding to the agent's visual field is projected upon the retina of the agent, which is the front-end visual perception system. The agent may also perform several actions that may cause environmental and agent parameters to change.

Component Schemas: Architecture

The detour model incorporates schemas (functional units) and neural modules (structural units) described in table 17.1 and shown in figure 17.2.

Table 17.1
Frog schemas according to their functional (schema level) and structural organization (neural level).

Function	Schema Level Modules	Neural Level Modules
Perceptual	Visual, Depth, Tactile, PreyRec, SoRec	Retina, T5_2layer, TH10layer
Sensorimotor	PreyApproach, SoAvoid	Motor Heading Map (MHM)
Motor	Forward, Orient, Sidestep, Backup	

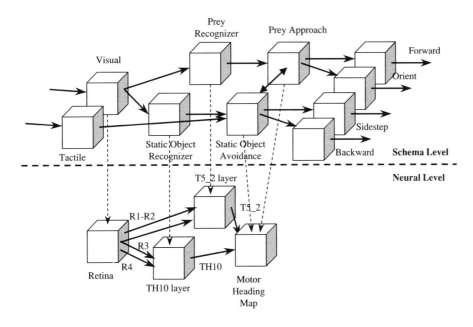

Figure 17.2
Schema Architecture for Detour Model consisting of two levels: a schema level and a neural networks level. The schema level consists of Perceptual Schemas: Visual and Tactile, Prey Recognition, Static Object Recognition (*SOR*); Sensorimotor Schemas: Prey Approach and Static Object Avoidance; and Motor Schemas Orient, Forward, Sidestep and Backup. The neural level consists of four modules: Retina, T5_2layer, TH10layer and the Motor Heading Map (*MHM*).

Perceptual Schemas

Perceptual schemas involve both sensors and recognizers based on these sensors.

Visual

The Visual schema simulates a visual sensor discriminating among different objects in the visual field, mainly prey and barrier in this model.

Depth

The Depth schema generates a depth map for the objects of interest, primarily barrier in order to avoid hitting it and generating appropriate responses according to how close the frog is to it.

Tactile

When the frog hits an object, in the current case the barrier, the Tactile schema gets triggered. The simulation environment checks when the frog comes level with the barrier (equal y-coordinates), and then checks whether there is a passable opening (we have chosen 3 cm wide or more for our simulations—this would change as the frog grows) at the frog's current x-coordinate. If the gap is not passable then the Tactile schema gets triggered:

$$Tactile = \begin{cases} 1 & \text{if } f_y = b_y \text{ and the closest to } f_x \text{ is less than 3cm wise} \\ 0 & \text{otherwise} \end{cases} \qquad (17.1)$$

where (f_x, f_y) are the (x,y) coordinates of the "snout" of the simulated frog in the 2D world, and b_y is the "depth" coordinate of the barrier.

Prey Recognizer

Cervantes-Perez et al. (1985) presented a detailed neural network implementation for prey recognition. Here we present a schema (PreyRec) that approximates this neural network mapping. The presence of prey within the visual field of the animal produces a 2D pattern of activity in the prey recognition system, while absence of prey leaves the system at rest. This is here implemented by simplified feature detectors but it is open to more detailed implementations.

Ewert (1971) found in toad's pretectum near the ventral part of the pct (postero-central thalamic nucleus), units that give continued discharge in the presence of a large dark stationary object. This occurred even when the stationary object was revealed by turning on the room lights without prior motion: Class th10 neurons—with an ERF of about 30–90°—exhibit prolonged discharge to large contrast stimuli that are stationary in their ERF.

Static Object Recognizer

A model of Stationary Object Recognition in anurans was proposed by Lee (1994) based on these findings. In this paper we provide a schema (SorRec) that approximates this model providing the output through the th10 cells map.

Sensorimotor Schemas

Sensorimotor schemas integrate between sensory perception and motor action.

Prey Approach

Epstein (1977) introduced, and Arbib & House (1987) refined, the notion of prey attractant field. A prey sets up a symmetric attractant field whose strength decays gradually with distance from the prey. Arbib & House (1987) described the mask for prey objects as projecting very broadly in the lateral direction and somewhat less broadly in the forward direction This "prey-attractant-field" represents the location of the stimulus accurately as the center of mass of the representation. It also provides the system with neighbor positions available as targets were the accurate position impossible to reach, thus providing the system with a coarse representation of prey location.

PreyApproach projects this excitatory field onto the MHM (motor heading map) explained below. We hypothesize the projection of activity giving rise to coarse coding of prey location.

$$prey(i,j,t)@kp(i,j) \qquad (17.2)$$

where i and j are indices for 2D arrays of neurons, t is time, k_p is a kernel, and @ denotes spatial convolution. In general, each kernel in the present model will be a truncated Gaussian of the general form

$$k(x, y, t) = \begin{cases} W \exp[-(x^2 + y^2)/2s^2] & \text{if } x^2 + y^2 \leq R^2 \\ 0 & \text{otherwise} \end{cases} \tag{17.3}$$

where R is the receptive field size.

Static Object Avoid

Analogously, the model also includes a repellent vector field associated with each fence post. Its effect is more localized to its point of origin than is that of the prey field.

$$th10(i,j,t)@k_s(i,j,\text{t}) \tag{17.4}$$

We hypothesize the inhibitory pattern of connectivity to be also Gaussian shaped.

Bump Avoid

The BumpAvoid schema produces a reorientation that triggers the projection of an activity pattern (with quite large eccentricity) to the *MHM*. This field gives rise to excitation on the neighbor regions thus encoding the reorientation under bumping. It takes the form of

$$reorient(i,t) \tag{17.5}$$

Motor Heading Map

Cobas and Arbib (1992) propose that a motor heading map (*MHM*) determines the direction to jump: i.e., prey-catching and predator avoidance systems share a common map for the heading of the responding movements (coded in body coordinates), as distinct from a common tectal map for the direction of the stimulus. Note that the direction of prey and the direction of prey catching are the same, but the directions of a predator and the escape are different. Thus, in the latter case, the sensory map and the motor map must be distinguished. Projections to the *MHM* must differ depending on whether a visual stimulus is identified as prey, predator or obstacle.

In our model, the outputs of the previously defined schemas (*th10* and *prey(T5_2)* respectively) are projected to *MHM* through kernels.

In the current study the "neural field" generated in the *MHM* will be 1D (vs. 2D *prey* and *th10* maps) - we restrict here to the eccentricity component since the elevation component is not important for the problem at hand. That is, the height of each fence-post (for fences high enough that the frog could not jump over them) does not affect the detour behavior. The eccentricity component which actually represents the target heading angle in the *MHM* will be the key "feature" in determining the sidestep to detour around the barrier.

In our model, then, the total input I_{in} to *MHM* becomes

$$I_{in}(i,t) = \sum_j th10(i, j, t) * k_s(i, j, t) + \sum_j prey(i, j, t) * k_P(i, j) \tag{17.6}$$

Thus the total input to *MHM* when including reorientation due to bumping becomes

$$I_{in}(i,t) = \sum_j th10(i, j, t) * k_s(i, j, t) + \sum_j prey(i, j, t) * k_P(i, j) + reorient(i,t) \tag{17.7}$$

Winner-take-all dynamics over *MHM* assure the selection of the strongest target angle, upon which a transformation from retinotopic to motor coordinates takes place. This is the input (besides different gating signals from the sensory apparatus) to the different motor schemas. The motor schemas are then selected based upon competition and cooperation dynamics. Corbacho and Arbib (1995) present a winner-take-all model (Amari & Arbib, 1977; Didday, 1976) which uses a competition mechanism to obtain a single winner in the network.

Heading Transform

The Heading Map in Cobas and Arbib (1992) is differentially connected with the Orient schema depending on the region represented. The more lateral the stimulus is, the more strongly the Orient schema will be activated. The central portion of the heading map has a very light projection onto the oriented schema, and thus a prey falling into that region will only elicit a weak activation and consequently a very small turning movement or perhaps no turn at all.

We have implemented the transformation from spatially coded to population coded in a similar manner. The output of the sensory motor transformation codes for the amplitude of the target-heading angle. To perform the transformation we use a gradient of weights with a "V" shape. The highest value corresponding to the highest eccentricity.

$$angle(t) = \sum_i gradient(i)^\wedge \Theta[I(i,t)] \tag{17.8}$$

where "$\wedge$" is a pointwise vector multiplication, and implements a thresholding function to avoid producing an orienting response until the motor heading map "settles down" on a target position. Before the winner-take-all dynamics settle down on a "winner" target heading angle several clusters of activity may coexist in MHM corresponding to the representation of several barrier gaps in *MHM*. We use (Eq. 17.8) so that during the winner-take-all dynamics, the cluster of activity with higher amplitude will reach this threshold first as it is growing faster than any of the other clusters of activity. This enables the model to avoid computing a heading angle that could be a linear combination of several clusters of activity in *MHM*.

Motor Schemas

In the current model, motor schemas are implemented as functional units/black boxes schematizing the neural interactions underlying behavior. The intrinsic motor patterns or muscle activations are not simulated. When active they simply change the coordinates of the agent (and/or environmental parameters) appropriately.

We postulate that each component of the behavior (sidestep, orient, approach, snap, etc.) is governed by a specific motor schema. We then see detour behavior as an example of the coordination of motor schemas. Ingle (1980, 1983) has offered some clues as to the possible neural correlates of the various schemas. Apparently, thalamic and tectal visual mechanism can operate somewhat independently (Ingle, 1973). Monocular frogs without a contralateral optic tectum can quite accurately localize barriers, and while visual input to the pretectal region of the caudal thalamus mediates barrier avoidance behavior, caudal thalamic lesions produce an inability to sidestep stationary barriers set in the frog's path during pursuit of prey.

Among other motor schemas we provide the system with forward movement and lateral (sidestep) movement. The forward schema when active produces a movement in the direction of the midsagittal axis of the body with frontal direction. The lateral sidestep movement is a movement orthogonal to the sagittal midline. Backup movement is similar to forward but in the opposite direction.

Cobas and Arbib (1992) proposed a general mechanism of motor pattern selection through the interaction of motor schemas. *MHM* contains target location but motor schema selection is the result of competition of many maps. Each of the motor schemas has a threshold so that its action on the controlled musculature is only enabled when its internal level of activation reaches or surpasses that threshold.

Schema Dynamics

Schemas consist of schema behavioral mappings and schema activity variables. The full formalization is beyond the scope of this chapter; here simply mention that schemas correspond formally to port automata with activity variables indicating the degree of confidence. The schema activity dynamics is described by the leaky integrator. The equation describing the dynamics of the schema activity variables is

$$\tau_i \frac{ds_i(t)}{dt} = -s_i(t) + \sum_j S_j(t) \cdot R_{i,j}(t)$$ (17.9)

where S is the result of a saturation by a sigmoid transfer function that guarantees that the activity variables remain within the interval [-1, 1],

$$S_i(t) = \Theta(s_i(t))$$ (17.10)

R is the matrix of support. It indicates how the activation of a schema supports the activation of another schema. The leaky integrators time constants may be different for different schema activation variables since some schemas may have a faster dynamics e.g. Tactile must reset quickly and with it BumpAvoid.

Schema Assertion

Schema assertion takes place when the schema activity variable surpasses certain threshold hence indicating enough confidence on the application of that particular schema to the particular context. Once asserted the schema mapping output is produced, this pattern may in turn become the input for other schema mapping output. For many schemas once they are asserted they must be reset to avoid successive unrealistic activations. For instance once a motor schema has been asserted its activity variable is reset to 0.

Schema Interactions

There are some "reflex" dynamics corresponding to fast pathways e.g. Tactile activates Backup in one step (instantiation and activation). Also Tactile must reset quickly and with it BumpAvoid. Tactile momentarily inhibits Forward since otherwise Forward would be too active and lower down Backup activity variable to the point where Backup could not get activated. In general many schemas will be simultaneously active interacting with each other, for instance Sidestep and Forward schemas are simultaneously active when "detouring" after learning.

17.3 Model Implementation

The **Detour** model is composed of the **World** module—a 3D input stimulus library, **Prey** and **Frog** modules, as shown in figure 17.3. The static objects, in this case the **Barrier**, are interactively specified from the scripting language as opposed to the other two.

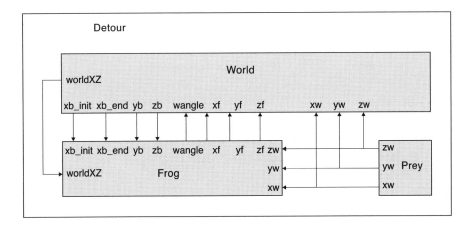

Figure 17.3
Schema Architecture showing the top-level world topology.

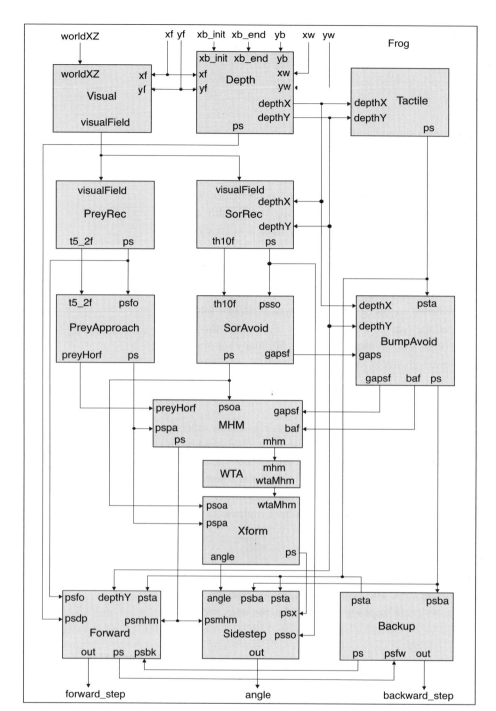

Figure 17.4
Schema Architecture showing the frog schemas topology.

World

We have provided for simple interactions with the *World* module. We simulate a simplified 3D environment by defining two different 2D projections or views: *worldXY* corresponding to the top down view only available to the user, and *worldXZ* corresponding to the view of an agent immersed in the environment. The *worldXZ* view is used as visual input to the frog.

The model takes advantage of the input layer components (see Appendix III for details) in generating external visual stimuli. A **NslInputFloat3** 3d input layer of **sizex1xsizex2** in the *x*-direction and **sizez1xsizez2** in the *z*-direction is instantiated by the *World* module as follows,

```
private NslInputFloat3 in(sizex1,sizex2,sizez1,sizez2);
```

Note that a the **NslInputFloat3** input layer actually involves two **NslInputFloat2** layers: an *xy*-matrix and a *xz*-matrix corresponding two the two different views in the 3d space. Input processing takes places as follows,

```
public void simRun(){
    ...
    in.run();
    worldXZ = in.get_xzview();
}
```

The *in* object is processed by applying a the *run* method to it. This generates a new *xy*-matrix together with a new *xz*-matrix assigned to *worldXZ* for further processing in the model.

Prey

The prey (worm in this case) is a static entity (although movement can be added to it, such as twiggling). In the current version the prey is described by its location and size.

Barrier

The obstacle (barrier in this case) is also a static entity composed of multiple posts separated by gaps, wide enough to let the frog see the prey behind it. The barrier gaps don't let the frog pass through it and are tall enough so the Frog won't jump over it. The size and gaps between barrier posts can be modified interactively as will be seen later on.

Frog

The agent (frog in this model) is the heart to the detour model. The frog model includes a number of perceptual, sensorimotor and motor schemas instantiated within the frog, as shown in figure 17.4, and described each in the following sections.

Perceptual Schemas

Perception for the frog in the model is based on **Visual** and **Tactile** sensors, where also **Depth** is computed. In particular, the frog perceives the prey, **PreyRec** (Prey Recognizer), and the barrier, **SoRec** (Static Object Recognizer).

Visual

The visual input to the frog correspond to 2D image projections of the virtual 3D world reflected on the eyes (or camera) of the agent. The model computes a *visualField* corresponding to the section of *worldXZ* that the frog can see at each time step. As the frog moves - frog coordinates *xf, yf* change - the *visualField* needs to be recomputed.

The **simRun** methods computes the new *visualField* from the complete *worldXZ* view depending on the size of its receptor field *recsize*

```
public void simRun()
{
    int recsize = visualField.getRows();
    int isize = worldXZ.getRows();
    int jsize = worldXZ.getCols();

    visualField = worldXZ.getSector(isize-recsize,isize-1,
        jsize/2-recsize/2,jsize/2+recsize/2-1);
}
```

The *getSector* method obtains the portion of the *worldXZ* view perceived by *visual-Field*.

Depth

The **Depth** module computes the distance in both *x* (*depthX*) and *y* (*depthY*) to the barrier or prey depending on the Frog's current position in the world. This information is passed to the static object recognition and bump avoidance modules as well as the Forward module in avoiding hitting the barrier. The module output *ps* is a confidence level describing when *depthY* is greater than *safeDistance*, where *safeDistance* corresponds to the minimum distance the Frog should be to avoid hitting the barrier.

The **simRun** method computes the dynamic location of the frog, and then calculates through simple subtractions the depth of the barrier and finally the *ps* confidence level that the frog is not too close to the barrier as output to other modules.

```
public void simRun()
{

...

if (depthY > safeDistance || depthX > safeDistance)
     ps = 2.0;                  // Go up fast
   else
     ps = 0.0;
}
```

Tactile

The **Tactile** module simulates the frog hitting the barrier from its current position to the barrier computed by **Depth**.

The **simRun** method computes the output confidence level *ps* depending on whether the frog is close enough, both *x* and *y*, to the barrier.

```
public void simRun()
{
   if (depthY > 0 && depthY <= safeDistance &&
    depthX <= safeDistance)
     ps = 2;             // Go up fast
   else
     ps = 0.0;
   ps = nslSigma(ps, -1.0, 1.0, -1.0, 1.0);
}
```

Prey Recognizer

The *Prey Recognizer* (**PreyRec**) module recognizes and localizes prey stimuli within the visual field of the frog. The *Prey* is defined as a set of features. In this particular implementation we have simplified this perceptual schema a great deal (see Corbacho and Arbib 1995 for a more detailed implementation). The module receives *visualField* input from the frog visual module and generates both an output confidence level and simulates the behavior of the *t5_2* neural cells.

The **simRun** method computes the prey recognizer output in terms of filtering the *visualField* for a prey stimulus.

```
public void simRun()
{
    t5_2 = DetourLib.filter(visualField,2);
    if (nslSum(t5_2) >= 1)
        ps=0.9;
    else
        ps=0;
    ps = nslSigma(ps,-1.0,1.0,-1.0,1.0);
    if (ps > th)
        t5_2f = nslRamp(t5_2);
    else
        t5_2f = 0;
}
```

In particular

$$t5\_2 = DetourLib.filter(visualField, 2); \qquad (17.11)$$

defines a prey in terms of a feature "2" corresponding to preys. The function filters out all elements in the matrix that do not have a corresponding value, in this case "2". This filtering function can be made more realistic including color, spatial frequency, complex shape filters, etc.

The output $t5\_2$ is still a 2D map representing the *retinotopic* position of the prey (vs. allocentric prey coordinates).

Since this is a "seed" perceptual schema it must also provide "seed support" for its schema activation variable *ps*.

$$ps = \begin{cases} 0.9 & \text{if nslSum}(t5\_2) >= 1 \\ 0 & \text{otherwise} \end{cases} \qquad (17.12)$$

Then, once the schema is asserted, $ps > th$,

$$t5\_2f = \text{nslRamp}(t5\_2); \qquad (17.13)$$

corresponding to the activation of the output port.

Static Object Recognizer

The *Static Object Recognizer* (**SoRec**) module recognizes and localizes static objects within the visual field of the frog. The *Static Object* is defined as a set of features. The module receives *visualField* input from the frog visual module and generates both an output confidence level and simulates the behavior of the *th10* neural cells.

The **simRun** method computes the prey recognizer output in terms of filtering the *visualField* for a barrier.

```
public void simRun()
{
    th10 = DetourLib.filter(visualField, 1);
    if (nslSum(th10) >= 1)
        ps=0.9;
    else
        ps=0;
    ps = nslSigma(ps,-1.0,1.0,-1.0,1.0);
    if (ps > th)
        th10f = nslRamp(th10);
    else
        th10f = 0;
}
```

Similarly to the *Prey Recognizer*, the stationary object recognition *filter stationary objects*,

$$th10 = DetourLib.filter(visualField, 1); \qquad (17.14)$$

corresponding to feature "1" defining stationary objects.

Then, once the schema is asserted, $ps > th$,

$$th10f = \mathrm{nslRamp}(th10); \qquad (17.15)$$

corresponding to the activation of the output port.

Sensorimotor Schemas

The frog model incorporates a number of sensorimotor schemas: **PreyApproach**, **SoAvoid**, **BumpAvoid**, Motor Heading Map (**MHM**) and Heading Transform (**Xform**).

Prey Approach

The **PreyApproach** module integrates the horizontal projection of $t5\_2$ cells generating a 1D representation (parcellation), since it is more efficient to make the 1D projection before convolving with the gaussian kernel. *preyHor* corresponds to the eccentricity component of the *prey attractant field* (horizontal component).

The **initSys** method reinitializes variables to 0, sets the confidence level input weight *rs* to 1, and initializes the excitatory gaussian kernel $t5\_2\_erf$,

```
public void initSys()
{
    preyHor = 0;
    preyHorf = 0;
    rsfo = 1.0; // Prey & Prey Approach.
    ps = 0;
    DetourLib.gauss2D(t5_2_erf,t5_2_erf_sig);
    t5_2_rf = t5_2_erf_wgt * t5_2_erf;
}
```

The **simRun** method computes the module activity,

```
public void simRun()
{
    preyF = t5_2_rf * t5_2f;
    preyHor = nslReduceRow(preyF); // Parcellation:
        horizontal comp
    ps = rsfo*psfo;
    ps = nslSigma(ps,-1.0,1.0,-1.0,1.0);
    if (ps > th) {
        float mx = nslMax(prey_hor);
        if (mx != 0.0)
            prey_hor_f = prey_hor/mx; // Normalize.
    }
    else
        prey_hor_f = 0;
}
```

Once the schema is asserted, *PreyHor* contains the field (normalized by the maximum value) to be projected to the other modules (e.g. *MHM*).

Static Object Avoid

The *SorAvoid* schema is implemented in a similar manner. IT integrates *th10Hor* as the 1D horizontal component corresponding to a parcellated representation (C&A95). *Gaps* corresponds to the inhibitory obstacle repellent field. Once the schema is asserted, *gapsf*, which is normalized by the maximum value, is projected to the other schemas (e.g. *MHM*).

The **initSys** method reinitializes variables to 0, sets the confidence level input weight *rs* to 1, and initializes the inhibitory gaussian kernel *tm_irf* and the final resulting kernel *tm_rf*

```
public void initSys()
{
    rsso = 1.0; // Obstacle & Obstacle Avoid
    ps = 0;
    DetourLib.gauss1D(tm_irf,tm_irf_sig);
    tm_rf = - tm_irf_wgt * tm_irf;
}
```

The **simRun** method computes the schema activity,

```
public void simRun()
{
    th10Hor = nslReduceRow(th10f); // Parcellation (from 2D to 1D)
    gaps = tm_rf * th10Hor;          // Convolve with kernel
    ps = rsso*psso;
    ps = nslSigma(ps,-1.0,1.0,-1.0,1.0);
    if (ps > th) {
        float mx = nslMax(gaps*-1);
        if (mx != 0.0)
        gapsf = gaps/mx;
    }
    else
        gapsf = 0;
}
```

Bump Avoid

The **BumpAvoid** schema contains two components: field projection *baf* for reorientation (avoid keeping bumping on the same point) and, tuning of the *SorAvoid* module.

The **simRun** method computes the activity as follows

```
public void simRun()
{
    if (depthY <= safeDistance && depthX <= safeDistance)
        //Bumping ps = 0;
    else
        ps = -1.0;          // Go down fast: -2.0
    if (tune_tm < 1.5)          // saturate tune_tm.
            tune_tm = tune_tm + tune_tm_base;
    tune_tm_layer = tune_tm;
    tune_tm_layer = tune_tm_layer ^ nslStep(-gaps);
    gaps = gaps - tune_tm_layer;
    gapsf = gaps;
    ps = ps + rsta*psta;
    ps = nslSigma(ps,-1.0,1.0,-1.0,1.0);
    if (ps > th){
        field_center = field_center + 2;
        baf[field_center.getValue()] = field_A;
    }
    else
        baf = 0;
}
```

The function modulates the kernel. Every time it bumps it increases *tune_tm* until it reaches a saturation point. It tunes the bump avoid field by increasing eccentricity, modulating only already active neurons. Every bump it increases *tune_tm* until it reaches a saturation point.

Motor Heading Map

The *Motor Heading Map (MHM)* schema then integrates the different fields *preyHorf*, *gapsf* and, *baf*. Another input to *MHM, in,* contains further modulating fields learned by the system. In particular, it will contain fields generated by newly constructed schemas (e.g. detour schema, at the moment the only one in the model).

The **simRun** method computes the schema activity,

```
public void simRun()
{
    if (d_mhm > d_norm && gapsf ! = 0)
    {
        baf[field_center.getValue()] = field_A;
        in = baf; // New Field "inserted"
    }
    else
        in = 0; // reset input (cf. antidromic
    mhm_hat = mhm;

    // Predictive MHM.
    mhm = gapsf + preyHorF + baf + in;
    // Fields over MHM.
    d_mhm = 0.03 * DetourLib.dist(mhm, mhm_hat);
    ps = ps + rspa*pspa + rsoa*psoa;
    ps = nslSigma(ps,-1.0,1.0,-1.0,1.0);
}
```

The above code computes the dynamics of Motor Heading Map (MHM), integrating several fields, while new fields can also be added while learning. The "if" section computes learning dynamics. It detects an incoherence and hence a trigger for a new schema.

Heading Transform

The *winner take all* selects a single target where *maxim* returns the vector normalized (subtraction) by its maximum, where only the maximum is above threshold (by 0.01).

```
public void simRun()
{
    wta_mhm = DetourLib.maxim(mhm);
}
```

Heading Transform

The *Xform* schema transforms from retinotopic (vector) to population code (scalar) the representation of the target.

The **simRun** method computes the schema activity,

```
public void simRun()
{
    int i = nslAvgMaxValue(wta_mhm);
    angle = 0;
    if (i != 0)
        angle = i - wta_mhm.getRows()/2;
    ps = ps + rspa*pspa + rsoa*psoa;
    ps = nslSigma(ps,-1.0,1.0,-1.0,1.0);
}
```

The method computes the transformation to population coding corresponding to

$$angle = \text{nslSum}(gradient \wedge wtaMhm); \tag{17.16}$$

coding the heading angle as a scalar (cf. population coding).

Motor Schemas

We have included three motor schemas as explained in the Model Description section, *forward*, *sidestep* and *backup*.

Forward

The **Forward** motor schema receives confidence contributions from other schemas as well as depth information to avoid hitting the barrier. *step* is a scalar coding the amplitude of forward movement. The **simRun** method computes the motor schema activity,

```
public void simRun()
{
    ps = ps + rsfo*psfo + rsta*psta + rsdp*psdp +
    rsmhm*psmhm + rsbk*psbk;
    ps = nslSigma(ps,-1.0,1.0,-1.0,1.0);
    if (ps > th) {
        ps = -1.0; // Reset
        out = step;
    }
    else
        out = 0;
}
```

Sidestep

The **Sidestep** motor schema receives confidence contributions from other schemas. *angle* is a scalar coding the amplitude of the sidesteps. The **simRun** method computes the motor schema activity,

```
public void simRun()
{
    ps = ps + rsso*psso + rsta*psta + rsba*psba + rsmhm*psmhm +
    rsx*psx;
    ps = nslSigma(ps,-1.0,1.0,-1.0,1.0);
    out = angle;
    if (ps > th) {
        ps = 0; // -1.0; // Reset
    }
}
```

Backup

The **Backup** motor schema receives confidence contributions from other schemas. *step* is a scalar coding the amplitude of the backup movement (we omit the sign). The **simRun** method computes the motor schema activity,

```
public void simRun()
{
    ps = ps + rsta*psta + rsba*psba + rsfw*psfw;
    ps = nslSigma(ps,-1.0,1.0,-1.0,1.0);
    if (ps > th) {
        ps = -1.0; // Reset
        out = step;
    }
    else
        out = 0;
}
```

Learning Dynamics

Schema dynamics previously presented are a simplification of Relaxation Labeling (Hummel & Zucker, 1983). Additionally, we provide a broad description of some of the learning mechanisms involved in both constructing a new schema and in tuning a existing schema. For the overall Schema-Based Learning (*SBL*) framework please refer to (Corbacho, 1998).

Schema Learning

We explain how a "new" field of activity over *mhm* is able to reproduce a previously successful pattern of interaction. Concretely the field of activity projected over *mhm* that caused the frog to reach the edge of the barrier.

Learning of a new schema is triggered when incoherence is detected. In this case the unexpected interaction when the frog gets to the edge of the barrier is reflected internally as incoherence in *mhm*. For every field projecting to *mhm* the predictive response is calculated by simply storing the previous value corresponding to the result of activating that field.

$$mhm\_hat(t+1) = mhm(t) \qquad (17.17)$$

The incoherence is measured as the distance between the current and the expected result,

$$d\_mhm(t+1) = Detour\_lib.dist(mhm(t+1), mhm\_hat(t+1)) \qquad (17.18)$$

when the incoherence is larger than a threshold it indicates "unexpected". In this case the "culprit" is the field of activity *baf* (triggered by the *BumpAvoid* schema in the first place), and hence this field is internally stored so that it can be "played back" in future interactions with the barrier.

$$\text{if } (d\_mhm > d\_norm) \qquad (17.19)$$
$$in = baf$$

On second presentation of the barrier *in* (reflecting a pattern of activity similar to *baf*) projects a field of activity over *mhm* which in turn gives rise to a large value in *angle* hence activating the *Sidestep* motor schema and detouring around the barrier.

Schema Tuning

In terms of schema tuning, the kernel for *SorAvoid* is tuned every time the *BumpAvoid* schema is asserted.

$$\text{if } (tune\_tm < 1.5) \qquad (17.20)$$
$$tune\_tm = tune\_tm + tune\_tm\_base$$

Additionally in *tuningField*

$$tune\_tm\_layer = tune\_tm \wedge nslStep(-gapsf) \qquad (17.21)$$
$$gapsf = gapsf - tune\_tm\_layer \qquad (17.22)$$

updates the field obstacle avoidance field (*gapsf*) by subtracting the modulation component.

17.4 Simulation and Results[1]

Different experiments were carried varying the barrier size (10cm and 20cm) as well as applying learning to the 20cm barrier experiment. The main simulation files are described in table 17.2:

File	Description
detour.nsl	contains all the model parameters
detour_sti.nsl	contains all the model stimulus specifications
detour_fields.nsl	displays different fields
detour_env.nsl	displays a top down and visual view of the environment

Table 17.2
NSLS script files needed to run the different simulations.

To execute the model do:

```
nsl source detour
nsl run
```

The stimuli specifications are done using the NSL input library described in Appendix III. The *detour_sti.nsl* file includes parameters for the input layer as follows,

```
nsl set detour.world.in.dx 1
nsl set detour.world.in.dy 1
nsl set detour.world.in.dz 1
nsl set detour.world.in.xz 0
nsl set detour.world.in.yz 0
nsl set detour.world.in.zz 0
```

The worm specification is given by an input stimulus defined from the NSL input library as follows,

```
nsl create BlockStim prey -layer detour.world.in -val 2 \
    -xc $xw -yc $yw -zc $zw -dx 1 -dy 1 -dz 1 -spec_type center
```

Note that all variables preceded by the "$" symbol corresponds to variable values from Tcl (see the NSLS scripting language description in chapter 7). The values for these variables are chosen according to the particular experiment selected through variables *learning* and *trial* as will be described next.

The frog specification is given similarly by an input stimulus defined from the NSL input library as follows,

```
nsl create BlockStim frog -layer detour.world.in -val 1 \
    -xc $xf -yc $yf -zc $zf -dx 3 -dy 3 -dz 3 -spec_type center
```

The barrier (or fence) specification is a little more involved given this time by a set of input stimuli defined from the NSL input library as follows,

```
for {set xb $xb_init} {$xb <= $xb_end} {incr xb $gap} {
    nsl create BlockStim fence -layer detour.world.in -val 1 \
        -x0 $xb -y0 $yb -z0 $zb -dx 1 -dy 1 -dz 100 -spec_type
            corner
}
```

Note that in the above specification the notation and expressions correspond to the NSLS scripting language extended from Tcl as described in chapter 7.

Experiment I

For experiment I (barrier 10 cm wide) set the following variable in *detour_sti.nsl*

```
set learning 0
set trial 10
```

After executing "nsl run" the system displays on one of the windows the different module fields as shown in figure 17.5.

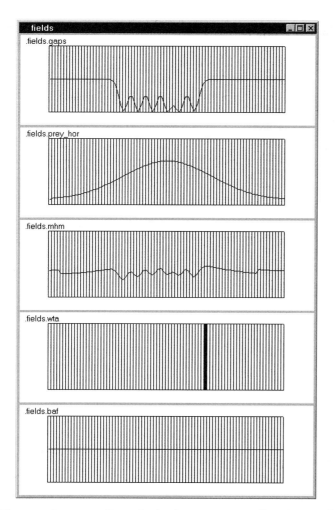

Figure 17.5
Different activity fields for the 10cm barrier experiment due to *visual_field* processing in the frog with the exception of the bottom one processed after the *tactile* field. The top display (*gaps*) shows the repulsive field generated from the barrier (note that it is negative). The next display down (*prey_hor*) represents the attraction field generated from the prey (note that it is positive). The next display down (*mhm*) represents the combined *gaps* and *prey_hor* fields. The next display down (*wta*) represents the winner-take-all element from the above *mhm* field. This winning element results in the heading or frog's orientation when moving forwards. The last display (*baf*) is currently empty and represents activity due to bumping against the barrier.

The most important factor in the frog movement direction results from the *wta* field, resulting itself from the combination of the prey attraction and barrier repulsion fields. In this experiment the direction of movement is towards the side of the barrier, heading towards the right since the frog was positioned just a bit to the right from the axis joining the center of the prey and barrier. The resulting path motion is shown in figure 17.6.

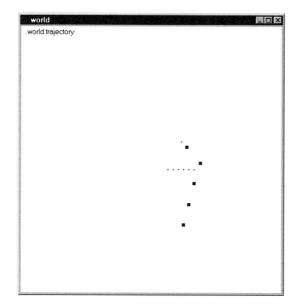

Figure 17.6
Rana Computatrix interacting with the 10 cm wide barrier. Note how the frog heads itself towards the side of the barrier.

Experiment II

For experiment II (barrier 20 cm wide) set the following variable in *detour_sti.nsl*

```
set learning 0
set trial 20
```

After executing "nsl run" the system displays on one of the windows the different module fields as shown in figure 17.7.

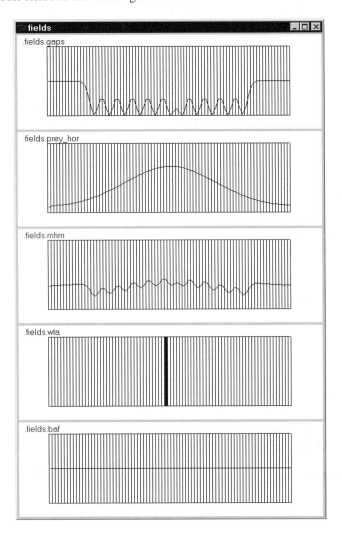

Figure 17.7

Different activity fields for the 20cm barrier experiment before bumping due to *visual_field* processing in the frog with the exception of the bottom one processed after the *tactile* field. The top display (*gaps*) shows the repulsive field generated from the barrier (note that it is negative). The next display down (*prey_hor*) represents the attraction field generated from the prey (note that it is positive). The next display down (*mhm*) represents the combined *gaps* and *prey_hor* fields. The next display down (*wta*) represents the winner-take-all element from the above *mhm* field. This winning element results in the heading or frog's orientation when moving forwards. The last display (*baf*) is currently empty and represents activity due to bumping against the barrier.

Again, the most important factor in the frog movement direction results from the *wta* field, resulting itself from the combination of the prey attraction and barrier repulsion fields. In this experiment the direction of movement before bumping into the barrier is towards the middle of the barrier. Once the frog hits the barrier a bumping (*baf*) field is generated. The purpose of this field is to redirect the movement towards a different heading. Before that occurs the frog will backup. The resulting field after bumping is shown in figure 17.8.

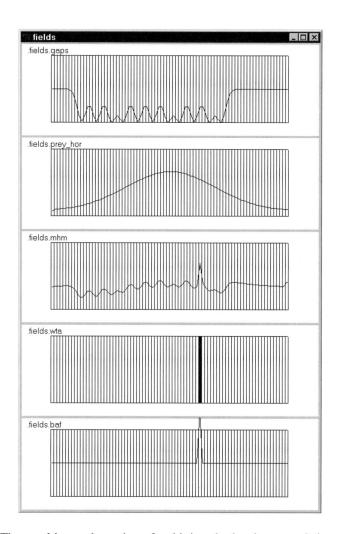

Figure 17.8
Different activity fields for the 20cm barrier experiment after bumping due to *visual_field* processing in the frog with the exception of the bottom one processed after the *tactile* field. The top display (*gaps*) shows the repulsive field generated from the barrier (note that it is negative). The next display down (*prey_hor*) represents the attraction field generated from the prey (note that it is positive). The next display down (*mhm*) represents the combined *gaps* and *prey_hor* fields. The next display down (*wta*) represents the winner-take-all element from the above *mhm* field. This winning element results in the heading or frog's orientation when moving forwards. The last display (*baf*) is represents activity due to bumping against the barrier.

The resulting path motion after hitting the barrier several times is shown in figure 17.9.

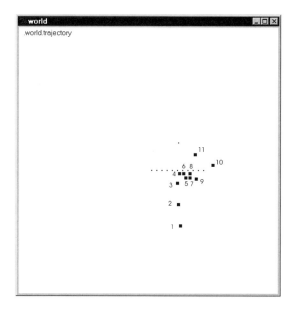

Figure 17.9
Rana Computatrix interacting with the 20 cm barrier before learning. We have added numbers corresponding to the frog's position in time. In this experiment the frog hits the barrier three times before perceiving the side of the barrier.

Experiment III

For experiment III (barrier 20 cm wide with learning) set the following variable in *detour_sti.nsl*

```
set learning 1
set trial 20
```

We change the threshold of *d_norm* to simulate that after one interaction with the 20cm barrier the frog would have learned and from then on it would detour when presented with the 20 cm barrier. The resulting behavior is shown in figure 17.10.

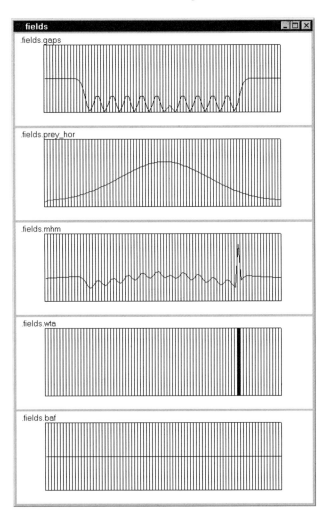

Figure 17.10

Different activity fields for the 20cm barrier experiment after learning due to *visual_field* processing in the frog with the exception of the bottom one processed after the *tactile* field. The top display (*gaps*) shows the repulsive field generated from the barrier (note that it is negative). The next display down (*prey_hor*) represents the attraction field generated from the prey (note that it is positive). The next display down (*mhm*) represents the combined *gaps* and *prey_hor* fields. The next display down (*wta*) represents the winner-take-all element from the above *mhm* field. This winning element results in the heading or frog's orientation when moving forwards. The last display (*baf*) is currently empty and represents activity due to bumping against the barrier.

Note that although no bumping occurs, the *mhm* field involves a similar integration where heading is explicitly generated, in this case by learning. The resulting behavior is shown in figure 17.11.

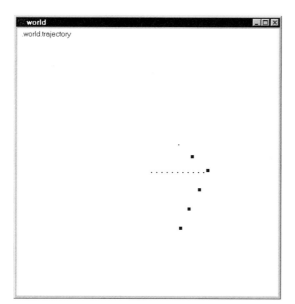

Figure 17.11
Rana Computatrix interacting with the 20 cm wide barrier after learning.

17.5 Summary

The model explains basic facts about detour behavior. If the retinotopic representation of the edge of the barrier in *SorRec* falls within the prey-attractant-field spread, then the summation of activity from the prey-attractant-field and from the *SOR*-repellent map on *MHM* at the retinotopic position just beyond the barrier's edge is stronger then the summation at the "center" of the barrier where the prey is located. Hence, the winner-take-all dynamics will select the cluster of activity corresponding to the retinotopic position of the edge of the barrier, thus predicting that frogs would detour around narrow barriers. On the other hand, for wide barriers the prey-attractant-field extent falls within a much wider barrier field. Hence, at the *MHM* retinotopic position corresponding to the barrier's edge there will be no input activity from the prey map. On the other hand, there will be a great projection of activity on *MHM* at the retinotopic position of the prey; and this in turn will trigger approach to a point within the barrier map, so long as the peak of prey attraction exceeds the trough of barrier inhibition. Thus, the model predicts that the naive frog would approach wide barriers rather than detour around them.

Notes

1. Preparation of this paper was supported in part by award number IBN-9411503 for Collaborative Research (M.A. Arbib and A. Weerasuriya, co-Principal Investigators) from the National Science Foundation.

2. A. Weitzenfeld developed the NSL3.0 version and extended the original NSL2.1 model implementation written by F. Corbacho as well as contributed Section 17.3 and part of 17.4 to this chapter.

3. The Detour model was implemented and tested under NSLC.

18 Face Recognition by Dynamic Link Matching[1]

L. Wiskott, C. von der Malsburg and A. Weitzenfeld[2]

We present here a biologically motivated system for invariant and robust recognition of objects from camera images. It originally arose from a homework assignment for a course of neural network self-organization at USC, and in a way it can be seen as a serious test of NSL's maturity as a (neural) simulation tool. Formulated as a large system of coupled non-linear differential equations comprising altogether approximately 3 million variables, its development required extensive series of experiments and continuous graphical monitoring of large sets of variables. Not only did NSL support this process, requiring just minor extensions, but it now makes our system directly accessible to students and colleagues for close inspection and for further development.

Our model is based on the principles of temporal feature binding and dynamic link matching. Objects are stored in the form of two-dimensional aspects. These are competitively matched against current images. During the matching process, complete matrices of dynamic links between the image and all models are refined by a process of rapid self-organization, the final state connecting only corresponding points in image and object models. As a data format for representing images we use local sets ("jets") of Gabor-based wavelets. We have tested the performance of our system by having it recognize human faces against databases of more than one hundred images. The system is invariant with respect to retinal position, and it is robust with respect to head rotation, scale, facial deformation, and illumination.

18.1 Introduction

For the theoretical biologist, the greatest challenge posed by the brain is its tremendous power to generalize from one situation to others. This ability is probably most concretely epitomized in terms of invariant object recognition—the capability of the visual system to pick up the image of an object and recognize that object later in spite of variations in retinal location (as well as other important changes such as size, orientation, changed perspective and background, deformation, illumination, and noise). This capability has been demonstrated by flashing the image of novel objects briefly at one foveal position, upon which subjects were able to recognize the objects in a different foveal position (and under rotation in depth) (B & Gerhardstein 1993).

The conceptual grandfather of many of the neural models of invariant object recognition is Rosenblatt's four-layer perceptron (Rosenblatt 1961). Its first layer is the sensory or retinal surface. Its second layer contains detectors of local features (that is, small patterns) in the input layers. Each one of these is characterized by a feature type and a position x. The third layer contains position-invariant feature detectors, each of which is characterized by a feature type and is to respond to the appearance of its feature type anywhere on the input layer. It is enabled to do so by a full set of connections from all of the cells of the same feature type in the second layer. Thus, the appearance of a pattern in any position of the input layer leads to the activation of the same set of cells in the third layer. Layer four now contains linear decision units which detect the appearance of certain sets of active cells in the third layer and thus of certain objects imaged into the input layer. A decision unit contains an implicit model of an object in the form of a weighted list of third-layer features to be present or absent.

The four-layer perceptron has to contend with the difficulty that a set of feature types has to be found on the basis of which the presence or absence of a given pattern becomes linearly separable on the basis of the un-ordered feature lists displayed by the third layer.

If the feature types employed are too indistinct, there is the danger that different patterns lead to identical third-layer activity, just because the only difference between the patterns is a different spatial arrangement of their features. The danger can be reduced or avoided with the help of feature types of sufficient complexity. However, this is a problematic route itself, since highly complex features are either very numerous (and therefore costly to install) or they are very specific to a given pattern domain (and have to be laboriously trained or hand-designed into the system and limit the system's applicability to the pattern domain). The difficulty arises from the fact that on the way from layer two to layer three position information is discarded for each feature individually (as is required by the condition of position invariance), so that also information on relative position of the features is lost (which creates the potential confusion).

In the study presented here we are solving the indicated problem using a double strategy. Firstly, we employ highly complex features which are constructed during presentation of individual patterns (and which are stored individually for each pattern later to be recognized), and secondly, we employ a data format and a pattern matching procedure (between our equivalent of Rosenblatt's layers two and three) which represent and preserve relative position information for features.

The features we employ are constructed from image data in a two-step process. First, elementary features in the form of Gabor-based wavelets of a number of scales and a number of orientations are extracted from the image (Daugman 1988), giving a set of response values for each point of the image, then the vector of those response values for a given point are treated as a complex feature, which we call a jet. Jets are extracted from an array of sample points in the image (the approach is described in detail in (Lades et al. 1993)).

Our system is explicit in its representation of analogs for layers two and three, which we call "image domain" and "model domain", respectively. The image domain is an array of (16x17) nodes, each node being labeled by a jet when an image is presented. The model domain is actually a composite of a large number (more than one hundred in some of our simulations) of layers ("models") composed of arrays of (10x10) nodes. To store the image of an object (e.g., a human face) a new model is created in the model domain and its nodes are labeled by copying an array of jets from the appropriate part of the image domain.

To recognize an object, the system attempts to competitively match all stored object models against the jet array in the image domain, a process which we call "Dynamic Link Matching." The winning model is identified as the object recognized. The two domains are coupled by a full matrix of connections between nodes, which is initialized with similarity values between image jets and model jets. (This can be seen as our version of Rosenblatt's feature-preserving connections.) The matching process is formulated in terms of dynamical activity variables for the image and model layers (forming localized blobs of activity in both domains), for the momentary strengths of connections between the domains (we assume that synaptic weights change rapidly and reversibly during the recognition process), and for the relative recognition status of each model. The matching process enforces the condition that neighboring nodes in the image layer link up with neighboring nodes in a model layer. In this way the system suppresses the feature rearrangement ambiguity of the Rosenblatt scheme.

Our model cannot be implemented (at least not in any obvious way) in conventional neural networks. Its implementation is, however, easily possible if two particular features are assumed to be realized in the nervous system, temporal feature binding and rapid reversible synaptic plasticity. Both features have been proposed as fundamental components of neural architecture in (von der Malsburg 1981). Temporal feature binding has in the mean time been widely discussed in the neuroscience literature and has received some

---

experimental basis (König and Engel 1995). Although rapid synaptic weight changes have been discussed (Crick 1982) and reported in the literature (Zucker 1989), the quasi-Hebbian control and the time course for rapid reversible plasticity which is implied and required here must still wait for experimental validation.

18.2 Model Description

Principle of Dynamic Link Matching

In Dynamic Link Matching (DLM), the image and all models are represented by layers of neurons, which are labeled by jets as local features (see figure 18.1). Jets are vectors of Gabor wavelet components (see Lades et al. 1993; Wiskott et al. 1997) and a robust description of the local gray value distribution. The initial connectivity is all-to-all with synaptic weights depending on the similarities between the jets. In each layer, neural activity dynamics generates one small moving blob of activity (the blob can be interpreted as covert attention scanning the image or model). If a model is similar in feature distribution to the image, its initial connectivity matrix contains a strong regular component, connecting corresponding points (which by definition have high feature similarity), plus noise in the form of accidental similarities. Hence the blobs in the image and that model tend to align and synchronize in the sense of simultaneously activating, and thus generating correlations, between corresponding regions. These correlations are used, in a process of rapid reversible synaptic plasticity, to restructure the connectivity matrix. The mapping implicit in the signal correlations is more regularly structured than the connectivity itself, and correlation-controlled plasticity thus improves the connectivity matrix. Iteration of this game rapidly leads to a neighborhood preserving one-to-one mapping connecting neurons with similar features, thus providing translation invariance as well as robustness against distortions.

Figure 18.1
DLM between image and model. The nodes are indicated by black dots, and their local features are symbolized by different textures. The synaptic weights of the initial all-to-all connectivity are indicated by arrows of different line widths. The net displays below show how correlations and connectivity co-develop in time. The image layer serves as a canvas on which the model layer is drawn as a net. Each node corresponds to a model neuron, neighboring neurons are connected by an edge. The nodes are located at the centers of gravity of the projective field of the model neurons, considering synaptic weights as physical mass. In order to favor strong links, the masses are taken to the power of three. The correlations are displayed in the same way, using averaged correlations instead of synaptic weights. It can be seen that the correlations develop faster and are cleaner than the connectivity. The rotation in depth causes a typical distortion pattern; the mapping is stretched on one side and compressed on the other.

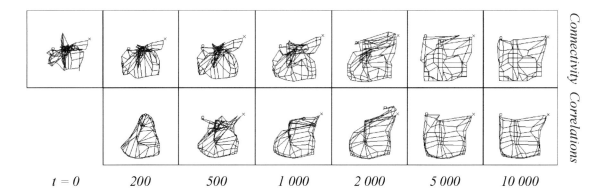

image layer

model layer

$t = 0$ 200   500   1 000   2 000   5 000   10 000

Connectivity   *Correlations*

For recognition purposes, DLM has to be applied in parallel to many models. The best fitting model, i.e. the model most similar to the image, will finally have the strongest connections to the image and will have attracted the greatest share of blob activity. A simple integrating winner-take-all mechanism detects the correct model (see figure 18.2).

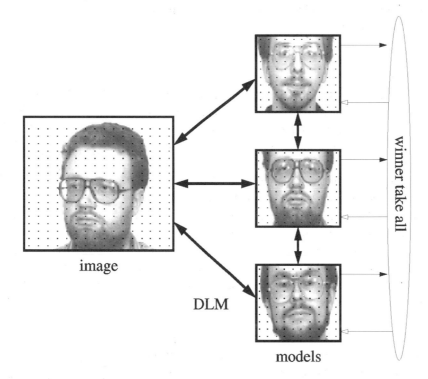

Figure 18.2
Architecture of the DLM face recognition system. Image and models are represented as neural layers of local features, as indicated by the black dots. DLM establishes a regular one-to-one mapping between the initially all-to-all connected layers, connecting corresponding neurons. Thus, DLM provides translation invariance and robustness against distortion. Once the correct mappings are found, a simple winner-take-all mechanism can detect the model that is most active and most similar to the image.

The equations of the system are given in table 18.1; the respective symbols are listed in table 18.2. In the following sections we will explain the system step by step: blob formation, blob mobilization, interaction between two layers, link dynamics, attention dynamics, and recognition dynamics.

Layer dynamics:

$$h_i^p(t_0) = 0$$

$$\dot{h}_i^p = -h_i^p + \sum_{i'} g_{i-i'} \max_{p'}\left(\sigma\left(h_{i'}^{p'}\right)\right) - \beta_h \sum_{i'} \sigma\left(h_{i'}^p\right) - \kappa_{hs} s_i^p$$

$$+ \kappa_{hh} \max_{qj}\left(W_{ij}^{pq}\sigma\left(h_j^q\right)\right) + \kappa_{ha}\left(\sigma\left(a_i^p\right) - \beta_{ac}\right) - \beta_\theta \Theta\left(r_\theta - r^p\right) \tag{18.1}$$

$$s_i^p(t_0) = 0$$

$$\dot{s}_i^p = \lambda_\pm\left(h_i^p - s_i^p\right) \tag{18.2}$$

$$g_{i-i'} = \exp\left(-\frac{(i-i')^2}{2\sigma_g^2}\right) \tag{18.3}$$

$$\sigma(h) = \begin{cases} 0 & h \leq 0 \\ \sqrt{h/\rho} & 0 < h < \rho \\ 1 & h \geq \rho \end{cases} \tag{18.4}$$

Attention dynamics:

$$a_i^p(t_0) = \alpha_N$$

$$\dot{a}_i^p = \lambda_a\left(-a_i^p + \sum_{i'} g_{i-i'}\sigma\left(a_{i'}^p\right) - \beta_a \sum_{i'} \sigma\left(a_{i'}^p\right) + \kappa_{ah} \max_{p'}\left(\sigma\left(h_i^{p'}\right)\right)\right) \tag{18.5}$$

Link dynamics:

$$W_{ij}^{pq}(t_0) = S_{ij}^{pq} = \max\left(S_\phi\left(J_i^p, J_j^q\right), \alpha_S\right) \tag{18.6}$$

$$\dot{W}_{ij}^{pq}(t) = \lambda_W\left(\sigma\left(h_i^p\right)\sigma\left(h_j^q\right) - \Theta\left(\max_{j'}\left(W_{ij'}^{pq}/S_{ij'}^{pq}\right) - 1\right)\right)W_{ij}^{pq}$$

Recognition dynamics:

$$r^p(t_0) = 1$$

$$\dot{r}^p(t) = \lambda_r r^p\left(F^p - \max_{p'}\left(r^{p'} F^{p'}\right)\right) \tag{18.7}$$

$$F^p(t) = \sum_i \sigma\left(h_i^p\right)$$

Table 18.1
Formulas of the DLM face recognition system

Variables:

h	internal state of layer neurons
s	delayed self-inhibition
a	attention
W	synaptic weights between neurons of two layers
r	Recognition variable
F	total activity of each neuron (fitness)

Indices:

$(p;p'\,;q;q')$	layer indices, -1 indicates image layer, 1,...,M indicate model layers
$=(-1;\,-1;\,1,...,M;\,1,...,M)$	if equations describe image layer dynamics
$=(1,...,M;\,1,...,M;\,-1;\,-1)$	if equations describe model layer dynamics
$(i;\,i';\,j;\,j')$	two-dimensional indices for individual neurons in layers $(p;\,p';\,q;\,q')$ respectively

Functions:

$g_{i\text{-}i'}$	Gaussian interaction kernel
$\sigma(h)$	nonlinear squashing function
$\Theta(\cdot)$	heavy side function
$S_\phi(J,J')$	similarity between feature jets J and J'

Parameters:

$\beta_h = 0.2$	strength of global inhibition
$\beta_a = 0.02$	attention blob global inhibition strength
$\beta_{ac} = 1$	global inhibition strength compensating for attention blob
$\beta_\theta = \infty$	model supression global inhibition strength
$\kappa_{hs} = 1$	self inhibition strength
$\kappa_{hh} = 1.2$	image and model layers interaction strength
$\kappa_{ha} = 0.7$	attention blob effect on running blob
$\kappa_{ah} = 3$	running blob effect on attention blob
$\lambda_\pm$	delayed self-inhibition decay constant
$= \lambda_+ = 0.2$	if $h\text{-}s > 0$
$= \lambda_- = 0.004$	if $h\text{-}s \leq 0$
$\lambda_a = 0.3$	attention dynamics time constant
$\lambda_W = 0.05$	link dynamics time constant
$\lambda_r = 0.02$	recognition dynamics time constant
$\alpha_N = 0.1$	attention blob initialization constant
$\alpha_S = 0.1$	minimal weight
$\rho = 2$	squashing function slope radius
$\sigma_g = 1$	excitatory interaction kernel Gauss width
$r_\theta = 0.5$	model suppression threshold

Table 18.2

Variables and parameters of the DLM face recognition system.

Blob Formation

Blob formation on a layer of neurons can easily be achieved by local excitation and global inhibition (consider equations 18.1, 18.3, and 18.4 with $\kappa_{hs} = \kappa_{hh} = \kappa_{ha} = \beta_\theta = 0$; cf. also Amari 1977). Local excitation is conveyed by the Gaussian interaction kernel g and generates clusters of activity. Global inhibition, controlled by β_h, lets the clusters compete against each other. The strongest one will finally suppress all others and grow to an equilibrium size determined by the strength of global inhibition.

Blob Mobilization

Generating a running blob can be achieved by delayed self-inhibition s, which drives the blob away from its current location to a neighboring one, where the blob generates new self-inhibition. This mechanism produces a continuously moving blob (consider equations 18.1 and 18.2 with $\kappa_{hh} = \kappa_{ha} = \beta_\theta = 0$; see also figure 18.3). In addition, the self-inhibition serves as a memory and repels the blob from regions recently visited. The driving force and the recollection time as to where the blob has been can be independently controlled by the time constants λ_+ and λ_-, respectively.

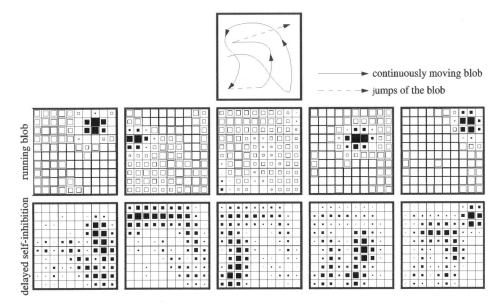

continuously moving blob
- - - jumps of the blob

running blob

delayed self-inhibition

Figure 18.3
A sequence of layer states. The activity blob h shown in the middle row has a size of approximately six active nodes and moves continuously over the whole layer. Its course is shown in the upper diagram. The delayed self-inhibition s, shown in the bottom row, follows the running blob and drives it forward. One can see the self-inhibitory tail, which repels the blob from regions just visited. Sometimes the blob runs into a trap (cf. column three) and has no way to escape from the self-inhibition. It then disappears and reappears again somewhere else on the layer. (The temporal increment between two successive frames is 20 time units.)

Layer Interaction and Synchronization

In the same way as the running blob is repelled by its self-inhibitory tail, it can also be attracted by excitatory input from another layer, as conveyed by the connection matrix W (consider equation 18.1 with $\kappa_{ha} = \beta_\theta = 0$). Imagine two layers of the same size mutually connected by the identity matrix, i.e. each neuron in one layer is connected only with the one corresponding neuron in the other layer having the same index value. The input then is a copy of the blob of the other layer. This favors alignment between the blobs, because then they can cooperate and stabilize each other. This synchronization principle hold also in the presence of the noisy connection matrices generated by real image data (see figure 18.4). (The reason why we use the maximum function instead of the usual sum will be discussed later on)

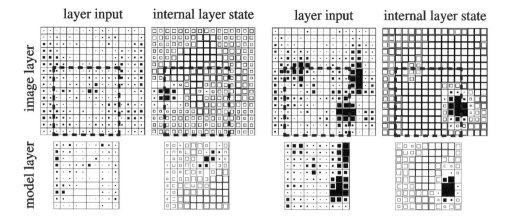

Figure 18.4

Synchronization between two running blobs. Layer input as well as the internal layer state h is shown at an early stage, in which the blobs of two layers are not yet aligned, left, and at a later state, right, when they are aligned. The two layers are of different size, and the region in Layer 1 which correctly maps to Layer 2 is indicated by a square defined by the dashed line. In the early non-aligned case one can see that the blobs are smaller and not at the location of maximal input. The locations of maximal input indicate where the actual corresponding neurons of the blob of the other layer are. In the aligned case the blobs are larger and at the locations of high layer input.

Link Dynamics

Links are initialized by the similarity S_ϕ between the jets J of connected nodes (see Wiskott 1995), with a guaranteed minimal synaptic weight of α_S Then, they become cleaned up and structured on the basis of correlations between pairs of neurons (consider equation 18.6; see also figure 18.1). The correlations, defined as $\sigma(h_i^p)\sigma(h_j^q)$, result from the layer synchronization described in the previous section. The link dynamics typically consists of a growth term and a normalization term. The former lets the weights grow according to the correlation between the connected neurons. The latter prevents the links from growing infinitely and induces competition such that only one link per neuron survives, suppressing all others.

Attention Dynamics

The alignment between the running blobs depends very much on the constraints, i.e. on the size and format of the layer on which they are running. This causes a problem, since the image and the models have different sizes. We have therefore introduced an attention blob a which restricts the movement of the running blob on the image layer to a region of about the same size as that of the model layers (consider equations 18.1 and 18.5 with $\beta_\theta = 0$). The basic dynamics of the attention blob is the same as for the running blob, except there is no self-inhibition. The model layers also have the same attention blob to keep the conditions for their running blobs similar to that in the image layer (only one attention blob is effectively used for all models for computational efficiency). This is important for the alignment. The attention blob restricts the region for the running blob via the term

$$\kappa_{ha}\left(\sigma\left(a_i^p\right)-\beta_{ac}\right) \tag{18.8}$$

with the excitatory blob

$$\sigma\left(a_i^p\right) \tag{18.9}$$

compensating the constant inhibition β_{ac}. The attention blob on the other hand gets excitatory input

$$\kappa_{ha}\left(\sigma\left(h_i^p\right)\right) \tag{18.10}$$

from the running blob and can thus be shifted into a region where input is especially large and favors activity. The attention blob therefore automatically aligns with the actual face position (see figure 18.5). The attention blob layer could be initialized based on preattentive segmentation cues, such as texture or color. However, we use a flat initialization and leave the alignment of the attention blob to an initial synchronization phase based purely on the similarity values of the image jets with the model jets in the gallery.

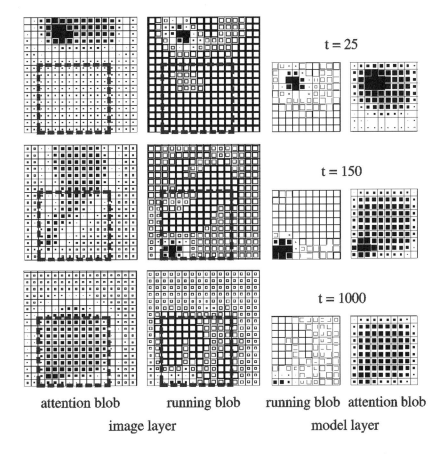

t = 25

t = 150

t = 1000

attention blob   running blob   running blob   attention blob

image layer   model layer

Figure 18.5
Function of the attention blob, using an extreme example of an initial attention blob manually misplaced for demonstration. At t=150 the two running blobs ran synchronously for a while, and the attention blob has a long tail. The blobs then lost alignment again. From t=500 on, the running blobs remained synchronous, and eventually the attention blob aligned with the correct face position, indicated by a square made of dashed lines. The attention blob moves slowly compared to the small running blob, as it is not driven by self-inhibition. Without an attention blob the two running blobs may synchronize sooner, but the alignment will never become stable.

Recognition Dynamics

We have derived a winner-take-all mechanism from Eigen's (1978) evolution equation and applied it to detect the best model and suppress all others (See equations 18.1 and 18.7). Each model cooperates with the image depending on its similarity. The most similar model cooperates most successfully and is the most active one. We consider the total activity of the model layer p as fitness F^p. The layer with the highest fitness suppresses all others (as can easily be seen if the F^p are assumed to be constant in time and the recognition variables r^p are initialized to 1). When a recognition variable r^p drops below the suppression threshold r_θ, the activity of layer p is suppressed by the term

$$-\beta_\theta \Theta\left(r_\theta - r^p\right) \tag{18.11}$$

Bidirectional Connections

The connectivity between two layers is bidirectional and not unidirectional as in the previous system (Konen and Vorbrüggen 1993). This is necessary for two reasons: Firstly, by this means the running blobs of the two connected layers can more easily align. With unidirectional connections one blob would systematically run behind the other. Secondly, connections in both directions are necessary for a recognition system. The connections from model to image layer are necessary to allow the models to move the attention blob in the image into a region which fits the models well. The connections from the image to the model layers are necessary to provide a discrimination cue as to which model best fits the image. Otherwise, each model would exhibit the same level of activity.

Blob Alignment in the Model Domain

Since faces have a common general structure, it is advantageous to align the blobs in the model domain to insure that they are always at the same position in the faces, either all at the left eye or all at the chin etc. This is achieved by connections between the layers, expressed by the term

$$+ \sum_{i'} g_{i-i'} \max_{p'} \sigma\left(h_{i'}^{p'}\right) \tag{18.12}$$

instead of

$$+ \sum_{i'} g_{i-i'} \sigma\left(h_{i'}^{p}\right) \tag{18.13}$$

in equation 18.1. If the model blobs were to run independently, the image layer would get input from all face parts at the same time, and the blob there would have a hard time to align with a model blob, and it would be uncertain. whether it would be the correct one. The cooperation between the models and the image would depend more on accidental alignment than on the similarity between the models and the image, and it would then be likely that the wrong model was picked up as the recognition result. One alternative is to let the models inhibit each other such that only one model would have a blob at a time. The models then would share time to match onto the image, and the best fitting one would get most of the time. This would probably be the appropriate setup if the models were of different structure, as is the case for arbitrary objects.

Maximum Versus Sum Neurons

The model neurons used here use the maximum over all input signals instead of their sum. The reason is that the sum would mix up many different signals, while only one can be correct, i.e. the total input would be the result of one correct signal mixed with many distractions. Hence the signal-to-noise ratio would be low. We have observed an example where even a model identical to the image was not picked as the correct one, because the sum over all the accidental input signals favored a completely different-looking person. For that reason we introduced the maximum input function, which is reasonable since the correct signal is likely to be the strongest one. The maximum rule has the additional advantage that the dynamic range of the input into a single cell does not vary much when the connectivity develops, whereas the signal sum would decrease significantly during synaptic re-organization and let the blobs loose their alignment.

18.3 Model Implementation

The **DlmModel** is made of a top level **Dlm** module as shown in figure 18.6. These sub-modules are related to the image/object domain (layer 1), model domain (layer 2) or their interconnection.

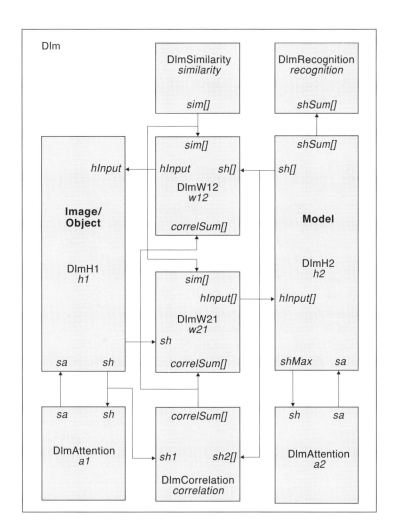

Figure 18.6
The **Dlm** module includes image or object domain modules (layer 1) and model domain (layer 2). The object domain comprises *h1* and *a1* modules, the model domain comprises *h2*, *a2*, *recognition* and *similarity*, while the interconnection modules are implemented by *w12*, *w21* and *correlation* modules. Note that some ports in the submodules have a "[]" (brackets) ending; these represent port arrays instead of the usual single value ports. The connections between such ports are actually multiple ones.

An important concern of this model is how to implement the fact that the model layer manipulates multiple faces, the ones stored in the database, as opposed to the image/object layer representing a single one to be compared against. We had the choice to create multiple model, recognition, attention, connection and correlation modules corresponding each to a single face transformation. This would have incremented the total number of modules in the system together with its complexity. Instead, we chose to have single model layer modules representing each multiple face transformations. To make this possible we implemented port arrays instead of single ports in each of these modules when appropriate (see the "[]" (brackets) port array notation in the figure). For example, the *sim* input port array in many of the modules, such as in *w12*, is defined as a **NslDinFloat4** array of size *gallerySizeMax* to make it really a 5-dimensional array,

```
public NslDinFloat4 sim()[gallerySizeMax];
```

Note that in this case we use dynamic memory allocation since no instantiation parameters were given above. For example, in the *w12* module, the *sim* port array is assigned memory space as follows (see Appendix I for further details),

```
for (int i=0; i<gallerySizeMax;i++)
    sim[i].nslMemAlloc(i2max,j2max,i1Rmax,j1Rmax);
```

Thus, module interconnections for port array interconnections require a "for loop" style format as follows,

```
for (int i=0; i<gallerySizeMax; i++)
    nslConnect(similarity.sim[i],w12.sim[i]);
```

Note that *gallerySizeMax* represents the maximum number of gallery faces used from the database for comparison purposes.

Similarity Module

The **Similarity** module performs the initial DLM model processing. The DLM database, implemented as special text and binary files (see Appendix I for a detailed description of text file manipulation and Appendix III for NSLC extensions to binary files), consists of objects and models in the form of stored graphs with the precomputed Gabor-wavelet transform coefficients. For the models they are taken from a grid of 10 x 10 nodes centered on the faces. For the objects the grids cover the whole image plane with 16 x 17 nodes. From these stored graphs a subgraph can be selected. From the 16 x 17 graph for example a 12 x 12 subgraph will automatically be selected if the size of layer 1 is 12 x 12. In addition one can choose the location of the subgraph by *Si1offset* and *Sj2offset* offsets given as integer numbers behind the model names in the gallery files.

Since the object and model layers vary in size a mapping must be created to match elements in both. This is achieved by using a connection patch in layer 1 corresponding to a single cell in layer 2, as shown in figure 18.7.

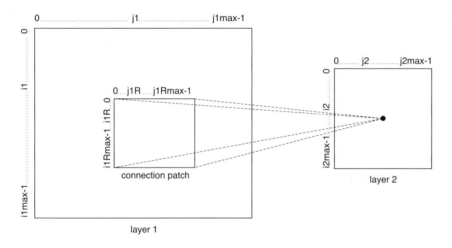

Figure 18.7
Matrix representation of layers 1 and 2, and the connectivity patch from a cell in layer 2 to layer 1.

The size of the patches in layer 1 is always *i1Rmax* x *j1Rmax*, but their position depends on the position of the corresponding cell in layer 2 (layer 2 can be as large as layer 1). If we consider only one dimension, for example the *i1*-index, the patches would have *i1max-i1Rmax*+1 different offsets varying in range from 0 to *i1max-i1Rmax*). These offsets should be equally distributed depending on the different positions in range from 0 to *i2max-1* in layer 2. Since $i2/(i2max-1)$ lies in the range [0..1], $(i1max-i1Rmax)*i2/(i2max-1)$ covers the correct range [0,..,(i1max-i1Rmax)]. In order to round it to the closest integer we define an index function named *i1Index* returning $(i1max-i1Rmax)*i2/(i2max-1)+0.5$. For example, given a layer 1 of size 7 and a patch size of 4, there are 4 different offsets, from 0 to 3.

In terms of actual computation, the **initSys** method initializes the *sim* array (order of five) corresponding to the module's output by computing the similarity between the original *DlmGImage* and the different *DlmGModel* library images, both read from external files (not shown here). For all models taken from the gallery (1 to *gallerySize*), for every element (*i2, j2*) in layer 2 (*i2max* and *j2max* are the 2-dimension sizes of the model layer), for every element (*i1R, j1R*) in the connection patch and for every offset element (*i1, j1*) in layer 1 (*i1Rmax* and *j1Rmax* represent the 2-dimension sizes of the patch while *i1max* and *j1max* represent the 2-dimension sizes of the object layer), compute the similarity as follows,

```
for (int model=1; model<=gallerySize; model++) {
  for (int i2=0; i2<i2max; i2++)
    for (int j2=0; j2<j2max; j2++)
      for (int i1R=0,int i1=i1Index
          (i2,0,frame,i1max,i1Rmax,i2max);
           i1R<i1Rmax; i1R++, i1++)
        for (int j1R=0,int j1=j1Index
            (j2,0,frame,j1max,j1Rmax,j2max);
             j1R<j1Rmax; j1R++, j1++) {
          sim[model][i2][j2][i1R][j1R] =
            nslMax(alpha_s,
              similarity(DlmGImage,i1,j1,DlmGModel,
                i2,j2));
        }
}
```

(Note that model=0 represents the average face model.) There are a few aspects to note in the above code. The *i1Index* (and *j2Index*) functions include a *frame* variable. The *frame*, whose elements are not connected to layers 2, is put around layer 1, the object layer, in order to give the attention blob space to move around the border of layer 1. If *i1max* and *j1max* are equal in size as *i2max* and *j2max* then no attention blob is required and the frame not necessary. The actual *i1Index* function (analogous to the *j2Index* function) is as follows,

```
int i1Index(int i2, int i1R, int frame,int i1max,int i1Rmax,
    int i2max){
        return i1R + frame + (i1max-2*frame-i1Rmax)*i2/
          (i2max-1)+0.5;
}
```

Note also in the similarity equation, that the value of *sim*, for each model, is assigned as the maximum value between parameter *alpha_s* and the resulting similarity value. This is done to restrict minimum values in *sim*.

Once the similarity computation has been completed, the average layer values (*model*=0) are set the maximum of all models.

```
for (int i2=0; i2<i2max; i2++)
    for (int j2=0; j2<j2max; j2++)
        for (int i1R=0; i1R<i1Rmax; i1R++)
            for (int j1R=0; j1R<j1Rmax; j1R++) {
            float s = 0;
            for (int model=1; model<=gallerySize; model++)
                s = nslMax(s,sim[model][i2][j2][i1R][j1R]);
            sim[0][i2][j2][i1R][j1R] = s;
            }
```

H Module

To take advantage of common functionality between the image and layer models, a *supermodule* **H** is defined containing aspects common to both **H1** and **H2**. At the structure level the two submodules **H1** and **H2** share a number of variables having the exact same dimension, corresponding to previously defined equation symbols, as shown in table 18.3 (we omit all scalar parameters from the table).

Symbol	Variable Name	Variable Type	Description
$G_i^p = \sum_{i'} g_{i-i'} \max_{p'}\left(\sigma\left(h_i^{p'}\right)\right)$	hTransE	NslFloat2	Gaussian lateral interaction
$\sigma\left(a_i^p\right)$	sa	NslDinFloat2	Input received from the attention module
$h_i^p - s_i^p$	d	NslFloat2	Delayed self inhibition argument

Table 18.3

Symbol and variable relationship defined in H and common to both H1 and H2 in dimension.

Additionally, the following method implements equation (18.3) and is used to initialize the Gaussian variable *g* used in both submodules,

```
protected void initGauss(){
    for (int k = 0; k < gSize; k++) {
        float x = (float) (k-gSigma/2);
        g[k] = nslExp(-x*x/(2*gSigma*gSigma));
    }
}
```

Additionally, the following method performs the convolution described in the second hand side element of equation (18.1) performed by both submodules,

```
protected NslFloat2 gaussConvolved(NslFloat1 g,NslFloat2 sh){
    return nslConvZero(nslFillRows(g,1),nslConvZero
        (nslFillCols(g,1),sh));
}
```

The above function generates a two dimensional array as result from this convolution. It first convolves *sh* against a matrix whose columns are replications (*nslFillCols*) of the gaussian vector *g*. The result of this convolution is applied to a matrix whose rows are replications (*nslFillRows*) of the gaussian vector *g*. We use a convolution function treating elements beyond the matrix border as zeroes (*nslConvZero*).

H1 Module

The image layer implementation defines a number of variables corresponding to previously defined equation symbols, as shown in table 18.4.

Table 18.4

Symbol and variable relationship defined in H1.

Symbol	Variable Name	Variable Type	Description
$I_i^p = \max_{qj}\left(W_{ij}^{pq}\sigma\left(h_j^q\right)\right)$	hInput	NslDinFloat2	Input received from *hInput* from *w12* layer
$\sigma\left(h_i^p\right)$	sh	NslDoutFloat2	Layer output
h_i^p	h	NslFloat2	Layer activity
s_i^p	s	NslFloat2	Delayed self inhibition

The **simRun** main computation, describing layer dynamics on h and s in module $h1$, is as follows:

1. Calculate the Gaussian lateral interaction *hTransE* in the image layer,

$$G_i^p = \sum_{i'} g_{i-i'} \max_{p'} \left(\sigma\left(h_{i'}^{p'} \right) \right) \tag{18.14}$$

corresponding to the second term of the right hand size of equation (18.1) where g has been computed in the **initRun** method during initialization,

```
hTransE = gaussConvolved(g,sh);
```

The maximum operation is not necessary since there is only one image layer p.

2. Integrate the differential equation for the image layer in correspondence to equation (18.1),

$$\dot{h}_i^p = -h_i^p + \sum_{i'} g_{i-i'} \max_{p'} \left(\sigma\left(h_{i'}^{p'} \right) \right) - \beta_h \sum_{i'} \sigma\left(h_{i'}^p \right) - \kappa_{hs} s_i^p$$

$$+ \kappa_{hh} \max_{qj} \left(W_{ij}^{pq} \sigma\left(h_j^q \right) \right) + \kappa_{ha} \left(\sigma\left(a_i^p \right) - \beta_{ac} \right) - \beta_\theta \Theta\left(r_\theta - r^p \right)$$

The equation is implemented as follows,

```
nslDiff(h,1.,- h + hTransE - beta_h*nslSum(sh)  - kappa_hs*s
     + kappa_hh*hInput + kappa_ha*(sa-beta_ac));
```

Note that *nslSum(sh)* corresponds to the following expression,

$$\sum_{i'} \sigma\left(h_{i'}^p \right)$$

Additionally notice that the strong inhibition term

$$- \beta_\theta \Theta\left(r_\theta - r^q \right)$$

is ineffective in the image layer since there are no competing image layers.

3. Compute the image layer output *sh* from current activity h as given by equation (18.4),

```
computeOutputFunc(sh,h,rho);
```

4. Integrate the differential equation (equation 18.2) given by,

$$\dot{s}_i^p = \lambda_\pm \left(h_i^p - s_i^p \right)$$

with *lambda* depending on the sign of the difference of h and s,

```
d = h - s;
for (i1=0; i1<i1max; i1++)
    for (j1=0; j1<j1max; j1++)
        if (d[i1][j1]>0)
            d[i1][j1] = d[i1][j1]*lambda_p;
        else
            d[i1][j1] = d[i1][j1]*lambda_m;
nslDiff(s,1.,d);
```

H2 Module

The image layer implementation defines a number of variables corresponding to previously defined equation symbols, as shown in table 18.5. Notice that these variables differ from those defined in module **H1** in that an additional dimension has been added in the form of an array (having its size correspond *gallerySizeMax*).

Symbol	Variable Name	Variable Type	Description
$I_j^q = \max\limits_{pi}\left(W_{ji}^{qp}\,\sigma\!\left(h_i^p\right)\right)$	`hInput`	`NslDinFloat2[]`	Input received from *hInput* from *w12* layer
$\sigma\!\left(h_j^q\right)$	`sh`	`NslDoutFloat2[]`	Layer output
$\sum\limits_j \sigma\!\left(h_j^q\right)$	`shSum`	`NslDoutFloat0[]`	Sum over *sh*
$\max\limits_{q'}\!\left(\sigma\!\left(h_j^{q'}\right)\right)$	`shMax`	`NslDoutFloat2[]`	Maximum activity of layer 2
h_j^q	`h`	`NslFloat2[]`	Layer activity
s_j^q	`s`	`NslFloat2[]`	Delayed self inhibition

Table 18.5

Symbol and variable relationship defined in H2. Notice that all types have an additional dimension specified by the "[]" array symbol.

The **simRun** main computation describing layer dynamics on *h* and *s* in module *h2*, is quite similar to module *h1*, being as follows:

5. Calculate the Gaussian lateral interaction *hTransE* in the model layer,

$$G_j^q = \sum_{j'} g_{j-j'} \max_{q'}\!\left(\sigma\!\left(h_{j'}^{q'}\right)\right)$$

Since the maximum operation is equal for all models it needs to be calculated only once.

```
hTransE = gaussConvolved(g,shMax,rho);
```

Notice that we have an additional variable *shMax* in **H2**.

6. Integrate the differential equation for the model layer in correspondence to equation (18.1),

$$\dot{h}_j^q = -h_j^q + \sum_{j'} g_{j-j'} \max_{q'}\!\left(\sigma\!\left(h_{j'}^{q'}\right)\right) - \beta_h \sum_{j} \sigma\!\left(h_{j\bullet}^{q}\right) - \kappa_{hs}\, s_j^q$$

$$+ \kappa_{hh} \max_{pi}\!\left(W_{ji}^{qp}\,\sigma\!\left(h_i^p\right)\right) + \kappa_{ha}\left(\sigma\!\left(a_j^q\right) - \beta_{ac}\right) - \beta_\theta \Theta\!\left(r_\theta - r^q\right)$$

The equation is implemented as follows and applied to each model,

```
nslDiff(h[model],1.0, - h[model] + hTransE
    - beta_h*shSum[model] - kappa_hs*s[model]
    + kappa_hh*hInput[model] + kappa_ha*(sa-beta_ac));
```

Notice that the strong inhibition term

$$- \beta_\theta \Theta\!\left(r_\theta - r^q\right)$$

is simulated simply by skipping over those layers that have too low recognition values r^q (skip statement in the source code), else continue processing the model layer.

Also notice that the output sum *shSum* is computed for each model as follows,

```
shSum[model] = nslSum(sh[model]);
```

7. Compute for each model layer output *sh* from current activity *h* as described in equation (18.4),

```
computeOutputFunc(sh[model],h[model],rho);
```

8. Integrate for each model the differential equation (equation 18.2) given by,

$$\dot{s}_j^q = \lambda_{\pm}\left(h_j^q - s_j^q\right)$$

with *lambda* depending on the sign of the difference of *h* and *s*,

```
d = h[model] - s[model];
for (i2=0; i2<i2max; i2++)
    for (j2=0; j2<j2max; j2++)
        if (d[i2][j2]>0)
            d[i2][j2] = d[i2][j2]*lambda_p;
        else
            d[i2][j2] = d[i2][j2]*lambda_m;
nslDiff(s[model],1.,d);
```

9. Compute the model layer output *shMax*

$$\max_{q'}\left(\sigma\left(h_j^{q'}\right)\right)$$

implemented by,

```
for (i2=0; i2<i2max; i2++)
    for (j2=0; j2<j2max; j2++) {
        shMax[i2][j2] = 0;
        for (int model=1; model<=gallerSizeMax; model++)
            shMax[i2][j2] = nslMax(shMax[i2][j2],sh[model]
                [i2][j2]);
    }
```

Attention Module

We take advantage of the similarity between the attention modules for image and model layers to define a single one instantiated twice, respectively. The **Attention** module defines equation symbols and variable names, as shown in table 18.5.

Symbol	Variable Name	Variable Type	Description
a_i^p	a	NslFloat2	Attention layer activity
$\sigma\left(a_i^p\right)$	sa	NslDoutFloat2	Attention layer output
$A_i^p = \sum_{i'} g_{i-i'}\sigma\left(a_i^p\right)$	aTransE	NslFloat2	Gaussian lateral interaction
$\sigma\left(h_i^p\right)$ or $\max_{p'}\left(\sigma\left(h_i^{p'}\right)\right)$	sh	NslDinFloat2	Layer input received from the image or model (max) layer, respectively.

Attention modules compute only if attention is set. The **initRun** method initializes the attention layer (**a1** and **a2**) as follows,

Table 18.5
Symbol and variable relationship.

```
a = alpha_N;
sa = computeOutputFunc(a);
```

The **simRun** method describes the attention dynamics for the two layers,

10. Calculate the Gaussian lateral interaction *aTransE* from its previous output *sa*,

$$A_i^p = \sum_{i'} g_{i-i'} \sigma\left(a_{i'}^p\right) \tag{18.15}$$

The implementation is as follows,

```
aTransE = gaussConvolved(g,sa);
```

Due to the maximum operation there is effectively only one attention layer for all models,

11. Integrate differential equation for the attention layer as described in equation (18.5) by obtaining inputs from the image or model layer outputs, respectively,

$$\dot{a}_i^p = \lambda_a\left(-a_i^p + \sum_{i'} g_{i-i'} \sigma\left(a_{i'}^p\right) - \beta_a \sum_{i'} \sigma\left(a_{i'}^p\right) - \kappa_{ah}\sigma\left(h_i^p\right)\right)$$

The equation is implemented as follows,

```
nslDiff(a,1.,lambda_a*(-a+aTransE-beta_a*nslSum(sa)+
    kappa_ah*sh)));
```

12. Compute the output function

$$\sigma\left(a_i^p\right)$$

The equation is implemented as follows,

```
computeOutputFunc(sa,a,rho);
```

W Module

To take advantage of common functionality between the image and layer model connectivity, a *supermodule* **W** is defined containing aspects common to both **W12** and **W21**. At the structure level the two submodules **W12** and **W21** share a number of variables having the exact same dimension, corresponding to previously defined equation symbols, as shown in table 18.6 (we omit all scalar parameters from the table).

Symbol	Variable Name	Variable Type	Description
W_{ij}^{pq}	w	NslFloat4[]	Connection weights
$C_{ij}^{qp} = \sigma\left(h_i^p\right)\sigma\left(h_j^q\right)$	correlSum	NslDinFloat4[]	Input from **Correlation** module
S_{ij}^{qp}	sim	NslDinFloat4[]	Input from **Similarity** module

Notice that since the link dynamics for both connection layers is simulated only after every *loops* iterations.

W12 Module

The connectivity layer from the model layer to the image layer is defined by module **W12**. The symbols particular to this layer are shown in table 18.7. In addition this layer inherits all symbols defined in supermodule **W**.

Table 18.6
Symbol and variable relationship defined in **W** and common to both **W12** and **W21** in dimension. Notice that all types have an additional dimension specified by the "[]" array symbol.

Symbol	Variable Name	Variable Type	Description
$I_i^p = \max\limits_{qj}\left(W_{ji}^{pq}\sigma\left(h_j^q\right)\right)$	hInput	NslDoutFloat2	Output to image layer
$\sigma\left(h_j^q\right)$	sh	NslDinFloat2[]	Input from model layer
$N_i^p = \min\limits_{qj}\left\{1, S_{ij}^{qp}\big/W_{ji}^{pq}\right\}$	normFactor	NslFloat2	Normalization matrix

Table 18.7

Symbol and variable relationship defined in **W12**. Notice the types having an additional dimension specified by the "[]" array symbol.

The **initRun** method computes the initialization values for the connection module given by the following equation (equation 18.6),

$$W_{ji}^{pq}\left(t_0\right) = S_{ij}^{qp} = \max\left(S_\phi\left(J_i^p, J_j^q\right), \alpha_S\right)$$

Taking out the nested "for" loops, the equation is implemented as follows,

```
w[model][i1R][j1R][i2][j2] = sim[model][i2][j2][i1R][j1R];
```

Notice how we switch subscripts since **W12** connects layer 2 elements to layer 1 patch elements. Also, the *max* function has already been applied in the similarity module. Additionally, the **initRun** method computes maximum values for the average layer (*model*=0).

```
float stmp = 0;
for (model=1; model<=gallerySize; model++)
    stmp = nslMax(stmp,sim[model][i2][j2][i1R][j1R]);
w[0][i1R][j1R][i2][j2] = stmp;
```

The **simRun** method describes connection dynamics on **W12**. Computation is as follows:

13. Calculate growth of the weight matrix *w* from model layers to image layer according to the first term in differential equation equation (18.6) based on the accumulated correlations and according to the equation

$$\dot{W}_{ji}^{pq}(t) = \lambda_W C_{ij}^{qp} W_{ji}^{pq} \qquad (18.16)$$

Since this integration switches scripts around we perform the integration directly as follows,

$$W_{ji}^{pq} = W_{ji}^{pq} + \lambda_W C_{ij}^{qp} W_{ji}^{pq} \Delta t$$

The latter is implemented by the following code,

```
w[model][i1R][j1R][i2][j2] += nslSystem.getSimDelta()
    *w[model][i1R][j1R][i2][j2]*lambda_W
    *correlSum[model][i2][j2][i1R][j1R];
```

Note the "+=" expression directly adding the left hand side variable to the right hand side. The "nslSystem.getSimDelta()" expression returns the system's "delta".

14. Although link dynamics is not simulated as a differential equation but by strict normalization, the outcome is the same. The normalization rule corresponding to the second term in equation (18.6) becomes an explicit and separate normalization rule in the program. The normalization factors by which the weights converging on the image layer need to be multiplied is

$$N_i^p = \min_{qj}\left\{1, S_{ij}^{qp}\Big/W_{ji}^{pq}\right\}$$

Notice that *sim* is symmetric and can be used for both directions. The variable *normFactor* is initialized to 1. Also notice that each model layer needs its own set of normalization factors for *w21* but not for *w12* (although we end up computing one for each anyway).

```
if (w[model][i1R][j1R][i2][j2]>sim[model][i2][j2][i1R][j1R])
   normFactor[i1][j1] = minimum(normFactor[i1][j1],
      sim[model][i2][j2][i1R][j1R]/w[model][i1R][j1R][i2][j2]);
```

15. Normalize the weights going from each model layer to the image layer by the normalization factors,

$$W_{ji}^{pq} = N_i^p W_{ji}^{pq}$$

```
w[model][i1R][j1R][i2][j2]  *= normFactor[i1][j1];
```

Note the "*=" expression directly multiplying the left hand side variable with the right hand side.

16. Skip computation if inhibition in model layer sh is too strong. (There is no competition between links going to different models while there is competition between links converging to the image layer from different models.)

17. Calculate the output *hInput* sent to the image layer calculated as the maximum of the input *sh* from the model layer multiplied by the connection *w* as described in equation (18.1),

$$\max_{pi}\left(W_{ji}^{pq}\,\sigma\!\left(h_i^p\right)\right)$$

The implementation is as follows,

```
hInput[i1][j1]  = nslMax(hInput[i1][j1],
      w[model][i1R][j1R][i2][j2]*sh[model][i2][j2]);
```

W21 Module

The connectivity layer from the image layer to the model layer is defined by module **W21**. The symbols particular to this layer are shown in table 18.8. In addition this layer inherits all symbols defined in supermodule **W**.

Symbol	Variable Name	Variable Type	Description
$I_j^q = \max_{pi}\left(W_{ij}^{qp}\,\sigma\!\left(h_i^p\right)\right)$	hInput	NslDoutFloat2[]	Output to model layer
$\sigma\!\left(h_i^p\right)$	sh	NslDinFloat2	Input from image layer
$N_j^q = \min_{pi}\left\{1, S_{ij}^{qp}\Big/W_{ij}^{qp}\right\}$	normFactor	NslFloat2[]	Normalization matrix

Table 18.8
Symbol and variable relationship defined in **W21**. Notice the types having an additional dimension specified by the "[]" array symbol, exactly the opposite from those specified in **W12**.

The **initRun** method computes the initialization values for the connection module given by the following equation (equation 18.6),

$$W_{ij}^{qp}(t_0) = S_{ij}^{qp} = \max\left(S_\phi\left(J_i^p, J_j^q\right), \alpha_S\right)$$

An important consideration here is that subscripts correspond to those in the similarity output. Taking out the nested "for loops" the equation is implemented as follows,

```
w[model] = sim[model]
```

Notice how we switch subscripts since **W21** connects layer 1 patch elements to layer 1 elements. Also, the *max* function has already been applied in the similarity module. Additionally, the **initRun** method computes maximum values for the average layer (*model*=0).

```
float stmp = 0;
for (model=1; model<=gallerySize; model++)
    stmp = nslMax(stmp,sim[model]);
w[0] = stmp;
```

The **simRun** method describes connection dynamics on **W21**. Computation is as follows:

18. Calculate growth of the weight matrix *w* from model layers to image layer according to the first term in differential equation equation (18.6) based on the accumulated correlations and according to the equation

$$\dot{W}_{ij}^{qp}(t) = \lambda_W C_{ij}^{qp} W_{ji}^{qp}$$

Since this integration switches scripts around we perform the integration directly as follows,

$$W_{ij}^{qp} = W_{ij}^{qp} + \lambda_W C_{ij}^{qp} W_{ij}^{qp} \Delta t$$

The latter is implemented by the following code,

```
w[model] += nslSystem.getSimDelta()
    *w[model][i2][j2]*lambda_W*correlSum[model];
```

Note the "+=" expression directly adding the left hand side variable to the right hand side. The "nslSystem.getSimDelta()" expression returns the system's "delta".

19. Although link dynamics is not simulated as a differential equation but by strict normalization, the outcome is the same. The normalization rule corresponding to the second term in equation (18.6) becomes an explicit and separate normalization rule in the program. The normalization factors by which the weights converging on the image layer need to be multiplied is

$$N_j^q = \min_{pi}\left\{1, S_{ij}^{qp} / W_{ij}^{qp}\right\}$$

Notice that *sim* is symmetric and can be used for both directions. The variable *normFactor* is initialized to 1. Also notice that each model layer needs its own set of normalization factors for *w21* but not for *w12* (although we end up computing one for each anyway).

```
if (w[model][i2][j2][i1R][j1R]>sim[model][i2][j2][i1R][j1R])
   normFactor[i1][j1] = minimum(normFactor[i1][j1],
      sim[model][i2][j2][i1R][j1R]/w[model][i2][j2][i1R][j1R]);
```

20. Normalize the weights going from each model layer to the image layer by the normalization factors,

$$W_{ij}^{qp} = N_j^q W_{ij}^{qp}$$

```
w[model][i2][j2][i1R][j1R] *= normFactor[i1][j1];
```

Note the "*=" expression directly multiplying the left hand side variable with the right hand side.

21. Skip computation if inhibition in model layer sh is too strong. (There is no competition between links going to different models while there is competition between links converging to the image layer from different models.)

Calculate the output *hInput* sent to the image layer calculated as the maximum of the input *sh* from the model layer multiplied by the connection *w* as described in equation (18.1),

$$\max_{qj}\left(W_{ij}^{qp}\sigma\left(h_j^q\right)\right)$$

The implementation is as follows,

```
hInput[i1][j1] = nslMax(hInput[i1][j1],
   w[model][i2][j2][i1R][j1R]*sh[model][i2][j2]);
```

Correlation Module

The correlation module between image-model connections and model-layer connections. The correlation symbols and variable names are shown in table 18.9.

Symbol	Variable Name	Variable Name	Description
$\sigma\left(h_i^p\right)$	Sh1	NslDinFloat2	Image layer input
$\sigma\left(h_j^q\right)$	Sh2	NslDinFloat2[]	Model layer input
C_{ij}^{qp}	correlSum	NslDoutFloat4[]	Accumulated correlation

The **initRun** method initializes variables to zero. The **simRun** method computes the link dynamics on the correlation module.

Table 18.9
Symbol and variable relationship.

22. Calculate the input received from the image layer output *sh1* and from the model layer output *sh2* multiplied to compute *correlSum* as described in the following equation,

$$C_{ij}^{qp} = \sigma\left(h_i^p\right)\sigma\left(h_j^q\right) \tag{18.17}$$

Notice that since the link dynamics is simulated only after every *loops* iterations, the correlations are accumulated over time, leading to the += operator. The correlations are symmetric and can be used for the weight matrices from image layer to model layers and vice versa.

```
correlSum[model][i2][j2][i1R][j1R] +=
   sh1[i1][j1]*sh2[model][i2][j2];
```

23. After the weights have been changed the accumulated correlations need to be reset to zero.

```
correlSum[model] = 0;
```

Recognition Module

The **recognition** module describes the recognition dynamics. If the recognition variable of a model drops below *r_theta*, the model becomes ruled out by a strong inhibition term. In the simulation it is just skipped in order to save cpu-time. The variables and symbols are shown in table 18.10.

Symbol	Variable Name	Variable Type	Description
r^p	rec	NslFloat0[]	Recognition activity
F^p	shSum	NslDinFloat0[]	Recognition sum value from model layers
$R = \max_{p'}\left(r^{p'} F^{p'}\right)$	recShSumMax	float	Recognition maximum sum value for the model layers

The **initRun** method initializes the recognition layer (winner-take-all mechanism). The **simRun** method processes the recognition layer (winner-take-all mechanism). Recognition dynamics are

Table 18.10
Symbol and variable relationship.

24. Calculate terms *shSum* and *recShSumMax* from equation (18.7),

$$R = \max_{p'}\left(r^{p'} F^{p'}\right)$$

The implementation is as follows,

```
float recShSumMax = 0;
for (model=1; model<=gallerySize; model++)
    recShSumMax = nslMax(recShSumMax,rec[model]*shSum[model]);
```

25. Integrate the recognition dynamics as described in equation (18.7),

$$\dot{r}^p(t) = \lambda_r r^p \left(F^p - \max_{p'}\left(r^{p'} F^{p'}\right) \right)$$

The implementation is as follows,

```
nslDiff(rec[model],1.,lambda_r*rec[model]^(shSum[model] -
    recshSumMax));
```

26. Compute which models to skip. This information is propagated back to other modules requiring this information through port interconnections not shown here.

```
if (model>0 && rec[model] <= r_theta)
    skipModel[model] = 1;
```

18.4 Simulation and Results[3]

Different experiments were carried out using different combinations of layer and patch sizes as shown in table 18.11.

Experiment	Layer and Patch Flags	frame	i1max	j1max	i2max	j2max	i1Rmax	j1Rmax
Blob, layer and link dynamics	*small_layer* = 1 *small_patch* = 0	0	10	10	10	10	10	10
Attention dynamics	*small_layer* = 0 *small_patch* = 0	2	17+4	16+4	10	10	17	16
Recognition dynamics	*small_layer* = 0 *small_patch* = 1	2	17+4	16+4	10	10	8	8

The first four experiments: Blob formation, blob mobilization, layer interaction and synchronization and link dynamics use the first combination where flags are set as *small_layer* = 1 and *small_patch* = 0. All modifications are made to the source file.

Table 18.11

Size combinations for layers and patches for the different experiments.

Blob Formation

Load the simulation file (*gallerySize* = 0, *attention* = 0)

```
nsl source DLMB
nsl init
nsl run
```

and observe how a blob arises.

Restart the simulation with different initial conditions

[Ctrl-C; nsl init; mouse clicks with left button on layer *h1*; nsl cont].

Vary also β_h, originally set to 0.2 e.g. [Ctrl-C; nsl set dlm.h1.beta_h 0.1; nsl set dlm.h2.beta_h 0.1; nsl cont].

What is a reasonable range for β_h?

Blob Mobilization

Load the simulation file (*gallerySize* = 0, *attention* = 0)

```
nsl source DLMR
nsl init
nsl run
```

and observe how a blob arises and moves over the layer.

Vary λ_+, λ_- and κ_{hs} (*lambda_p, lambda_m, kappa_hs*), originally set to 0.2, 0.004, and 1, respectively, to e.g. [Ctrl-C; nsl set dlm.h1.lambda_m 0.001; nsl set dlm.h2.lambda_m 0.001; nsl cont].

Why should λ_- be larger for smaller layers? Is the shape of the blob speed-dependent?

Layer Interaction and Synchronization

Load the simulation file (*gallerySize* = 1, *attention* = 0, *workOnAverage* = 0)

```
nsl source DLMS
nsl init
nsl run
```

observe how the two blobs synchronize and align with each other. Try different runs (for each run a new object is selected randomly and some synchronize easier than others) and use different object galleries [edit the file *DLMobjects* and exchange the *pose1* (= 15 degrees rotated faces) block with the *pose2* (= 30 degrees rotated faces) or *pose3* (= different facial expression) block]. Vary κ_{hh} (*kappa_hh*), originally set to 1.2. What happens if κ_{hh} is too large or too small?

Link Dynamics

Load the simulation file (*gallerySize* = 1, *attention* = 0, *workOnAverage* = 0)

```
nsl source DLMM
nsl init
nsl run
```

observe how the connectivity develops in time.
Vary λ_w (*lambda_W*). What happens if λ_w is too large?

Attention Dynamics

Load the simulation file (*gallerySize* = 1, *attention* = 1, *workOnAverage* = 0)

```
nsl source DLMR
nsl source DLMA
nsl init
nsl run
```

observe how an attention blob arises and restricts the region in which the small blob is allowed to move.
Vary κ_{ah} and κ_{ha} (*kappa_ah*, *kappa_ha*), originally set to 3 and 0.7, respectively.
Now restart the simulation with

```
nsl source DLMS
nsl init
nsl run
```

and see whether the two blobs on the layers of different size can synchronize without an attention blob.
Then add the attention blob [Ctrl-C; nsl load DLMA; nsl init; nsl run]
and see how the alignment between the blobs can become more stable (notice that for each run a new object is selected randomly, which can be suppressed by

[nsl set dlm.similarity.ObjectSelectionMode 1] in which case always the object indicated by preferredObject is used; with [nsl set dlm.similarity. ObjectSelectionMode 3] objects are selected randomly again).

You can also experiment with the attention blob misplaced in the beginning [Ctrl-C; nsl init; mouse clicks with the left button near the border on layer a1; nsl cont]. Vary κ_{ah} and κ_{ha}.

Recognition Dynamics

Load the simulation file (*gallerySize* = 5, *attention* = 1, *workOnAverage* = 1)

```
nsl source DLMG
nsl source DLMA
nsl init
nsl run
```

observe the recognition process. In the first 1000 time units only the average layer with index 0 is simulated. The correct model has index 1. Shown are, for all models, the total layer activity, the recognition variable, and the sum over all synaptic weights (cf. also figure). The connectivity and the layer 2 internal state as well as its input is shown only for the currently most active layer. The time, the index of the most active layer, and the values of the recognition parameters are given as usual output. Asterisks indicate layers that have been ruled out.

Data Base

As face database we used galleries of 111 different persons. For most persons there is one neutral frontal view, one frontal view of different facial expression, and two views rotated in depth by 15 and 30 degrees respectively. The neutral frontal views serve as model gallery, and the other three are used as test images for recognition. The models, i.e. the neutral frontal views, are represented by layers of size 10X10. Though the grids are rectangular and regular, i.e. the spacing between the nodes is constant within each dimension, the graphs are scaled horizontally and vertically and are aligned manually: The left eye is always represented by the node in the fourth column from the left and the third row from the top, the mouth lies on the fourth row from the bottom, etc. The x- (that is, horizontal) spacing ranges from 6.6 to 9.3 pixels with a mean value of 8.2 and a standard deviation of 0.5. The y-spacing ranges from 5.5 to 8.8 pixels with a mean value of 7.3 and a standard deviation of 0.6. An input image of a face to be recognized is represented by a 16X17 layer with an x-spacing of 8 pixels and a y-spacing of 7 pixels. The image graphs are not aligned, since that would already require recognition. The variations of up to a factor of 1.5 in the x- and y-spacings must be compensated for by the DLM process.

Technical Aspects

DLM in the form presented here is computationally expensive. We have performed single recognition tasks with the complete system, but for the experiments referred to in table 18.12 we have modified the system in several respects to achieve a reasonable speed. We split up the simulation into two phases. The only purpose of the first phase is to let the attention blob become aligned with the face in the input image. No modification of the connectivity was applied in this phase, and only one average model was simulated. Its connectivity was derived by taking the maximum synaptic weight over all real models for each link:

$$W_{mn}^{a}(t_0) = \max_{pq} W_{mn}^{pq}(t_0)$$

This attention period takes 1000 time steps. Then the complete system, including the attention blob, is simulated, and the individual connection matrices are subjected to DLM. Neurons in the model layers are not connected to all neurons in the image layer, but only to an 8X8 patch. These patches are evenly distributed over the image layer with the same spatial arrangement as the model neurons themselves. This still preserves full translation invariance. Full rotation invariance is lost, but the jets used are not rotation invariant in any case. The link dynamics is not simulated at each time step, but only after 200 simulation steps or 100 time units. During this time a running blob moves about once over all of its layer, and the correlation is integrated continuously. The simulation of the link dynamics is then based on these integrated correlations, and since the blobs have moved over all of the layers, all synaptic weights are modified. For further increase in speed, models which are ruled out by the winner-take-all mechanism are no longer simulated; they are just set to zero and ignored from then on ($\beta_\theta = \infty$). The CPU time needed for the recognition of one face against a gallery of 111 models is approximately 10-15 minutes on a Sun SPARCstation 10-512 with a 50 MHz processor.

In order to avoid border effects, the image layer has a frame with a width of 2 neurons without any features or connections to the model layers. The additional frame of neurons helps the attention blob to move to the border of the image layer. Otherwise, it would have a tendency to stay in the center.

Results

Figure 18.8 shows a sample recognition process using a test face strongly differing in expression from the model. The gallery contains five models. Due to the tight connections between the models, the layer activities show the same variations and differ only little in intensity. This small difference is averaged over time and amplified by the recognition dynamics, which rules out one model after the other until the correct one survives. The example was monitored for 2000 units of simulation time. An attention phase of 1000 time units had been applied before, but is not shown here. We selected a sample run which had exceptional difficulty to decide between models. The sum over the links of the connectivity matrices was even higher for the fourth model than for the correct one. This is a case where the DLM is actually required to stabilize the running blob alignment and recognize the correct model. In some other cases the correct face can be recognized without modifying the connectivity matrix.

Recognition rates for galleries of 20, 50, and 111 models are given in table 8.12. As is already known from previous work (Lades et al. 1993), recognition of depth-rotated faces is in general less reliable than, for instance, recognition of faces with an altered expression. It is interesting to consider recognition times (measured in arbitrary units). Although they vary significantly, a general tendency is noticeable: Firstly, more difficult tasks take more time, i.e. recognition time is correlated with error rate. This is also known from psychophysical experiments (see for example Bruce et al. 1987; Kalocsai et al. 1994). Secondly, incorrect recognition takes much more time than correct recognition. Recognition time does not depend very much on the size of the gallery.

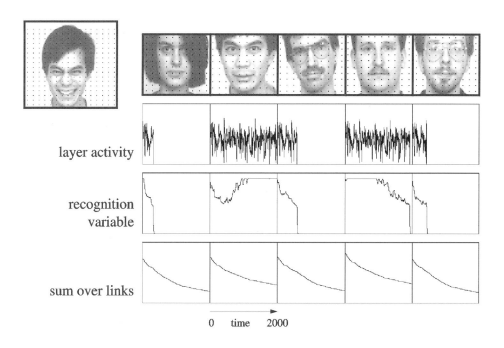

layer activity

recognition variable

sum over links

0   time   2000

Figure 18.8

DLM recognition: A sample run. The test image is shown on the left, with 16x17 neurons indicated as black dots. The models have 10x10 neurons and are aligned with each other. The corresponding total layer activities, i.e. the sum over all neurons of one model, are shown in the upper graph. The most similar model is usually slightly more active than the others. On that basis the models compete against each other, and eventually the correct one survives, as indicated by the recognition variable. The sum over all links of each connection matrix is shown in the lower graphs. It gives an impression of the extent to which the matrices self-organize before the recognition decision is made.

Gallery Size	Test Images	Correct Recognition Rate		Recognition Time	
		#	%	Correct Recognition	Incorrect Recognition
20	111 rotated faces (15 degrees)	106	95.5	320±490	4110±2860
	110 rotated faces (30 degrees)	93	84.5	990±1900	2480±2580
	109 frontal views (grimace)	100	91.7	290±530	5610±7480
50	111 rotated faces (15 degrees)	104	93.7	390±500	3770±2120
	110 rotated faces (30 degrees)	83	75.5	930±1010	2080±1440
	109 frontal views (grimace)	95	87.2	440±1290	4480±6190
111	111 rotated faces (15 degrees)	101	91.0	420±460	3770±3130
	110 rotated faces (30 degrees)	69	62.7	1350±3017	4600±3720
	109 frontal views (grimace)	92	84.4	380±410	3380±4820

18.5 Summary

We routinely use NSL for homework assignments in class as well as for our own research, and we found it appropriate for both. It is very easy to get started with NSL. It provides a reasonable set of basic structures and functions to create a neural model with just a few lines of code. Moreover, when a more complex model requires more than this basic functionality, additional functions and data structures can conveniently be added. As a matter of fact, the model presented here used very little of the NSL-specific algorithms and functions and profited mainly from NSL's graphic display facilities and interactive control structures.

The model presented here deviates in some very fundamental ways from other biological and neural models of vision or of the brain. Foremost among these is its extensive exploitation of rapid reversible synaptic plasticity and temporal feature binding. Since these features, although first presented a decade and a half ago (von der Malsburg 1981), have not received wide acceptance in the community yet, we have expended great effort to demonstrate the functional superiority of the dynamic link architecture over more conventional neural models by using it to solve a real-world problem, object recognition. We are presenting here our best achievement so far in this venture.

The model presented here is closely related to a more technically oriented system (the "algorithmic system" in contrast to the "dynamical system" described here). It has also been developed in our group and is described in (Lades et al. 1993; Wiskott et al. 1997). Essential features are common to the two systems, among them the use of jets composed of Gabor-based wavelet features, and of dynamic links to establish a mapping between the image domain and individual models.

Our model for object recognition is successful in emulating the performance and operational characteristics of our visual system in some important aspects. As in the biological case, the flexible recognition of new objects can be installed simply by showing them once. Our system works with a type of standard feature detector, wavelets, which dominates much of the early visual cortical areae (Jones & Palmer 1987). The sensitivity of our system to changes in the stimulus, as for instance head rotation and change in facial expression, is strongly correlated with that of human subjects (Kalocsai et al. 1994; this study involved a version of our algorithmic system). And, above all, our model is superior in its object discrimination ability to all biologically motivated models known to us, and is at least one of the top competitors among technical systems for face recognition (in a blind test of face recognition against large galleries, performed by the American Army Research Lab, our algorithmic system came out as one of the top

Table 18.12

Recognition results against a gallery of 20, 50, and 111 neutral frontal views. Recognition time (with two iterations of the differential equations per time unit) is the time required until all but one models are ruled out by the winner-take-all mechanism.

competitors). Moreover, our system goes beyond mere recognition of objects, providing the basis for a detailed back-labeling of the image with interpretations in terms of explicit object or pattern models which are linked to the image by dynamic links and temporal feature binding.

In spite of this success, there are still some difficulties and discrepancies. One concern is processing time. The reorganization of the connectivity matrix between the image domain and the model domain requires that the two domains be covered at least twice by the running blob. The speed of this blob is limited by the time taken by signal transmission between the domains and by the temporal resolution with which signal coincidence can be evaluated by dendritic membranes and rapidly plastic synapses. Assuming a characteristic time of a few milliseconds we estimate that our model would need at least one second to create a synaptic mapping. This is much too long compared to the adult's speed of pattern recognition (Subramaniam et al. 1995). We therefore see our system as a model for processes that require the establishment of mappings between the image and object models. This is often the case whenever the absolute or relative placement of parts within a figure is important, and is very likely to be also required when a model for a new object is to be laid down in memory. The actual inspection times required by subjects in such cases are much longer than those required for mere object recognition and can easily be accommodated by our model. We believe that mere recognition can be speeded up by short-cuts. Potential for this we see in two directions, a reduction of the ambiguity of spatial feature arrangement with the help of trained combination-coding features, and a more efficient way (than our running activity blobs) of installing topographically structured synaptic mappings between the image domain and the model domain. A possible scheme for this would be the switching of whole arrays of synapses with the help of specialized control neurons and presynaptic terminals (Anderson & van Essen 1987).

Another as yet weak point of our model is the internal organization of the model domain and the still semi-manual mode in which models are laid down. It is unrealistic to assume completely disjoint models, for several reasons, not the least of which economy in terms of numbers of neurons required. Also, it is unrealistic to see the recognition process as a competition between the dozens of thousands of objects that an adult human may be able to distinguish. Rather, pattern similarities within large object classes should be exploited to give the recognition process hierarchical structure and to support generalization to new objects with familiar traits. The existence of such hierarchies is well supported by neurological observations (Damasio & Damasio 1992) and is implicit in psychophysical results (Biederman 1987) showing that many objects are recognized as simple arrays of shape primitives which are universally applicable. In a system closely related to the one presented here (von der Malsburg & Reiser 1995), a model domain was dynamically constructed as one comprehensive fusion graph containing as sub-graphs models for different objects, and in fact for different aspects of these objects, with different models sharing many nodes. Further research is required in this direction.

Another limitation of the present system is its inability to deal with alterations of size and orientation of the object image beyond a few percent and beyond a few degrees. For this it would be necessary that the connections between the image domain and the model domain linked also features of different size and orientation. Size and orientation invariance has been successfully demonstrated in the context of the algorithmic system (Buhmann et al. 1990; Lades 1995). Direct implementation in the present model would, however, make the DLM process slower and much more difficult or perhaps even impossible, because the system would have to start with a connectivity matrix with many more non-zero entries. The problem may have to be solved with the help of a two-step DLM process, the first step installing an expectation as to size and orientation of the image, specializing the dynamic links accordingly, the second step organizing the match as described here. In many cases, estimates of size and orientation of an object's image can be derived from available cues, one of which being the object's outline as found by a segmentation mechanism.

In the set of simulations presented here we simplified the recognition problem by presenting the objects to be recognized against a homogeneous background. More difficult scenes may require separate segmentation mechanisms which first identify an image region or regions as candidates for recognition (although a version of the algorithmic system was able to recognize known objects in spite of a dense background of other objects and of partial occlusion (Wiskott & von der Malsburg 1993)). Our model is ideally suited to implement image segmentation mechanisms based on temporal feature binding, as proposed in (von der Malsburg 1981), implemented in (von der Malsburg & Buhmann 1992; Vorbrüggen 1995) and supported by experimental data as reviewed in (König & Engel 1995). According to that idea, all neurons activated by a given object synchronize their temporally structured signals to express the fact that they are part of one segment. This coherent signal, suitably identified with our attention variable a_i^p, equation (5), could focus the recognition process on segments.

In summary, we feel that in spite of some remaining difficulties and discrepancies we may have, with our model, a foot in the door to understanding important functional aspects of the human visual system. The environment provided by NSL has proved to be of great help in the development of our system, and we are extremely pleased that with NSL's help we can share our system with students and research groups, both for didactic purposes and as a cutting-edge research tool.

Notes

1. This work has been funded by grants from the German Federal Ministry of Science and Technology (413-5839-01 IN 101 B/9), from AFOSR (F49620-93-1-0109), from the EU (ERBCHRX-CT-930097), and a grant by the Human Frontier Science Program.

2. A. Weitzenfeld developed the NSL3.0 version from the original NSL2.1 model implementation written by L. Wiskott and he contributed Section 18.3 to this chapter.

3. The DLM model was implemented and tested under NSLC.

Appendix I – NSLM Methods

We describe in this appendix a number of library methods in addition to those already introduced in chapter 6.

A.I.1 System Methods

NSLM provides a number of system methods for getting and setting the NSL system variables and for manipulating the simulation. These methods are accessed using the "system" prefix as follows:

```
system.methodCall();
```

We mention the most important system methods in the following sections. Note that chapter 7 commands that begin with the "nsl" prefix all have an equivalent method call in NSLM.

In general, setting parameter values at the system level may be overridden by each module, i.e. system method calls to set parameter value are used as a default, such as setting the value for a "delta" for the complete system while each module may assign its own particular value.

Data Access

The **nslSetAccess** method sets the default NSL access of the entire system:

```
system.nslSetAccess('W');
```

This is an important statement since all model variables get their default access from the system, similarly all module variables get their default access from either the model or their corresponding parent modules and so on. The **nslSetAccess** method takes a single character as argument, either 'W', 'R' or 'N' for write/read, read, and no-access, respectively. The system default setting is 'W'. (We hope to change the default access to 'R' in a future version.) The **nslGetAccess** method will retrieve the default access value for the system,

```
char cur_access = system.nslGetAccess();
```

Simulation Parameters

Simulation parameters are usually set from a model's **initSys** method. It is important to remember that simulation time starts at 0, cycles start at 1, and epochs start at 1. Code segment A.I.1. shows the most important simulation parameters that may be set at the system level,

```
system.setTrainEndTime(dval);
system.setRunEndTime(dval);
system.setTrainDelta(dval);
system.setRunDelta(dval);
system.setNumTrainEpochs(ival);
system.setNumRunEpochs(ival);
```

Code Segment A.I.1: Methods for setting simulation parameter values for the entire system where dval corresponds to a double value and ival corresponds to an int (integer) value.

Getting the simulation parameters with a **double** or **int** type *var* as shown in the following methods in code segment A.I.2.

```
dval = system.getTrainEndTime();
dval = system.getRunEndTime();
dval = system.getTrainDelta();
dval = system.getRunDelta();
ival = system.getNumRunEpochs();
ival = system.getNumTrainEpochs();
ival = system.getCurrentTime();
ival = system.getCurrentCycle();
ival = system.getCurrentEpoch();
ival = system.getTrainEpoch();
ival = system.getRunEpoch();
```

Code Segment A.I.2: Methods for getting simulation parameter values from the entire system where *dval* corresponds to a **double** value and *ival* corresponds to an **int** (integer) value.

Incrementing, Breaking and Continuing

This section describes methods for incrementing, breaking and continuing with system defined loops. Note that unless otherwise specified, the method can be applied in either the training phase or the run phase. Methods that increment counters are:

```
system.incCycle();
system.incRunEpoch();
system.incTrainEpoch();
system.incTime();
```

Methods that break the simulation between modules, cycles, or epochs are:

```
system.breakModules();
system.breakCycles();
system.breakEpochs();
```

Methods continuing with the next module, cycle, or epoch after a break are:

```
system.continueModule();
system.continueCycle();
system.continueEpoch();
```

Model Variables

NSL lets the user set and get a number of parameters from existing model variables.

To set the name of an object instance we use:

```
obj.nslSetName(charString);
```

To get the NSL instance name of an module or class object we use:

```
charString name=obj.nslGetName();
```

The user may obtain or assign values to and from arbitrary variables in a model using the **nslSetValue** and **nslGetValue** methods, respectively. Note that all value setting and getting using these functions requires a corresponding data access similar to NSLS script data accessing. To set the value of a variable *var1* to a variable *var2* the user may use the following functions (*cast* represents a NSLM object type where variables, *var1* and *var2*, are object types as well),

```
var1=(cast)system.nslGetValue("var1");
system.nslSetValue("var2", var1);
```

Note that in the above methods the user must know each variable's absolute name starting at the tree hierarchy root, i.e. the model name. For example, if we wanted to get the value of a variable named *w1* located in module *m1* of model *modelA* and assign it to a variable *foo*, we would type,

```
NslFloat1 foo(10);
foo=(NslFloat1)system.nslGetValue("modelA.m1.w1");
```

or

```
NslFloat1 foo(10);
system.nslSetValue("modelA.m1.w1", foo);
```

In some cases the user may want to convert some of the above object type values into primitive types. This is accomplished using the **nslGetValue** method applied directly to an object type. This applies only to scalar object types using an appropriate cast. For example for a scalar **NslFloat0** *w0* object we could do the following,

```
NslFloat0 doo;
doo=(NslFloat0)system.nslGetValue("modelA.m1.w0");
double d;
d=(double)doo.nslGetValue();
```

Note that simple assignment wouldn't work since a primitive type cannot be directly assigned from an object type unless such method is present.

There are a number of methods that obtain values from objects of higher dimensions. The **getDimensions** method returns an integer specifying whether the object has 0, 1, 2, 3, or 4 dimensions.

```
int dim=obj.getDimensions();
```

The **getSizes** method obtains the different dimensions of an object where *obj1* is of dimension 1, *obj2* is of dimension 2 and so on:

```
obj1.getSizes(int);
obj2.getSizes(int,int);
obj3.getSizes(int,int,int);
obj4.getSizes(int,int,int,int);
```

We can also get the size of each dimension individually.

```
int size1=obj1.getSize1();
int size2=obj2.getSize2();
int size3=obj3.getSize3();
int size4=obj4.getSize4();
```

One more note about the different *getSizes* methods is that they can be used to control the looping for say initialization of a variable. For example, to assign a value to each element in the two-dimensional NSL object we could use the **for** control statement as follows,

```
NslFloat2 y(2,3);
int i,j;
for (i=0; i<y.getSize1(); i++)
    for (j=0; j<y.getSize2(); j++)
        y[i][j] = i+j;
```

where the functions *y*.**getSize1**() and *y*.**getSize2**() get the *rows* and *columns* sizes, respectively.

We include as well the following methods returning different sectors of multidimensional objects. For example, to get the jth column (1 dimensional object) of a 2 dimensional object we would do:

```
obj2.nslGetColumn(j);
```

(Recall that a row is simply obtained using squared brackets, e.g. obj[*i*].) To obtain a 2 dimensional sector from a 2 dimensional object we would do

```
obj2.nslGetSector(start1, start2, end1, end2);
```

Similarly, for 3 dimensional objects we would do:

```
obj3.nslGetSector(start1, start2, start3, end1, end2, end3);
```

For a 4 dimensional object we would do:

```
Obj4.nslGetSector(start1, start2, start3, start4,
    end1, end2, end3, end4);
```

Dynamic Memory Allocation

As introduced in chapter 6 NSL lets the user set the size of an object in a dynamic fashion. This applies to other than scalar types having dimensions higher than 1. The user first instantiates the variable as follows without specifying its actual size:

```
VisibilitySpec ObjectType obj();
```

Then a call to the dynamic memory allocation routine is done where *sizeList* depends on the particular *ObjectType* chosen:

```
obj.nslMemAlloc(sizeList);
```

For example, in chapter 18, the "Face Recognition by Dynamic Link Architecture" model defines almost all the variables in such a way as *NormFactor*:

```
private NslFloat2 normFactor();
```

Since the dimensions of the variable type is 2 then two arguments are passed to the memory allocation routine:

```
normFactor.nslMemAlloc(i1max,j1max);
```

Printing

Printing data in NSL takes the form of **nslPrint** and **nslPrintln** (print on a new line) for output of any string or variable. Note that we do not preface them with "system". For example, to print the value of a variable we would do (note the use of the "+" string concatenation operator),

```
nslPrint("x="+ x);
```

The above represents an implicit conversion from any variable type into a string equivalent to the explicit form:

```
nslPrint("x="+ x.toString());
```

Additionally, to print the name of an object we type:

```
nslPrint("x="+ x.getName());
```

Since every class should have a "**toString**" method, we provide one for the "system". The system **toString** method returns the current model name if it is set and an error string if it is not set:

```
nslPrintln(system.toString());
```

Another useful method is **nslPrintAllVariables**. This method prints out the name and value of all variables in the system; however, this method is very time consuming and we recommend using it sparingly.

```
system.nslPrintAllVariables();
```

Also the **nslPrintStatistics** is very useful, printing the current model name, the current phase (initialization, train, run, or end), the current epoch, the current time and the current cycle.

```
system.nslPrintStatistics();
```

File Manipulation

NSL supports reading and writing into external files.[1] NSLM defines a **NslFile** object class for doing the corresponding input and output manipulations. For example, to access a file named "file.dat" (suffix is not relevant), the user must first define an object holding the reference to the file as follows,

```
NslFile file("file.dat");
```

To open a file we use the following function specifying the type of interaction we want to use: '**R**' for read only, '**A**' (all) for both read and write or '**W**' for write only. For example, to opening "file.dat" for both read and write,

```
file.open('A');
```

To close the file we simply do,

```
file.close();
```

Also since the text files we use are buffered, we provide the flush command to immediately flush the buffer:

```
file.flush();
```

To write string values into the file one line at a time, we use the method **puts** just as in the NSL script language that is based on TCL. Note that the **puts** method write one line at a time, and will convert numerical objects to strings of characters:

```
file.puts(obj);
```

To read a value into a charString object named **obj**, we would use the method **gets** which gets one line of text and puts the whole line into **obj:**

```
file.gets(obj);
```

To write string values into the file one lexeme at a time, we use the method **write**. Note values are separated by *white-space* (space, tab, carriage return, linefeed). The method **write** will also convert numerical objects to strings of characters:

```
file.write(obj);
```

To write a value into the file with a new line at the end,

```
file.writeln(obj);
```

To read a value into a charString object named **obj**, we would use the method **read** , which gets one lexeme of text and puts the whole lexeme into **obj:**

```
file.read(obj);
```

In addition, what we have defined as *white-space*, may not be what the user desires; thus we provide two more methods that allow the user to define what *white-space* is, where *char1* specifies one character to put between lexemes and *array10* specifies a native array of 10 characters defining white-space

```
file.write(obj,char1);
file.read(obj,array10);
```

For example, the *Backpropagation* model of chapter three uses the readFile method described in the code segment A.1.3 to read training data from a file.

```
public int readFile(CharString fname,NslInt1 nPats,
NslFloat2 pInput, NslFloat2 pOutput, int iSize, int oSize)
{
    int pat=0;
    int i,j =0;
    status=-1;
    NslFile file(fname);

    if (file.open('R') <0) {
        nslPrintln("Bad File Name: "+fname);
        return(status);
    } else {
        file.gets(nPats);

        for (pat = 0; pat < nPats; pat++) {
            for (i = 0; i < iSize; i++) {
            file.read(pInput[pat][i]);
        }
        for (j = 0; j < oSize; j++) {
                file.read(pOutput[pat][j]);
        }
        file.close();
    }
}
```

Code Segment A.1.3
Example of the readFile method within the Backpropagation mode.

Display Step

The following display and protocol methods are provided for manipulation of the displays and creation and selection of the protocols. The value of a variable t representing the display delta or update time can be set or get as follows,

```
system.setDisplayDelta(t);
double var = system.getDisplayDelta();
```

A.I.2 Mathematical Methods

Numerical methods/functions supported by NSLM can be applied to any numerical object of any dimension (**NslInt**, **NslFloat**, **NslDouble**, dimensions 0,1,2,3,4 unless otherwise specified) or primitive type (**int**, **float**, **double**). They consist of *arithmetic*, *threshold*, *differential approximation* methods as well as some additional miscellaneous functions. Some of these functions have a corresponding operator, see section 6.2. There are two general formats for methods, the first one where the resultant is passed as return value and the second where the resultant is passed as the first parameter to the method as shown next,

```
z = method(x,y);
method(z,x,y);
```

While the first style is more elegant the second one is more efficient since a return value requires additional memory allocation, a relatively slow operation that should be avoided if possible. In particular, this becomes critical when dealing with higher level object dimensions.

Basic Arithmetic Methods and Operators

NSLM provides a number of numerical functions taking either a single or two arguments and returning a value.

- The arithmetic functions shown in table A.I.1 are defined for x, y and z of similar NSL type and dimensions

Operator Expression	Method Expression	Description
$z = x + y$	$z = \text{nslAdd}(x,y)$	element by element addition
$z = x - y$	$z = \text{nslSub}(x,y)$	element by element subtraction
$z = x \wedge y$	$z = \text{nslElemMult}(x,y)$	element by element multiplication
$z = x / y$	$z = \text{nslElemDiv}(x,y)$	element by element division

If both operands are of the same dimension, the operation will apply to corresponding object elements. For example, in the case of 2D arrays if x and y are 4-by-4 matrices, the expression "$z=x+y$" will add elements $x[i][j]$ with $y[i][j]$ and store the resulting $x[i][j]+y[i][j]$ into $z[i][j]$, for $0 \leq i,j < 4$. Additionally, if one argument of the operation is an array and the other one is a scalar, the operation will apply to every object element with the scalar number. For example, if x is a scalar, y is 4-by-4 matrix, the expression "$z=x+y$" will add element $y[i][j]$ with x and store the resulting $x+y[i][j]$ into $z[i][j]$, for $0 \leq i,j < 4$.

- The "*" product operator works for scalars, a vector and a scalar, a scalar and a vector, a vector and a vector, a vector and a two dimensional matrix, and two, two dimensional matrices. In the case where a scalar is involved, the "*" operator will call **nslElemMult**. In the case of two vectors, then the "*" operator will call

Table A.I.1
Basic arithmetic operators and methods.

nslElemMult as well. In the case where two matrices are involved, then the "*" operator will call **nslProduct** and return a matrix.

In table A.I.2 **nslProduct** assumes x is a matrix and y is matrix having the same number of rows as the number of columns in x. The size and dimension of resultant, z, is constructed from the number of rows in x and the number of columns in y.

Operator Expression	Method Expression	Description
$z = x * y$	$z = \text{nslProduct}(x,y)$	vector/matrix product

Table A.I.2
Multiplication method.

In the case where x is a matrix or a vector and y is a vector, we should use the **nslTrans** vector transpose method (see following sections) on the vector to make it a *column vector*.

The convolutions operators and methods shown in table A.I.3 are defined for both vectors and matrices of two dimensions. The type and dimension of z corresponds to that of y.

Operator Expression	Method Expression	Description
$z = x @ y$	$z = \text{nslConv}(x,y)$	zero-edge convolution
	$z = \text{nslConvW}(x,y)$	wrap-edge convolution
	$z = \text{nslConvC}(x,y)$	copy-edge convolution

Table A.I.3
Multiplication method.

For example, for the zero-edge effect and two matrices x, and y we have:

$$y = \begin{Bmatrix} 1 & 1 & 1 \\ 1 & 2 & 1 \\ 1 & 1 & 1 \end{Bmatrix} \qquad x = \begin{Bmatrix} 1 & 1 & 1 & 1 & 1 \\ 1 & 2 & 2 & 2 & 2 \\ 1 & 2 & 4 & 4 & 4 \\ 1 & 2 & 4 & 8 & 8 \\ 1 & 2 & 4 & 8 & 0 \end{Bmatrix}$$

will result in "z = x@y"as follows:

- First a larger matrix is created with 0 values for the edges (the size of the new matrix depends on both the size of the mask and the convolved matrix; for example for a (2d+1)x(2d+1) mask, the border of zeroes must be d-deep):

$$xc = \begin{Bmatrix} 0 & 0 & 0 & 0 & 0 & 0 & 0 \\ 0 & 1 & 1 & 1 & 1 & 1 & 0 \\ 0 & 1 & 2 & 2 & 2 & 2 & 0 \\ 0 & 1 & 2 & 4 & 4 & 4 & 0 \\ 0 & 1 & 2 & 4 & 8 & 8 & 0 \\ 0 & 1 & 2 & 4 & 8 & 0 & 0 \\ 0 & 0 & 0 & 0 & 0 & 0 & 0 \end{Bmatrix}$$

- Second we overlap y on the left top corner of xc with y [0,0] on top of xc[0,0] so the first convolution will be given by:

```
z[0,0] = (0*1 + 0*1 + 0*1) + (0*1 + 1*2 + 1*1) +
         ( 0*1 + 1*1 + 2*1) = 6
```

and so on for the other elements. For the wrap around edge effect and copy edge effect please see the website.

Additional Arithmetic Methods

NSL offers a number of additional arithmetic functions. We describe the most important of these in table A.I.4.

Method Expression	Description
z=nslAbs(x);	absolute value
z=nslDistance(x,y);	calculates the distance to a point x,y.
z=nslGaussian($x,mean,stddev$);	*guassian* distribution for x with defaults of mean 0, and standard deviation 1.
z=nslRandom($x,lower, upper$);	Calculates a random value for every element of var9 between the bounds of lower and upper. The defaults for lower and upper are 0 and 1.
z=nslRint(x);	rounds every element of x to an integer value but returns the values in the same native type of array as x. The variable z must be of the same native primitive type as the value stored by x (int, float, double).
z=nslExp(x);	calculates e to the power x.
z=nslLog(x);	calculates the *log* of x.
z=nslPow(x,n);	calculates x to the power of n. The variable n must be of the same native primitive type as the value stored by x (int, float, double).
z= nslSqrt(x);	calculates the square root of x.

For example, the **nslDistance** function calculates the distance to a point x,y using the following formula:

```
z=sqrt(pow(x,2)+pow(y,2));
```

Table A.I.4

Abs,Distance,Gaussian,Random,Rint,Exp,Log,Pow, and Sqrt methods.

In table A.I.5 we include different forms of the maximum and minimum methods.

Method Expression	Description
z=nslMaxValue(x);	finds the element with the maximum value throughout all of x and returns it in z. Variable z must be of the same native primitive type as the values of x.
z=nslMinValue(x);	finds the element with the minimum value throughout all of x and returns it in z. Variable z must be of the same native primitive type as the values of x.
nslMaxElem(nj,x);	finds the maximum value in a vector x returning the index of the element
nslMinElem(nj,x);	finds the minimum value in a vector x returning the index of the element
nslMaxElem(ni,nj,x);	finds the maximum value in a matrix x returning the index of the element
nslMinElem(ni,nj,x);	finds the minimum value in a matrix x returning the index of the element
nslMaxElem(,nh,ni,nj,x);	finds the maximum value in a 3d array x returning the index of the element
nslMinElem(nh,ni,nj,x);	finds the minimum value in a 3d array x returning the index of the element
nslMaxElem(ng,nh,ni,nj,x);	finds the maximum value in a 4d array x returning the index of the element
nslMinElem(ng,nh,ni,nj,x);	finds the minimum value in a 4d array x returning the index of the element
z=nslMaxMerge(x,y);	Calculates the maximum between the two elements of x and y returning it in z.
z=nslMinMerge(x,y);	Calculates the minimum between the two elements of x and y returning it in z.

Table A.I.5

Maximum and minimum methods.

Since we have up to four dimensions, the **nslMaxElem** method is overloaded and can have 2, 3, 4, or 5 parameters. For example, in the case where x is a four-dimensional object we use the return variables ng, nh, ni, and nj which are indexes of type **NslInt0** and are returned as well as the element they point to which is z. z must be of the same native primitive type as the values of x. We perform a similar task for function **nslMinElem**.

In table A.I.6 we include different forms of the sum methods.

Method Expression	Description
$z =$ nslSum(x);	sums all of the values in x and returns it in z. Variable z must be of the same native primitive type as the values of x.
$z =$ nslSumColumns(x);	sums the columns of matrix x and returns a native vector of the same type as the values of x and returns it in z. Variable z must be of the same native primitive type as the values of x.
$z =$ nslSumRows(x);	sums the rows of matrix x and returns a native vector of the same type as the values of x and returns it in z. Variable z must be of the same native primitive type as the values of x.

Table A.I.6
Sum methods.

In table A.I.7 we include different forms of the fill method.

Method Expression	Description
$z =$ nslFillColumns(x,y);	the method takes a y vector and fills every column of matrix x with it. The length of y and the number of rows in x must match. Also the values of x and y should be of similar types, and z should all be of the same type as x.
$z =$ nslFillRows(x,y);	the method takes a y vector and fills every row of matrix x with it. The length of y and the number of columns in x must match. Also the values of x and y should be of similar types, and z should all be of the same type as x.

Table A.I.7
Fill methods.

In table A.I.8 we include different forms of the set and get method.

Method Expression	Description
$z=$ nslGetColumn(x,n);	the method takes a matrix x and returns a vector z made of the n-th column of x The length of z and the number of rows in x must match. Also the values of x and z should be of similar types.
$z=$ nslGetRow(x,n);	the method takes a matrix x and returns a vector z made of the n-th row of x. The length of z and the number of columns in x must match. Also the values of x and z should be of similar types.
$z=$ nslGetSector(x,*start1*,*start2*, *end1*,*end2*);	returns the specified sector of matrix x. Variables *start1* through *end2* should be **int** or **NslInt0**.
$z=$ nslGetSector(x,*start1*,*start2*, *start3*, *end1*,*end2*,*end3*);	returns the specified sector of 3d array x. Variables *start1* through *end3* should be **int** or **NslInt0**.
$z=$ nslGetSector(x,*start1*,*start2*, *start3*,*start4*,*end1*,*end2*, *end3*,*end4*);	returns the specified sector of 4d array x. Variables *start1* through *end4* should be **int** or **NslInt0**.
nslSetColumn(z,x,n);	set a vector z with a vector made of the n-th column of x The length of z and the number of rows in x must match. Also the values of x and z should be of similar types.
nslSetRow(z,x,n);	set a vector z with a vector made of the n-th row of x. The length of z and the number of columns in x must match. Also the values of x and z should be of similar types.
nslSetSector(z,x,*start1*,*start2* ,*end1*,*end2*);	sets the specified sector of z with a matrix x. Variables *start1* through *end4* should be **int** or **NslInt0**.
nslSetSector(z,x,*start1*,*start2*, *start3*,*end1*,*end2*, *end3*);	sets the specified sector of z with a 3d array x. Variables *start1* through *end4* should be **int** or **NslInt0**.
nslSetSector(z,x,*start1*,*start2*, *start3*,*start4*,*end1*,*end2*, *end3*,*end4*);	sets the specified sector of z with a 4d array x. Variables *start1* through *end4* should be **int** or **NslInt0**.

Table A.I.8
Set and Get methods.

In table A.I.9 we include matrix transformation methods.

Method Expression	Description
$z=$ nslTrans(x);	the method transposes a vector or matrix x into z.
$z=$ nslInverse(x);	the method computes the inverse of a matrix x into z.

Table A.I.9
Fill methods.

Trigonometric Methods

In table A.I.10 we include a number of trigonometry methods.

Method Expression	Description
$z=$ nslCos (x);	compute cosine of the values in x and returns it in z.
$z=$ nslSin (x);	compute sine of the values in x and returns it in z.
$z=$ nslTan (x);	compute tangent of the values in x and returns it in z.
$z=$ nslArcCos (x);	compute arc cosine of the values in x and returns it in z.
$z=$ nslArcSin (x);	compute arc sine of the values in x and returns it in z.
$z=$ nslArcTan (x);	compute arc tangent of the values in x and returns it in z.

Table A.I.10
Trigonometry methods.

Threshold Methods

NSLM provides with a number of threshold functions: *ramp, step, saturation, bound,* and *sigmoid*, as shown in figure A.I.1. All these functions are considered *pointwise* operations similar to addition, being applied to corresponding elements in the object independent of dimension.

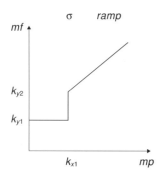

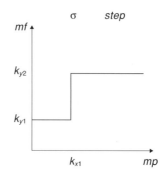

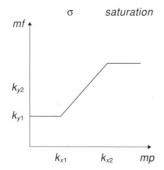

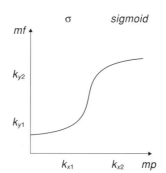

Figure A.1.2
Common Threshold Functions.

The functions are defined as follows:

- *Step* function is defined for x and y of similar NSL type and dimensions

$$y = \mathbf{nslStep}(x, k_{x_1}, k_{y_1}, k_{y_2})$$

corresponding to the pointwise application of

$$y = \begin{cases} k_{y2} & x \geq k_{x1} \\ k_{y1} & x < k_{x1} \end{cases}$$

with defaults $k_{x1} = 0$, $k_{y1} = 0$, and $k_{y2} = 1$.

- *Ramp* function is defined for x and y of similar NSL type and dimensions

```
y = nslRamp(x,k_x1,k_y1,k_y2)
```

corresponding to the pointwise application of

$$y = \begin{cases} x - k_{x1} + k_{y2} & x \geq k_{x1} \\ k_{y1} & x < k_{x1} \end{cases}$$

with defaults $k_{x1} = 0$, $k_{y1} = 0$, and $k_{y2} = 0$.

- *Saturation* function is defined for x and y of similar NSL type and dimensions

```
y = nslSaturation(x,k_x1,k_x2,k_y1,k_y2)
```

corresponding to the pointwise application of

$$y = \begin{cases} k_{y2} & x \geq k_{x2} \\ \dfrac{(k_{y2} - k_{y1})(x - k_{x1})}{(k_{x2} - k_{x1})} + k_{y1} & k_{x1} \leq x < k_{x2} \\ k_{y1} & x < k_{x1} \end{cases}$$

with defaults $k_{x1} = 0$, $k_{x2} = 1$, $k_{y1} = 0$, and $k_{y2} = 1$.

- *Bound* function is defined for x and y of similar NSL type and dimensions

```
y = nslBound(x,k_x1,k_x2,k_y1,k_y2)
```

corresponding to the pointwise application of

$$y = \begin{cases} k_{y2} & x \geq k_{x2} \\ x & k_{x1} \leq x < k_{x2} \\ k_{y1} & x < k_{x1} \end{cases}$$

with defaults $k_{x1} = 0$, $k_{x2} = 1$, $k_{y1} = 0$, and $k_{y2} = 1$.

- *Sigmoid* function is defined for x and y of similar NSL type and dimensions

```
y = nslSigmoid(x,slope,offeset)
```

corresponding to the pointwise application of

$$y = \begin{cases} \dfrac{1}{\left(1 + \exp^{(-slope(x-offset))}\right)} \end{cases}$$

with defaults $x = 1$, *slope* $= 1$, *and offset=0,* and

```
y = nslSigmoid(x, k_{x1}, k_{x2}, k_{y1}, k_{y2, inverseErrorConst});
```

corresponding to the pointwise application of the above function but with the following substitutions:

```
offset=(kx1+kx2)/2;
slope=(inverseErrorConst /(kx2-kx1));
result=nslSigmoid(x,slope,offset) * (ky2-ky1) + ky1;
```

with defaults $k_{x1} = 0$, $k_{x2} = 1$, $k_{y1} = 0$, and $k_{y2} = 1$, error_const=10.

Notes

1. In the current version only ascii (text) files are supported. The NSLC system supports extensions to binary files as exemplified in chapter 18 with the DLM model.

Appendix II – NSLJ Extensions

This section describes the features of the NSLJ simulation environment that are not present in the standard system. We expect that these extensions will be incorporated into NSL3_0 in the future.

A.II.1 Additional NslModule Types

The NslOutModules and NslInModules are import within the NSLJ system since they allow for the special processing of display data and are a core part of the user interface. It is important to note that NslInModules and NslOutModules are scheduled by the scheduler while NslInFrames and NslOutFrames are not. NslInFrames and NslOutFrames are just one variable within a NslInModule or a NslOutModule. The NslOutModule is used to control the output going to a NslOutFrame. Every NslOutModule has one and only one NslOutFrame. (The frame's title is generated from the NslOutModule's instance name.) Every NslOutModule has one and only one NslOutFrame. (The frame's title is generated from the NslOutModule's.) Each NslOutModule must specify to which protocols it belongs and all NslOutModule are assumed to belong to the "manual" protocol unless specifically removed. If a NslOutModule is enabled by selection of a protocol, it is executed by the scheduler at the frame's specified DisplayDelta times. The same holds true for NslInModules as well: the module has one and only one NslInFrame, each NslInModule must specify to which protocols it belongs, and it executes at the frame's specified DisplayDelta time.

To define a module of type NslOutModule, type the following:

```
nslOutModule Foo (int size) {
    public void initModule() {
      nslAddProtocolRecursiveUp("Jumping");
      nslAddAreaCanvas(outpu,-1,1);
      nslAddTemporalCanvas(energy,-1-,10);
    }
}
```

In the code above, we have declared the nslOutModule "Foo" and have subscribed to the protocol "Jumping". In addtion, we have also declared that two plots shall appear on this NslOutModule's NslOutFrame—namely one Area graph and one temporal graph. All standard output plots can be added in this way.

To define a module of type NslInModule, type the following:

```
nslInModule Moo (int size) {
    public void initModule() {
      nslAddProtocolRecursiveUp("Learn");
      nslAddPanel("controlBar");
      nslAddButton("clear","Clear image","controlBar");
    //stuff
    }
public void clearPushed() {//the name "clear" came from
    nslAddButton
    //stuff
    }

}
```

In the NslInModule we have added a few of the NSLJ widget types. For a complete list of these, please see our website at http://www-hbp.usc.edu/Projects/nsl.htm. Here are the ones we used above.

NslAddPanel is used to add a blank panel to the canvas

```
public void nslAddPanel(charString name){}
```

where name is the variable name of the panel. The size of the panel will grow with each new button added to the panel.

NslAddButton is used to add a button to the panel.

```
public void nslAddButton(charString name, charString label,
charString panel name){}
```

where name is the name of the button. A corresponding method must be written in the user's code with the name "buttonnamePushed" ("buttonname" concatenated with "Pushed".). The label name is the name that will appear on the button, and the panel name is the name of the panel in which to place the button.

nslAddInputImageCanvas looks like that shown in figure 5.18. NslInputImage-Canvas is placed directly on NslInFrames. Clicking the box of the element desired within the grid will cause that box to become shaded and take on the ymax value. All boxes not selected will have the ymin value.

```
public void nslAddInputImageCanvas(NslNumeric variable, int
ymin, int ymax){}
```

where the NslNumeric can have one or two dimensions; ymin is the lower bound on y; and ymax is the upper bound on y.

NslAddNumericEditorCanvas allows the user to see the values of a zero, one, or two-dimensional array displayed in a grid like fashion.

```
public void nslAddNumericEditorCanvas(NslNumeric variable, int
ymin, int ymax){}
```

where the NslNumeric can have zero, one or two dimensions; ymin is the lower bound on y, and ymax is the upper bound on y. For an example of the NumericEditor widget please see figure 5.17. In that example we add three NumericEditor Widgets to one frame. The NumericEditor widget can be used both as an input widget and an output widget. If used as an output widget, the values are updated every Display Delta increment.

A.II.2 NSLM Extensions

Additional System Methods
Two convenient methods in neural simulation are "nslGetValue" and "nslSetValue." These methods can act as **probes** (system.**nslGetValue**, system.**nslSetValue**-(*foo*, *"modelA.m1.w1"*) and as **injectors** (system.**nslSetValue**(*"modelA.m1.w1"*, *foo*)). We can use them in a **NslModule** or a **NslClass** without having to put the "system" in front of the method name. Thus we would just type:

```
foo=(NslFloat1)nslGetValue( "modela.m1.w1");
```

The method **nslGetModelRef** is also convenient for manipulating the model instance by returning a reference to a variable of type **NslModel**. The syntax is:

```
var1=system.nslGetModelRef();
```

The **nslGetRefOfModuleOrClass** method is similar to the **getModelRef** method. It returns a reference to a NslHierarchy class object, thus you will need to cast it to the appropriate type:

```
var2=(NslModule)system.nslGetRefOfModuleOrClass
("modelA.m1",'R');
var3=(NslClass)system.nslGetRefOfModuleOrClass
("modelA.c1",'R');
```

Note that "*modelA.m1*" is m1's *long-name* or *real-name*. *long-names* or *real-names* start with the model instance names and each child module or class instance is appended from there.

Differential Approximation

To add a new approximation method we type:

```
system.addApproximationMethod(NslDiff);
```

To set or get the system approximation method we use:

```
system.setApproximationMethod(NslDiff);
NslDiff diffObj;
diffObj=system.getApproximationMethod();
```

Currently only **NslDiffEuler** and **NslDiffRungeKutta2** are available as parameters to the **setApproximationMethod**. The default approximation method is Euler.

To set or get the current approximation delta we type:

```
system.setApproximationDelta(double);
double var=system.getApproximationDelta();
```

The default delta is 0.1.

To set or get the current approximation time constant we type:

```
system.setApproximationTimeConstant (double);
double var=system.getApproximationTimeConstant();
```

The default time constant is 1.0.

DisplayDelta

To set or get *t5* as a double representing the display delta or update time. The current default display delta is set to every cycle.

```
system.setDisplayDelta(t5); );
double var = system.getDisplayDelta();
```

Additional NslBase Methods

The **NslBase** class is the most primitive class in the NSL class hierarchy tree. Every NSL object inherits this class (except for system) and thus can use these methods. Since these classes could be *subclassed*, we prefix their names with "nsl" so that the model builder does not override our methods accidentally.

To set the parent of an object instance we can use:

```
obj.nslSetParent(NslHierarchy parent);
```

To get the parent objects reference we can type:

```
NslHierarchy objParent;
    objParent = objChild.nslGetParent();
```

To get the parent objects reference of type NslModule we can type:

```
NslModule objParent;
    objParent = objChild.nslGetParentModule();
```

To get the parent objects reference of type NslClass we can type:

```
NslClass objParent;
    objParent = objChild.nslGetParentClass();
```

Additional NslData Methods

The **NslData** class provides the backbone for the classes **NslNumeric**, **NslString** and **NslBoolean**. Half of the methods are abstract or virtual meaning that they must be overridden in all of the subclasses. In all of the following examples we assume that *objX* is of some **NslData** type, such as **NslBoolean0**, **NslString0**, **NslDouble0**, **NslDinDouble0**, or **NslDoutDouble0**.

The first method we will discuss is **duplicateData**. This method is abstract/virtual, and it copies or clones the value of *obj1* and places it in the parameter.

```
NslFloat2 obj1(4,4);
NslFloat2 obj2(4,4);
obj1.duplicateData(obj2);
```

The **duplicateThis** method is abstract/virtual, and it returns a copy of itself.

```
obj2=(NslFloat2)obj1.duplicateThis();
```

where *obj2* is of type and will probably need to be cast to the same type that obj1 is.

The next method is also abstract and called **setReference**. This method sets the reference pointer of this object to the data value of the parameter. (It is similar to two pointers pointing to a same object in C/C++.) Whenever the data value of one side is changed, the other side is changed as well. It is used only in NslPorts.

```
obj3.setReference(obj1);
```

The **isDataSet** method is also used within the NSL system. This method checks whether the object value is null or not. (This method is also abstract/virtual.) A **NslData**'s value can be null if the **NslData** object was created without instantiations, and the user was planning to use **nslMemAlloc** to allocate the space for the value.

```
obj4.isDataSet();
```

The next method is a complement to **isDataSet**. It is called **resetData**. It sets the objects value back to null. (This method is also abstract/virtual.)

```
obj5.resetData();
```

The methods which are not abstract/virtual but which can be overridden are:

```
int sizes[4];
sizes=obj8.getSizes();
```

The last statement returns the sizes for all dimensions. If *obj8* is a scalar, then the *sizes* array will contain all zeros. If *obj8* is a vector (dimension1), then *sizes*[0] will contain the length of the vector, etc.

Additional NslNumeric Methods

The numeric methods involve the following classes: **NslNumeric** (only abstract /virtual), **NslNumeric*X*** (mostly abstract/virtual), **NslDouble*X*, NslFloat*X*, NslInt*X*, NslDinDouble*X*, NslDinFloat*X*, NslDinInt*X*, NslDoutDouble*X*, NslDoutFloat*X*, NslDoutInt*X*** where *X* represents 0, 1, 2, 3, or 4. The class hierarchy of the NslDinDouble4 class is shown in figure A.1.1.

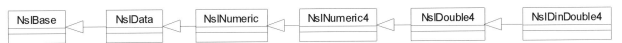

Since there are so many **NslNumeric** associated classes, we will just mention two of them here: **NslNumeric0**, and **NslDouble2**. We feel that this will give most readers an overview of the methods they are interested in and if the user would like more information, he/she can see our website for the full details on each class.

Figure A.II.1
Class Hierarchy of the NslDinDouble4 Class using UML notation.

Additional NslNumeric0 Methods

In this section we will not reiterate the methods that were covered in **NslBase** and **NslData**, we will just assume that the abstract methods mentioned in those classes were implemented correctly in this class or in one of its subclass. In addition to the abstract/virtual type methods, this class also contains pseudo templates for several methods that return a different type based on the type of object the method is associated with. We do this since Java does not let us return different types when a method is declared abstract. In all of the following we assume *obj0* is of some **NslNumeric** type such as **NslDouble0**, **NslDinDouble0**, or **NslDoutDouble0**.

The first of these pseudo abstract methods is **get,** returning a native primitive value or native primitive array reference.

```
var1=obj0.get();
```

The next set of methods are all abstract/virtual, meaning they are all overridden in one of the subclasses NslDouble0, NslFloat0, or NslInt0.

```
doubleVar= obj0.getdouble() ;
floatVar = obj0.getfloat() ;
intVar = obj0.getint() ;
NslDouble0 var = obj0.getNslDouble0() ;
NslFloat0 var = obj0.getNslFloat0() ;
NslInt0 var = obj0.getNslInt0() ;
```

In the next statement value is a either **double**, **float**, **int**, or **NslNumeric0**; notice the set method is *overloaded*

```
obj0.set(value);
```

This last method is not abstract/virtual. It is called **getSize** and is only implemented in **NslNumeric0**, **NslNumeric1**, **NslBoolean0**, and **NslBoolean1**.

```
int someint=obj0.getSize();
```

where *obj0* is either a **NslNumeric0**, **NslNumeric1**, **NslBoolean0**, and **NslBoolean1** type.

Additional NslNumeric2 Methods

Note that in this class we do not declare any abstract/virtual methods since this is a leaf class. However, the methods within the **NslDinDouble2** and **NslDoutDouble2** classes can override these methods. And again we will not repeat the methods covered in **NslBase** or **NslNumeric**. In the following examples, *obj2* is of type **NslDouble2** returning either a reference to the original object's value in the case where no casting is needed, and returning a reference to an object of the appropriate type where casting is indicated.

```
double[][] somedouble2d=obj2.get();
double[] somedouble1d=obj2.get(int);
double somedouble=obj2.get(int,int);
double[][] somedouble2d=obj2.getdouble2();
float[][] somefloat2d=obj2.getfloat2();
int[][] someint2d=obj2.getint2();
double[] somedouble1d=obj2.getdouble1(int);
float[] somefloat1d=obj2.getfloat1(int);
int[] someint1d=obj2.getint1(int);
double somedouble=obj2.getdouble(int,int);
float somefloat=obj2.getfloat(int,int);
int someint=obj2.getint(int,int);
NslDouble2 someNslDouble2(4,4);
NslFloat2 someNslFloat2(4,4);
NslInt2d someNslInt2(4,4);
someNslDouble2=obj2.getNslDouble2();
someNslFloat2=obj2.getNslFloat2();
someNslInt2d=obj2.getNslInt2();
```

Code Segment A.II.5
NslDouble2 Methods Using Get.

Next we have the set methods. All set methods copy the value passed in before assigning to the value of the object. The set methods are overloaded so that they can take a variety of parameters. The first method is:

```
obj2.set(value);
```

where *value* is a native **double**, **float**, **int** array of dimension 2 or **NslNumeric2**; *obj2* is **NslDouble2.** The next method is:

```
obj2.set(int,int,value);
```

where *value* is of type **double**, **float**, **int**, or **NslNumeric0**. This method sets a particular element within the array. The next method is:

```
obj2.set(value);
```

where *value* is of type **double**, **float**, **int** or **NslNumeric0**. This method sets all of the elements of the matrix to the value specified.

Finally, we need to mention the **memAlloc** method. We use this method when we want to dynamically allocate the size of a matrix sometime later on in the simulation. A typical use is to set the dimensions of a variable from a script file or from the NSLS script window. The *Backpropagation* model from chapter 3 set the sizes of some of its NSL objects this way. While a NSL numeric object must be initially specified with an appropriate dimension type, the user may delay specifying the corresponding dimension sizes. For example, a two-dimensional object may have its corresponding sizes specified during object instantiation as follows,

```
NslDouble2 a(size1,size2);
```

or could be specified in two steps using the **memAlloc** function as follows

```
NslDouble2 a();
a.memAlloc(size1,size2);
```

The above memory allocation expression can take place anywhere in the program. Just beware that if the object is used before doing the memory allocation call, errors may result in the program. In addition, NSL port types can only use the **memAlloc** method within the **callFromConstructorBottom** method, or the top of the **makeConn** method. This is due to the fact that **makeConn** wants to make sure the ports are well defined before it connects them to other modules. Remember the dimensions and the sizes of the dimensions on the port types must match to make a connection. If the sizes are not know, then **makeConn** cannot make a connection.

Additional NslBoolean Methods

The **NslBoolean** class inherits from **NslData** and **NslBase**; thus we will not cover the methods from those classes again. However, **NslBoolean** and **NslBoolean***N* have some methods unique to the **boolean** class. For this example we will look at the **NslBoolean2** class.

In all examples *obj2* is of type **NslBoolean2**. Also the methods that convert from **boolean** to native primitive types, convert true to the value 1 or 1.0, and false to 0 or 0.0.

```
boolean[][] someboolean2d=obj2.get();
boolean[] someboolean1d=obj2.get(int);
boolean someboolean=obj2.get(int,int);
boolean[][] someboolean2d=obj2.getboolean2();
boolean[] someboolean1d=obj2.getboolean1(int);
boolean someboolean=obj2.getboolean(int,int);
NslBoolean2 someNslBoolean2(4,4);
someNslBoolean2=obj2.getNslBoolean2();
```

Next we have the **set** methods. All **set** methods copy the value passed in before assigning to the value of the object. The set methods are overloaded so that they can take a variety of parameters where *value* is a native **double**, **float**, **int** array of dimension 2 or **NslNumeric2**; *obj2* is **NslBoolean2**.

```
obj2.set(value);
```

In the following statement *value* is of type **double**, **float**, **int**, **NslNumeric0** or **NslBoolean0**.

```
obj2.set(int,int,value);
```

In the following statement *value* is of type **double[]**, **float[]**, **int[]**, **NslNumeric1**, or **NslNumeric1**.

```
obj2.set(int, value);
```

Finally we have the **memAlloc** method, and just as in the **NslDouble2** case above, we can dynamically set the sizes of the dimensions of the arrays at run time in any method. However, NSL port types and their dimensions sizes must be defined before the first *nslConnect* statement is made using one of these ports.

```
NslBoolean2 b();
b.memAlloc(size1,size2);
```

Additional NslString0 Methods

The **NslString** or the **NslString0** class was covered somewhat in section 6.2. However, we will describe its unique method in more detail here. Again note, that since **NslString** is a subclass of **NslData** and **NslBase** we will not cover those methods here.

In all of the following examples, the *obj0* is of type *NslString0*.

```
charString somestring=obj0.get();
charString somestring= obj0.getstring() ;
NslString0 someNslString0();
someNslString0 = obj0.getNslString0() ;
```

In the following statement *value* is either a **double**, **float**, **int**, **boolean**, **charString**, **NslNumeric0**, **NslBoolean0**, or **NslString0**; notice the set method is *overloaded*

```
obj0.set(value);
```

In the following statement *obj0* is of type **NslString0**. **getLength** is only implemented in **NslString0** and it returns the length of the string.

```
int someint=obj0.getLength();
```

Additional NslHierarchy Methods

The NSLJ class NslHierarchy is the parent class for NslModule and NslClass. Its original name was NslThingsWithChildren but we felt the name was too long. Many of the **NslHierarchy** methods have already been discussed in the **NslSystem** methods earlier in this appendix. We will mention some of them here but will refer you to the **NslSystem** section for a more in depth description of these functions. When the set methods are used in relation to a **NslModule** or NslClass object, the setting of a value only change the value of the current module or class and not the entire system. When the get methods are used in relation to a **NslModule** or NslClass object, the getting of a value only returns the default for that module or class, and not the system default.

The methods that are also in **NslSystem** are:

```
value=(cast)mod1.nslGetValue(name);
mod1.nslSetValue(target,data);
```

where *target* is a **charString** and *data* is of type **NslData**

```
mod1.nslSetValue(target, num);
```

where *target* is of type **NslData** and *num* is a **charString.**

```
mod1.nslSetAccessRecursive(char1);
```

where *char1* is either 'R', 'W', or 'N'.

The **NslHierarchy** class also contains the following methods (note that all of these methods begin with "nsl" to avoid accidental overrides by subclasses). The following gets the long-name or real-name of the module or class,

```
somestring=mod1.nslGetRealName();
```

To print the name of the current module/class and the name of its parent module

```
charString=nslGetNameAndParent();
```

To print the name of the current module/class and all ancestors

```
charString=nslGetNameAndParentRecursive();
```

This method gets a reference to the variable with the specified name. This method works as long as the named variable has NSL read access; otherwise it returns null. Note: only NSL types are stored as data variables.

```
var2=nslGetDataVar(name);
```

where name is of type **charString** and *var2* is of type **NslData**. And also

```
var2=nslGetDataVar(name,'R');
```

where *name* is of type **charString** and *var2* is of type **NslData**. This method gets a reference to the variable with the specified name. This method works as long as the named variable has the specified NSL access; otherwise it returns null. Additional methods, where *name* is **charString** and *status* is boolean are given below:

```
status=nslHasChildClass(name);//true if has instance of
    NslClass
nslPrintChildClasses();// prints all child classes
```

Additional NslModule Methods

All NSL modules inherit from this class. This class contains many methods that we manipulate internally to NSL, and it also contains many classes for the flow of execution, such as the **initSys**, **initModule**, **initRun**, **simRun**, and **endRun** methods that were covered in chapter 6. Since this class is meant to be subclassed we begin all method names with "nsl" and all public attribute variables with underscore. (The exceptions to this rule are the simulation control methods, the setting and getting of delta values, and the getting and setting of the buffering flag.) Also, these methods are typically called from within a NslModule and thus we do not need to put the module instance name in front of the method name. However, if we were to call one of these methods from a different **NslModule** or **NslClass**, then we would need to use the syntax:

```
somemodule.method(param1);.
```

The first set of methods we would like to discuss are the methods that augment the automatic constructor "makeInst". These methods are meant to be built by the model builder and are described in table A.II.1.

Constructor Methods	Description
callFromConstructorTop	Allows the user to instantiate special objects before the NSL types are instantiated in makeInst. callFromConstructorTop is called immediately upon instantiating a new module; right after any parent attributes are instantiated.
callFromConstructorBottom	Allows the user to instantiate special objects before makeConn called. The callFromConstructorBottom is called immediately after instantiating a new module.
makeInst	makeInst is not overridable and is not callable from the user's code. We use makeInst to instantiate all NSL type parameters and native arrays that were declared in the attribute section of the code. In object-oriented programming terms, makeInst is the heart of the constructor for the module. We could have called it callFromConstrutorMiddle but did not.

There are no arguments to **callFromConstructorTop** or **callFromConstructor-Bottom** method. Also, NSL type variables defined in the attribute section of the NslModule, are instantiated after **callFromConstructorTop** and before **callFromConstructorBottom**. Thus, if you need to manipulate one of these attributes, it is best to put the code in **callFromConstructorBottom**. For example, in code segment A.II.1 the **callFromConstructorBottom** method will print the *name* stored for the object as well as the *size* parameter passed to the class during instantiation. This will be done for every new object created of type **MemoryCalc**.

Table A.II.1
Module constructor methods.

```
public void callFromConstructorBottom()
{
    nslPrint("MemoryCalc instance name: ", nslName);
    nslPrint("MemoryCalc size: ", size);
}
```

Code Segment A.II.1
callFromConstructorBottom
for NslClasses.

The next method adds a *child* NslModule to the list:

```
nslAddToModuleChildren(child1);
```

The next method gets a reference to the named child module where *name* is of type **charString**:

```
NslModule foo;
foo=nslGetModuleRef(name);
```

To set the access for module and all below it where *char1* is 'R,' 'W,' or 'N' we use:

```
nslSetAccessRecursive(char1);
```

nslHasChildModule will tell you if a module has submodules. Note *status* is of type **boolean** and *name* is of type **charString**.

```
status=nslHasChildModule(name);
```

nslPrintChildModules prints all of the submodules.

```
nslPrintChildModules();
```

nslGetPort will retrieve the reference to the named port.

```
NslDinFloat2 port1(5,5);
port1=nslGetPort(name);
```

The **getDelta** method returns the current simulation delta either Train or Run for this module.

```
double d1=getDelta();
double d1=getTrainDelta();
double d1=getRunDelta();
```

The setTrainDelta method sets the current simulation train delta for this module where *d1* is of type **double.** And the getRunDelta method gets the runDelta value.

```
setTrainDelta(d1);
double var1=getRunDelta(d1);
```

The next methods reset the train delta to the system train delta or the system run delta for all modules :

```
nslResetTrainDelta();
nslResetRunDelta();
```

In the next method, *flag* indicates whether the current module is in the schedule for the training or running phase. We provide this method since sometimes protocols leave out certain modules.

```
boolean status=nslGetTrainEnableFlag();
boolean status=nslGetRunEnableFlag();
```

The next methods sets or gets the currently set approximation delta or methods used in the **nslDiff** methods for this module.

```
double d2=getApproximationDelta();
setApproximationDelta(d2);
NslDiff m2=nslGetApproximationMethod();
nslSetApproximationMethod(m2);
```

Buffering was discussed in chapter 6. However, there are some additional methods. The next method resets the buffering to the system buffering default for all modules below this one.

```
nslResetBuffering ();
```

To add the following protocol name to the system list of protocols and add this name to the module's list of protocols, and add this *name* to all of the protocol lists within the child.

```
nslAddProtocolRecursiveDown(name);
```

To add the following protocol name to the system list of protocols and add this name to the module's list of protocols, and add this name to all of the protocol lists of the ancestors of this module. This is the method typically used by users.

```
nslAddProtocolRecursiveUp(name);
```

To remove the following name from the modules protocol list.

```
nslRemoveFromLocalProtocols(name);
```

To add the name to the system list of protocols and add it also to the NSL Executive list of protocol names.

```
nslDeclareProtocol(name,label);
```

The following methods return the value of the named variable within the parent module. This method is not encouraged since the variable should have been passed to the child.

```
NslData var1;
var1=nslValParent(name);
```

Additional NslClass Methods

NslClass exists because **NslClasses** cannot contain **NslModules**. It inherits from **NslHierarchy** and **NslBase**. Thus, all of the methods available from **NslClass** have already been discussed.

The following method is generated by the preparser and initializes the invisible temporary variables the NSL system uses to in mathematics expressions. It initializes the variables in the specified methods so that it does not have to reinitialized them every cycle.

```
initTempClass();
```

Logical Methods

The following logical methods can be applied pointwise to the variables of either **NslNumeric**, **NslBoolean** or native primitive variables and arrays/matrices.

If *var1* and *var2* are of equal value, the method returns true; else false.

```
nslEqu(var1,var2);
```

If *var1* is greater than or equal to *var2*, the method returns true; else false.

```
nslGeq(var1,var2);
```

If *var1* is greater than to *var2*, the method returns true; else false.

```
nslGtr(var1,var2);
```

If *var1* is less than or equal to *var2*, the method returns true; else false.

```
nslLeq(var1,var2);
```

If *var1* is less than *var2*, the method returns true; else false.

```
nslLes(var1,var2);
```

If *var1* is not equal to *var2*, the method returns true; else false.

```
nslNeq(var1,var2);
```

The following logical methods can be applied to the variables of type **NslBoolean** or native primitive variables and arrays/matrices of type **boolean**. All logical methods are applied pointwise except for **nslAll**, **nslNone** and **nslSome**.

If *var1* and *var2* are both true, the method returns true, else false.

```
nslAnd(var1,var2);
```

If none of the values in *var1* are true, then returns true, else false.

```
nslNone(var1);
```

The following function returns the opposite **boolean** value as that stored in *var1*.

```
nslNot(var1);
```

If *var1* or *var2* is true, the method returns true, else false.

```
nslOr(var1,var2);
```

If all of the values in *var1* are true, then return true, else false.

```
nslAll(var1,);
```

If some of the values in *var1* are true, then return true, else false.

```
nslSome(var1);
```

A.II.3 Displays and Protocols

NSL Protocols

As mentioned in chapter 5 protocols provide an easy way for the model builder to set up predetermined parameters and windows for a particular protocol. We make the distinction between experiment and protocol in that many experiments can be executed for one protocol. For instance if the model builder has a random number generator in the model, then the results of the "run" will be different each time the protocol is executed. The **default protocol** is "**manual**" which means that the model does not have any particular protocols. All modules and the script window subscribe to the manual protocol initially.

Adding Protocols

The user is free to add new protocols via on of the following statements:

```
system.addProtocolToAll("protocolName")
nslAddProtocolRecursiveUp("protocolName")
```

The first statement will subscribe all known modules to the specified protocol; the second will only subscribe the current module and all its ancestors to the protocol. Both statements will add the protocol name to the Executive's menu list of protocols as well as the systems internal list of protocols. The addition of protocols should occur as early as possible in the model creation process; thus we recommend that they be placed in the top module's **initModule** method although they can be placed in any of the initialization methods other than initSys. Also to change the name of protocol in the Executive windows menu, we can use:

```
nslDeclareProtocol("protocolName", "protocolLabel")
```

where only the protocol label will appear in the menu.

Removing Protocols

It is also important to note that a module can remove itself from a particular protocol within an any of the initialization methods (other than initSys) via one of the statements

```
nslRemoveFromLocalProtocols("protocolName")
nslRemoveProtocolRecursiveUp("protocolName")
```

The difference between the two statements is that the first will unsubscribe only that module from the protocol; the second will unsubscribe the current module and all of it ancestors (even the model module) from the protocol. For instance, in code segments 5.1 and 5.2 we see that these display windows or frames should not appear if the protocol is the default "manual". If we do not want a particular NslInFrame or NslOutFrame to appear when the NSL system is first started, then we should add a **nslRemoveFrom-LocalProtocols("manual")** statement or a **nslRemoveProtocolRecur-siveUp("name")** statement to the NslOutModule's or NslInModule's initModule method.

Setting the Default Protocol
To set the model up with a particular protocol on start up we can add the statement

```
system.setProtocol("protocolName")
```

to any of the initialization methods (other than the initSys) but should be added after all the other protocol statements (if any) have been issued. The statement **system.set-Protocol("protocolName")** first disables any module not subscribed to the protocol, and then enables any module that is subscribed to the protocol. Next it reconnects all of the subscribed modules. Since this is a very expensive operation, we recommend that it be use sparingly and that it only be called from initModule. Also we should note that the setting of the protocol name would only happen after the completion of the initialization cycle or epoch that the statement appears in.

Menu Selection of a Protocol
From the Executive menu we can select a particular protocol that the model builder has provided for us. The new protocol may or may not bring up a new NslInFrame or NslOutFrame (to be discussed below); however, it will almost certainly set different parameter inputs to the model. This is demonstrated in Dominey's model in chapter 14 and by Jacob Spoelstra's model in chapter 16.

Getting the Schedule Associated with a Protocol
If curious, the modeler can also query the NSL system to retrieve the schedule of NSL modules that will run under the selected protocol. The call to do this is:

```
nslShowSchedule("protocolName");
```

This statement should only be executed only after a protocol has been selected either via the menu system, or via the "system.setProtocol" statement.

Protocol Associated Methods
We can also declare methods associated with the protocol in the same module file that the protocol was declared in. If a protocol is selected, then its associated protocol method will also be called. These methods are not necessary but are a convenient for printing status messages or setting certain variables. Associated protocol methods should be declared in the following way:

```
public void procolnameProtocol() {
      //code
}
```

As can be seen above, the associated protocol method should have a name such as "protocolnameProtocol" where protocol name matches one of the protocols declared concatenated with the word "Prococol".

The following protocol methods are provided for manipulation of the displays and creation and selection of the protocols. We note here that all of the following commands usually are placed in the **initModule** method of the model.

To check if the following protocol exists in the any module use:

```
system.protocolExist(charString);
```

To set or get the current protocol specified by the string name use:

```
system.setProtocol(name);
charString var = system.getProtocol();
```

Another useful method for adding the protocol name to the Executive's menu is:

```
NslDeclareProtocol("name");
```

defined within the NslModule class.

A.II.4 Command Line Parameters

The following methods where designed to get some of the values of the parameters that can be passed into the main model at execution time from the shell window.

Set or get the flag stating whether debug is set or not; default=0. This method can take any integer value and it is up to the user as to its interpretation; debug=0 means no debug.

```
Command line: nslj ModelA -debug int
system.setDebug(int);
int var=system.getDebug();
```

Set or get the flag indicating whether the any graphics should be displayed. If no graphics are to be displayed, the operating system shell window is used as the script window. The default is false. The *noDisplay* option is nice when your are running from a remote machine.

```
Command line: nslj ModelA -noDisplay
system.setNoDisplay(true);
boolean var=system.getNoDisplay();
```

Redirect standard input and output to the console or script window and retrieve whether the *stdio* is to going either the console or script window.

```
Command line: nslj ModelA -stdio script
system.setStdio(charString);
charString var = system.getStdio();
```

Redirect standard error to the console or script window and retrieve whether the *stderr* is going to either the console or script window.

```
Command line: nslj ModelA -stderr console
system.setStderr(charString);
charString var = system.getStderr();
```

Set or get the flag indicating this is a batch job—meaning no graphics and a default script should be provided. The default is false. Batch jobs are convenient for timing a simulation.

```
Command line: nslj ModelA -batch fileName
system.setBatch(boolean);
boolean var=system.getBatch() ;
```

A.II.5 The Interactive System

One of the features left out of chapter 5 was NSLJ's ability to save temporal plot data in the Mathworks Matlab format. To export the data from a Canvas Window first select the canvas and then select "Canvas→Export Data". A pop-up window will appear that looks like that in figure A.II.3. The only plot output currently supported is Matlab from Math-Works. The file specified by the user should end with the ".m" extension. The other files needed to view the NSL data in Matlab are available in NSLJ's "copyme/matlab" directory.

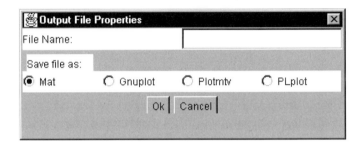

A.II.2 Figure
The Export Data Popup Window

Appendix III – NSLC Extensions

The NSL C++ (NSLC) version includes a number of extensions not included at the moment in NSLM, the common language to both C++ and Java versions. We expect that these extensions will be incorporated into NSLM in the future.

A.III.1 Object Type Extensions

NSLC adds a number of extensions to NSLM object types. Among these the most important ones are the addition of object type arrays, new object types and a number of extensions on module connectivity.

Arrays

NSLC adds a *dimSpec* array specification to any object type definition as follows:

```
VisiblitySpec ObjectType varName(paramList)dimSpec;
```

For example a single dimension 10 element private array of *ObjX* named *x* can be defined as follows:

```
private ObjX x()[10];
```

where no instantiation parameters are provided in this example. Additional dimensions are provided by simply adding new brackets with their corresponding element number specification. An extended example of array usage is shown in the "Face Recognition by Dynamic Link Matching" model in chapter 18.

Defined Types

NSLC adds additional defined types besides those described in chapter 6.

Table A.III.1
Additional charString object types defined in NSLC.

String

NSL defines two additional **charString** object types as shown in table A.III.1.

Dimension Type	0	1	2	3	4
charString		NslString1	NslString2		

Ports

NSLC defines additional **charString** port object types as shown in table A.III.2.

Dimension Type	0	1	2	3	4
charString		NslDoutString1	NslDoutString2		
		NslDinString1	NslDinString2		

Convolution

NSLC adds two additional convolutions methods as shown in table A.III.3 defined for both vectors and matrices of two dimensions. The type and dimension of z corresponds to that of y.

Table A.III.2
Additional charString port object types defined in NSLC.

Method Expression	Description
$z = $ **nslConvW**(x,y)	wrap-edge convolution
$z = $ **nslConvC**(x,y)	copy-edge convolution

Table A.III.3

Multiplication method.

Connect

NSLC provides additional **nslConnect** statements enabling *fan-out* and *fan-in* connections between multiple ports at once (NSLM as described in chapter 6 permits single port interconnections). *Fan-out* enables the output of a particular port to be sent out to a number of input ports at the same time using the following format,

```
nslConnect (port-out, port-in-list);
```

where *port-out* specifies an output port and *port-in-list* specifies a list of input ports separated by commas. Each input port is connected to the same output port. Analogous, *fan-in* enables the output of a list of port to be sent out to a particular input port using the following format,

```
nslConnect (port-out-list, port-in);
```

where *port-out-list* specifies a list of output ports separated by commas and *port-in* specifies a particular input port. Each output port is connected to the same input port. Note that in this case the input port would queue data from the different output ports according to the order in which they are received.

More generally, a list of output ports may be connected to a list of input ports using the following format,

```
nslConnect (port-out-list, port-in-list);
```

where *port-out-list* specifies a list of output ports and *port-in* specifies a list of input ports port both separated by commas.

Disconnect

NSLC provides an additional construct, **nslDisconnect**, to delete existing connections. The basic format is as follows,

```
nslDisconnect (port-out, port-in);
```

where *port-out* specifies an output port and *port-in* specifies an input port.

Similarly to connections, NSLC provides *fan-out*, *fan-in* and the more general disconnection formats as follows,

```
nslDisconnect (port-out, port-in-list);
nslDisconnect (port-out-list, port-in);
nslDisconnect (port-out-list, port-in-list);
```

Relabel

NSLC provides additional **nslRelabel** statements enabling *fan-out* and *fan-in* relabels between multiple ports at once (NSLM as described in chapter 6 permits single port relabels). *Fan-out* enables either a particular output or input port to be relabeled to a number of output or input ports at the same time, respectively. We use either of the following formats,

404   APPENDIX III

```
nslRelabel (port-out, port-out-list);
nslRelabel (port-in, port-in-list);
```

Analogous, *fan-in* enables either a list of output or input ports to be relabeled to a particular output or input port at the same time, respectively. We use either of the following formats,

```
nslRelabel (port-out-list, port-out);
nslRelabel (port-in-list, port-in);
```

More generally, a list of either output or input ports may be relabeled to a list of output or input ports, respectively, using the following formats,

```
nslRelabel (port-out1-list, port-out2-list);
nslRelabel (port-in1-list, port-in2-list);
```

Delabel

Analogous to **nslDisconnect** NSLC supports a delabeling (deleting a relabel) construct **nslDelabel**. The basic formats are as follows,

```
nslDelabel (port-out1, port-out2);
nslDelabel (port-in1, port-in2);
```

where *port-out1* and *port-out2* specify output port and *port-in* specifies an input port.

Similarly to disconnections, NSLC provides *fan-out*, *fan-in* and the more general delabel formats as follows,

```
nslDelabel (port-out, port-out-list);
nslDelabel (port-in, port-in-list);
nslDelabel (port-out-list, port-out);
nslDelabel (port-in-list, port-in);
nslDelabel (port-out1-list, port-out2-list);
nslDelabel (port-in1-list, port-in2-list);
```

File Manipulation

As described in Appendix I NSL supports reading and writing into external text files. NSLC additionally supports reading and writing into binary files as shown in chapter 18 with the "Face Recognition with Dynamic Link Architecture" model.

NSLC uses the same basic file manipulation methods described in Appendix I with an additional optional second argument in the **open** method describing the type of file (*file-type*) being manipulated, **text** or **binary**, as shown next:

```
file.open(interaction-spec,file-type);
```

As previously discussed in Appendix I *interaction-type* corresponds to any of the following: '**R**' for read only, '**A**' (all) for both read and write or '**W**' for write only. Note that binary files do not separate values with spaces thus the user must read each byte or character at a time such as in the model described in chapter 18. Since NSLC is based on C++ the user may take advantage of **char** and **unsigned char** types when reading binary files.

A.III.2 Script Extensions

NSLC adds the following script extensions.

Logs

Log files contain the history of previous user model interaction. This is quite useful in generating a previous interaction that has not been stored. Scripts can be logged and saved automatically at the end of the simulation (however, the default is logging false).

```
nsl set system.log true
```

There is one default log for the complete simulation. The log file name corresponds to the model name followed by a dot and a numeric suffix corresponding to the log version followed by a "log" and it may be specified with a different name by the user. For example,

```
nsl set system.logfile maxSelectorModel.1.log
```

Besides being able to review the log file, it is possible to reload it and execute it as any other NSLS script.

A.III.3 Input Facility

NSLC includes predefined object classes for the generation of temporal visual stimuli. These types are usually instantiated inside a special visual input module such as the **Visin** module used in the "Retina" model (chapter 10) and the **World** module used in the "Learning to Detour" model (chapter 17). Using these object types different stimuli may be set, with constrains on their location and time when they should appear and disappear. In the following sections we explain these in more detail.

Object Types

Input object types extend their basic semantics from NSLM numeric types while adding special functionality for processing visual stimuli. These types vary according to their dimension and types as shown in table A.III.4.

Dimension Type	0	1	2	3
float	NslInputFloat0	NslInputFloat1	NslInputFloat2	NslInputFloat3
double	NslInputDouble0	NslInputDouble1	NslInputDouble2	NslInputDouble3
int	NslInputInt0	NslInputInt1	NslInputInt2	NslInputInt3

Table A.III.4
Input layer object types defined in NSLC.

Since the input layer object types are derived from the regular numeric layer types have the same instantiation parameters as regular layers. The only exception is the 3-dimensional input array taking four instead of three instantiation arguments. This difference corresponds to the fact that a 3-dimensional input layer is actually a combination of two 2-dimensional input layers corresponding to the *xy* and *xz* space views (see the "Learning to Detour" model in chapter 17 as an example of its usage). Thus input layers may be added with regular layers, and so on. On the other hand the input layer is able to map visual stimulus objects onto the layer. For example, figure A.III.1 shows an **AreaLevel** graph view of a **NslInputFloat2** input layer made of 40x40 elements, containing an object of size 8x4. This example is taken from the **Visin** module in the **Retina** model in chapter 10.

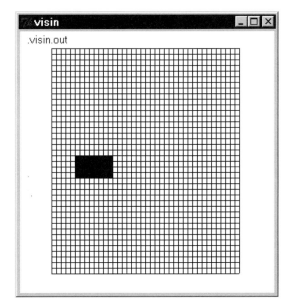

Figure A.III.1
A **NslInputFloat2** input layer of 40x40 elements containing a 8x4 stimulus.

Figure A.III.2 shows a **Temporal** graph view of a **NslInputFloat0** input layer, containing an stimulus appearing at two different time intervals.

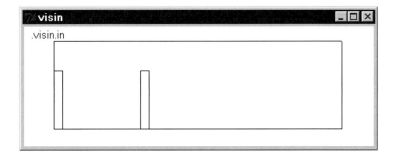

Figure A.III.2
A **NslInputFloat0** with a time varying stimulus.

Input Processing

Actual input layer processing involves "running" the stimuli specified for the particular layer. We show how to interactively specify stimuli in the next section. Input layer processing is achieved by including the following statement inside a module,

```
input_layer = 0;
input_layer.run();
```

where *input_layer* specifies the name of the layer, and *run* is the method processing any existing stimuli specification. For example, in the "Retina" model the visual input *in* is processed in the *Visin* module as follows,

```
in = 0;
in.run();
```

Note that the input layer is first reset to "0". This is optional since in some case the user may want to leave a trail or history of previous stimuli locations as in the "Learning to Detour" model in chapter 17.

Input Specification

In the current NSLC version all input and stimuli specification takes place interactively using the NSLS script interpreter. Before being able to specify any stimuli one must understand the coordinate system used in the input layer and stimuli, shown in figure A.III.3.

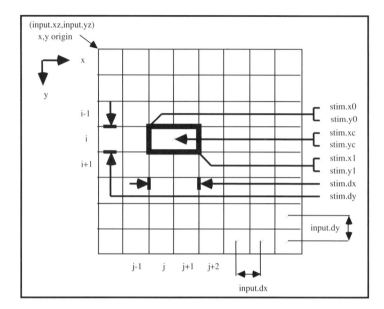

There are two aspects to input specification. First the coordinate system in the input layer must be specified. This involves specifying the origin of the coordinate system, (*input.xz,input.yz*) and the distance among adjacent elements in the input layer, (*input.dx,input.dy*) as shown in figure A.III.3.

These parameters are specified as follows where *input* in this figure represents the *input_layer* name,

```
nsl set input_layer.par-name par-value
```

where the different alternatives for *par-name* with their corresponding *par-value* types and descriptions are given in table A.III.5. Note that the input library supports up to 3-dimensional specifications.

Parameter	Type	Description
xz	int	coordinate system *x*-axis origin element
yz	int	coordinate system *y*-axis origin element
zz	int	coordinate system *z*-axis origin element
dx	numeric	distance among adjacent elements in the *x*-axis
dy	numeric	distance among adjacent elements in the *y*-axis
dz	numeric	distance among adjacent elements in the *z*-axis

For example, in the "Retina" model the input layer coordinate system is specified as follows,

```
nsl set retinaModel.retina.visin.input.xz 0
nsl set retinaModel.retina.visin.input.yz 20
nsl set retinaModel.retina.visin.input.dx 2.0
nsl set retinaModel.retina.visin.input.dy 2.0
```

Once the input layer coordinate system has been specified it is necessary to add stimuli specifications. The general stimulus specification format is as follows,

```
nsl create stim-type stim-name -layer input-name -val val \
    [-x0 x0 -y0 y0 -z0 z0] [-xc xc -yc yc -zc zc] \
-dx dx -dy dy -dz dz -vx vx -vy vy -vz vz -spec_type spec-type
```

These parameters are those shown in figure A.III.3 and specified in more detail in table A.III.6. In the current NSLC version *stim-type* can only be set as **BlockStim**, while *stime-name* and *input-name* are the names of the stimulus and input layer, respectively.

Parameter	Type	Description
val	numeric	value taken for the complete stimulus
spec_type	string	specification format: **center** [xc,yc] or **corner** [x0,y0]
x0	numeric	stimulus upper left corner *x*-coordinate
y0	numeric	stimulus upper left corner *y*-coordinate
z0	numeric	stimulus upper left corner *z*-coordinate
xc	numeric	stimulus center *x*-coordinate
yc	numeric	stimulus center *y*-coordinate
zc	numeric	stimulus center *z*-coordinate
dx	numeric	stimulus width in *x*-direction
dy	numeric	stimulus depth in *y*-direction
dz	numeric	stimulus height in *z*-direction
vx	numeric	stimulus speed in *x*-direction
vy	numeric	stimulus speed in *y*-direction
vz	numeric	stimulus speed in *z*-direction

Table A.III.6
Stimulus parameter options.

The location of the stimulus may be specified either by setting *spec_type* to either corner or center and specifying [*x0,y0,z0*] or [*xc,yc,zc*], respectively. For example, the stimulus shown in figure A.III.1 was specified with the following script,

```
nsl create BlockStim stim -layer retinaModel.retina.visin.in -
val 1.0 \
    -spec_type center -xc 2.0 -yc 0.0 -dx 4.0 -dy 4.0 -vx 7.6
```

Note that the actual figure shows the stimulus situated in a new location according to its initial position, current speed and simulation time elapsed.

Additionally, NSL lets the user define time intervals when a stimulus should appear using the following format,

```
nsl create TimeInterval -stim stim-name -t0 t0 -t1 t1
```

Table A.III.7 describes the two parameters in more detail.

Parameter	Type	Description
t0	numeric	interval starting time
tz	numeric	Interval ending time

For example, the stimulus shown in figure A.III.2 was created using the following script:

```
nsl create BlockStim stim1 -layer tectum11Model.tectum.in
nsl create TimeInterval -stim stim1 -t0 0.0 -t1 0.3
nsl create TimeInterval -stim stim1 -t0 3.0 -t1 3.3
```

This creates a time interval between 0.0 and 0.3 and a second one for the same stimulus between 3.0 and 3.3. Notice that in this example the input layer was actually a scalar thus no other stimulus parameters were given, including stimulus size or location).

A.III.4 Distribution

One additional extension to the NSLC system currently in development is the distributed execution environment to make processing more efficient. See the NSLC web site (*http://www.cannes.itam.mx/*) for the latest developments.

Appendix IV – NSLJ and NSLC Differences

There are several small differences between the NSLC and NSLJ implementations.

A.IV.1 Ports

One such difference is the way in which the input and output ports are implemented on a module. In the NSLJ version, output ports allocate memory whereas input ports do not. In the NSLC version both input and output ports allocate memory.

A.IV.2 Read/Write Script Access

Another difference, is the fact that the NSLJ system actually implements the "nslSetAccess" methods and thus variables that do not have a 'W' access associated with them are not manipulatable from the scripting environment nor from the other modules. The current NSLC version does not implement "nslSetAccess," thus providing a default 'W' access for all variables.

A.IV.3 Frames and Modules

Another difference is the fact that in NSLJ all **NslOutFrames** and **NslInFrames** automatically create a **NslOutModule** or **NslInModule** respectively. This is due to the fact that the modules are the objects that actually get scheduled by the scheduler and not the frames.

A.IV.4 NslBoolean

Another difference is the NslBoolean class. NSLJ allows boolean arrays from dimension 0 to 4 and provides a number of methods to manipulate and compare boolean arrays. NSLC treats the NslBoolean class as NslInt.

A.IV.5 Methods

One important thing to note about the NSLJ mathematical methods is that since it is not possible to provide every combination of parameters when parameters can be one of six different types, it was decided to implement the most "logical" combinations. Typically this means that if the method takes more than one parameter, the parameters and result should be of all the same base type (**int, float, double, NslInt, NslFloat, NslDouble**). NSLC implements the different combintations as templates.

Appendix V – NSLJ and NSLC Installation Instructions

All installation instructions and extensions can be found at *www.neuralsimulationlanguage.org*, the official NSL web site. At the time of book impression, different NSL locations exist, one for NSLJ and the other for NSLC.

A.V.1 NSLJ Version

The NSL Java Version can be download from the following site:

http://www-hbp.usc.edu/Projects/nsl.htm

A.V.2 NSLC Version

The NSL C++ Version can be download from the following site:

http://www.cannes.itam.mx/English/Simulators/Nsl.htm

Bibliography

Abu-Mustafa, Y., and St. Jacques, J. 1989. "Information Capacity of the Hopfield Model," *IEEE Transactions on Information Theory* **31**(**4**), 461–464, July.

Albus, J. S. 1971. A theory of cerebellar function. *Mathematical Bioscience* **10**, 25–61.

Alexander, G. E., Crutcher, M. R., and DeLong, M. R. 1990. "Basal ganglia-thalamo-cortical circuits: Parallel substrates for motor, oculomotor, "prefrontal" and "limbic" functions." *Prog. Brain Res.* **85**, 119–146.

Alexander G. E., DeLong, M. R., Strick, P. L. 1986. Parallel Organization of Functionally Segregated Circuits Linking Basal Ganglia and Cortex. *Ann. Rev. Neurosci.* **9**, 357–381.

Alexander, G. E., and Fuster, J. M. 1973. Effects of cooling prefrontal cortex on cell firing in the nucleus medialis dorsalis. *Brain Res.* **61**, 93–105

Amari, S. 1977. Dynamics of pattern formation in lateral-inhibition type neural fields. *Biol. Cybern.* **27**, 77–87.

Amari, S., and Arbib, M. A. 1977. Competition and cooperation in neural nets. In *Systems Neuroscience*, ed. J. Metzler, pp. 119–165, Academic Press.

Andrade, M. A., and Morán, F. 1996. Structural study of the development of ocularity domains using a neural network model. *Biol. Cybern.* **74**, 243–254.

an der Heiden, U., and Roth, G. 1987. Mathematical model and simulation of retina and tectum opticum of lower vertebrates. *Acta Biotheoretica* **36**, 179–212.

Anderson, C. H., and Van Essen, D. C. 1987. Shifter circuits: A computational strategy for dynamic aspects of visual processing. *Proc Natl. Acad. Sci. USA* **84**, 6297–6301.

Andrade, M. A., and Morán, F. 1997. Receptive field map development by anti-hebbian learning. *Neural Networks* **10**, 1037–1052.

Arbib, M. A. 1987. Levels of modeling of mechanisms of visually guided behavior. *Behavioral and Brain Sciences* **10**, 407–465.

Arbib, M. A. 1989. The Metaphorical Brain 2, *Neural Networks and Beyond*. Wiley.

Arbib, M. A. 1990. Programs, Schemas, and Neural Networks for Control of Hand Movements: Beyond the RS Framework. In *Attention and Performance XIII. Motor Representation and Control*, ed. M. Jeannerod. Hillsdale, NJ: Lawrence Erlbaum Associates.

Arbib, M. A. 1992. Schema Theory. In the *Encyclopedia of Artificial Intelligence*, 2nd Edition, ed. Stuart Shapiro. **2**, 1427–1443, Wiley.

Arbib, M. A., Schweighofer, N., and Thach, W. T. 1994. Modeling the role of cerebellum in prism adaptation. In *From Animals to Animats 3,* ed. D. Cliff, P. Husbands, J.-A. Meyer, and S. W. Wilson, pp.–44. The MIT Press.

Bartha, G. T., and Thompson, R. F. 1995. Cerebellum and conditioning. In *The Handbook of Brain Theory and Neural Networks,* ed. M. A. Arbib, pp.169–172. The MIT Press, Cambridge, MA.

Barto, A. G., Sutton, R. S., and Brouwer, P. S. 1981. Associative search networks: A reinforcement learning associative memory. *Biological Cybernetics* **40**, 201–211.

Barto, A. G., and Sutton, R. S. 1981. Landmark learning: An illustration of associative search. *Biological Cybernetics* **42**, 1–8.

Barto, A. G., Sutton, R. S., and Anderson, C. W. 1983. Neuronlike Adaptive Elements That Can Solve Difficult Learning Control Problems. *IEEE Transactions on Systems, Man, and Cybernetics*, SMC-5, 834–46.

Berns, G. S., and Sejnowski, T. J. 1995. A model of basal ganglia function unifying reinforcement learning and action selection. Joint Symposium on Neural Computation. 129–148.

Berthoz A., and Droulez, J. 1991. The concept of Dynamic Memory in Sensorimotor Control. *Motor Control: Concepts and Issues,* ed. D. R. Humphrey and H.-J. Freund. John Wiley & Sons Ltd.

Biederman, I. 1987. Recognition-by-components: A theory of human image understanding. Psychological Review **94**, 115–147.

Biederman, I., and Gerhardstein, P. C. 1993. Recognizing depth-rotated objects: Evidence and conditions for three-dimensional viewpoint invariance. *J. Exp. Psychology* **19**, 1162–1182.

Boussaoud, D., and Wise, S. P. 1993. "Primate frontal cortex: Effects of stimulus and movement." *Exp. Brain Res.* **95**, 28–40.

Booch, G., Rumbaugh, J., and Jacobson, I. 1999. The Unified Modeling Language, User Guide, Addison-Wesley.

Bower, J. M., and Beeman, D. 1998. *The Book of GENESIS, Exploring Realistic Neural Models with the GEneral NEural SImulation System,* Telos, Springer-Verlag, 2nd Edition.

Braun, D., Breitmeyer, B. G. 1988. Relationship between directed visual attention and saccadic reaction times. *Exp. Brain Res.* **73**, 546–552.

Bruce, C. J., and Goldberg, M. E. 1984. Physiology of the frontal eye fields. *Trends Neurosci.* **7**, 436–441.

Bruce, V., Valentine, T., and Baddeley, A. 1987. The basis of the 3/4 view advantage in face recognition. *Applied Cognitive Psychology* **1**, 109–120.

Buhmann, J., Lades, M., and von der Malsburg, C. 1990. Size and distortion invariant object recognition by hierarchical graph matching. In *Proceedings of the IJCNN International Joint Conference on Neural Networks,* pages II 411–416, San Diego. IEEE.

Carey, R. G. 1975. *A quantitative analysis of the distribution of the retinal elements in frogs and toads with special emphasis on the Area Retinalis.* Masters Thesis, University of Massachusetts at Amherst, Amherst Massachusetts.

Carlson, A. 1990. Anti-Hebbian learning in a non-linear neural network. *Biol. Cybern.* **64**, 171–176.

Carpenter G. A., and Grossberg S. 1987. A Massively Parallel Architecture for a Self-Organizing Neural Pattern Recognition Machine. *Computer Vision. Graphics and Image Processing* **37**, 54–115.

Carpenter G. A., and Grossberg S. 1987. ART2: Self-Organization of Stable Category Recognition Codes for Analog Input Patterns. *Applied Optics* **26**, 4919–4930.

Carpenter G. A., Grossberg S., and Mehanian S. 1989. Invariant Recognition of Cluttered Scene by a Self-Organizing ART Architecture: CORT-X Boundary Segmentation. *Neural Networks* **2**, 1169–1181.

Carpenter G. A., and Grossberg S. 1990. ART3: Hierarchical Search Using Chemical Transmitters in Self-Organizing Pattern Recognition Architectures. *Neural Networks* **3**, 129–152.

Carpenter G. A., Grossberg S., and Rosen D. B. 1991. Fuzzy ART: Fast Stable Learning and Categorization of Analog Patterns by an Adaptive Resonance System. *Neural Networks* **4**, 759–771.

Cervantes-Pérez, F., Lara, R., and Arbib, M. A. 1985. Neural Model of Interactions Subserving Prey-Predator Discrimination and Size Preference in Anuran Amphibia. *J. Theor. Biol.* **113**, 117–152

Chevalier, G., Vacher, S., Deniau, J. M., and Desban, M. 1985. Disinhibition as a Basic Process in the Expression of Striatal Functions. I. The Striato-Nigral Influence on the Tecto-spinal/Tecto-diencephalic Neurons. *Brain Res.* **334**, 215–226

Cobas, A., and Arbib, M. A. 1992. Prey-catching and Predator-avoidance in Frog and Toad: Defining the Schemas. *J. Theor. Biol.* **157**, 271–304.

Collett, T. 1983. Picking a route; Do toads follow rules or make plans? In *Advances in Vertebrate Neuroethology,* ed. J. P. Ewert, R. R. Capranica, and D. J. Ingle, pp.321 – 330.

Corbacho, F. J., and Arbib, M. A. 1995. Learning to Detour. *J. Adaptive Behavior* **3(4)**, 419–468.

Corbacho, F., Khort, B., Lin, B., Nothis, A., and Arbib, M. A. 1996. Learning to Detour: Behavioral Experiments with Frogs. *Proceedings of the Workshop on Sensorimotor Coordination: Amphibians, Models, and Comparative Studies.* Sedona, Arizona.

Corbacho, F. 1998. Commentary: Schema-based Learning. *Artificial Intelligence* **101**, 370–373.

Cote, L., and Crutcher, M. D. 1991. The Basal Ganglia. Principles of Neuroal Science. New York, Elsevier.

Crick, F. 1982. Do dendritic spines twitch? Trends in Neurobiology, February:44–46.

Damasio, A. R., and Damasio, H. 1992. Cortical systems underlying knowledge retrieval: Evidence from human lesion studies. In *Neurobiology of Neocortex.* John Wiley.

Dassonville, P., Schlag, J., and Schlag-Rey, M. 1990. Oculomotor Localization Relies On a Damped Representation of Saccadic Eye Displacement in Human and Nonhuman Primates. *Vis Neurosci* **9**, 261–269.

Daugman, J. G. 1988. Complete discrete 2-D Gabor transform by neural networks for image analysis and compression. IEEE Transactions on Acoustics, Speech and Signal Processing, **36(7)**, 1169–1179.

Deniau, J. M., and Chevalier, G. 1985. Disinhibition as a basic process in the expression of striatal functions. II. The striato-nigral influence on thalamocortical cells of the ventromedial thalamic nucleus. *Brain Res.* **334**, 227–233

Dev, P. 1975. Perception of Depth Surfaces in Random-dot Stereograms: A Neural Model. *Int J. Man-Machine Studies* **7**, 511–528.

Didday, R. L. 1976. A model of visuomotor mechanisms in the frog optic tectum, *Math. Biosci.* **30**, 169–180.

Dominey P. F., and Arbib, M. A. 1991. Multiple Brain Regions Cooperate in Sequential Saccade Generation. In *Visual Structures and Integrated Functions,* ed. M. A. Arbib and J.-P. Ewert. Springer-Verlag pp.281–295.

Dominey, P. F., and Arbib, M. A. 1992. "A cortico-subcortical model for generation of spatially accurate sequential saccades." *Cerebral Cortex.* **2**, 153–175.

Eckmiller, R. 1975. Electronic simulation of the vertebrate retina. *IEEE Transactions on Biomedical Engineering,* BME-22(4), 305–311.

Eigen, M. 1978. The hypercycle. Naturwissenschaften, **65**, 7–41.

Erwin, E., Obermayer, K., and Schulten, K. 1995. Models of orientation and ocular dominance columns in the visual cortex: a critical comparison. *Neural Computation* **7**, 425–468.

Ewert, J. P. 1971. Single unit response of the toad's (*Bufo americanus*) caudal thalamus to visual objects. *Z. vergl. Physiol.* **74**, 81–102.

Ewert J.–P. 1976. The visual system of the toad: Behavioral and physiological studies on a pattern recognition system. In *The Amphibian Visual System,* ed. K. V. Fite. Academic Press : New York. pp. 142–202.

Ewert J.-P., and Hock, F. 1972. Movement-sensitive neurons in the toad's retina. *Experimental Brain Research* **16**, 41–59.

Földiak, P. 1990. Forming sparse representations by local anti-Hebbian learning. *Biol. Cybern.* **64**, 165–170.

Frégnac, Y., and Imbert, M. 1984. Development of neuronal selectivity in primary visual cortex of cat. *Physiol. Rev.* **64**, 325–434.

Funahashi S., Bruce, C. J., and Goldman-Rakic, P. S. 1989. Mnemonic Coding of Visual Space in Monkey's Dorsolateral Prefrontal Cortex. *J Neurophysiol.* **61**, 331–349.

Fuster, J. M., and Alexander, G. E. 1973. Firing changes in cells of the nucleus medialis dorsalis associated with Memory response behavior. *Brain Res.* **61**, 79–91.

Gaillard, F., Arbib, M. A., Corbacho, F., and Lee, H. B. 1998. Modeling the Physiological Responses of Anuran R3 Ganglion Cells. *Vision Research* **38**, 1282–1299.

Gerfen, C. R. 1992. "The neostriatal mosaic: Multiple levels of compartmental organization in the basal ganglia." *Ann. Rev. Neurosci.* **15**, 285–320.

Gilbert, P. F. C., and Thach, W. T. 1977. Purkinje cell activity during motor learning. *Brain Research* **128**, 309–328.

Gnadt J. W., and Andersen, R. A. 1988. Memory related motor planning activity in posterior parietal cortex of macaque. *Exp Brain Res.* **70**, 216–220.

Goldberg M. E., and Bruce, C. J. 1990. Primate Frontal Eye Fields. III. Maintenance of a Spatially Accurate Saccade Signal. *J Neurophysiol.* **64**, 489–508.

Goldman-Rakic, P. S. 1987. Circuitry of primate prefrontal cortex and regulation of behavior by representational memory. In *Handbook of Physiolog, Chap V. The Nervous System* **9**, 373–417.

Grossberg, S. 1976. A Theory of Visual Coding, Memory, and Development: Part 1. Parallel Development and Coding of Neural Feature Detectors. *Biological Cybernetics* **23**, 121–134.

Grüsser O.-J., and Grüsser-Cornehls, U. 1976. Neurophysiology of the anuran visual system. In *Frog Neurobiology,* ed. R. Llinás and W. Precht. Springer: New York. pp. 297–385.

Grüsser-Cornehls, U. 1988. Neurophysiological properties of the retinal ganglion cell classes of the Cuban treefrog, Hyla septentrionalis. *Exp Brain Res.* **73**, 39–52.

Häussler, A. F., and von der Malsburg, C. 1983. Development of retinotopic projections: an analytical treatment. *J. Theo. Biol.* **2**, 47–73.

Hebb, D. O. 1949. *Organization of Behavior.* John Wiley & Sons, New York.

Hikosaka, O. 1989. Role of Basal ganglia in Initiation of Voluntary Movement. In *Dynamic Interactions in Neural Networks: Models and Data,* ed. M. Arbib and S. Amari. Springer-Verlag, New York, pp 153–168.

Hikosaka, O., and Wurtz, R. 1983a. Visual and Oculomotor functions of Monkey Substantia Nigra Pars Reticulata. I. Relation of visual and Auditory Responses to Saccades. *J Neurophysiol.* **49**, 1230–1253.

Hikosaka, O., and Wurtz, R. 1983b. Visual and Oculomotor functions of Monkey Substantia Nigra Pars Reticulata. II. Visual Responses Related to Fixation of Gaze. *J Neurophysiol.* **49**, 1254–1267.

Hikosaka, O., and Wurtz, R. 1983c. Visual and Oculomotor functions of Monkey Substantia Nigra Pars Reticulata. III. Memory-Contingent Visual and Saccade Responses. *J. Neurophysiol.* **49**, 1268–1284.

Hikosaka, O., and Wurtz, R. 1983d. Visual and Oculomotor functions of Monkey Substantia Nigra Pars Reticulata. IV. Relation of Substantia Nigra to Superior Colliculus. *J. Neurophysiol.* **49**, 1285–1301.

Hines, M., and Carnevale, T. 1997. The NEURON Simulation Environment, *Neural Computation* **9**, 1179–1209.

Hinton, G. E, and Sejnowski, T. J. 1986. Learning and Relearning in Boltzmann Machines. In *Parallel Distributed Processing: Explorations in the Microstructure of*

Cognition, Volume 1: Foundations, ed. J. L. McClelland and D. E. Rumelhart, pp. 282–317. Bradford Book/The MIT Press.

Hodgkin, A. L., and Huxley, A. F. 1952. A quantitative description of membrane current and its application to conduction and excitation in nerve. *Journal of Physiology* **117**, 500–544.

Hopfield, J. 1982. "Neural Networks and Physical Systems with Emergent Collective Computational Abilities," *Proc. of the National Academy of Sciences* **79**, 2554–2558, April.

Hopfield, J. J., and Tank, D. W. 1985. Neural Computation of Decisions in Optimization Problems. *Biological Cybernetics* **52**, 141–152.

House, D. 1985. Depth Perception in Frogs and Toads: A study in Neural Computing, *Lecture Notes in Biomathematics 80*, Springer-Verlag.

Hubel, D. H., and Wiesel, T. N. 1963. Receptive fields in cells in striate cortex of very young visually inexperienced kittens. *J. Neurophysiol.* **26**, 994–1002.

Ilinsky, I. A., Jouandet, M. L., and Goldman-Rakic, P. S. 1985. Organization of the Nigrothalamo-cortical system in the Rhesus Monkey. *J. Comp Neurol.* **236**, 315–330.

Ito, M. 1984. *The Cerebellum and Neural Control.* Raven Press, New York.

Ingle, D. 1983. Brain mechanisms of visual localization by frogs and toads. *Advances in Vertebrate Neuroethology,* ed. J.-P. Ewert, R. R. Capranica, and D. J. Ingle, 177–226.

Jones, J. P., and Palmer, L. A. 1987. An evaluation of the two dimensional Gabor filter model of simple receptive fields in cat striate cortex. *J. of Neurophysiology* **58**, 1233–1258.

Kalocsai, P., Biederman, I., and Cooper, E. E. 1994. To what extent can the recognition of unfamiliar faces be accounted for by a representation of the direct output of simple cells. In *Proceedings of the Association for Research in Vision and Ophtalmology*, ARVO, Sarasota, Florida.

Keating, E. G., and Gooley, S. C. 1988. Saccadic disorders caused by cooling the superior colliculus or the frontal eye fields or from combined lesions of both structures. *Brain Res.* **438**, 247–255.

Kitai, S. T., Kocsis, J. D., Preston, R. J., and Sugimori, M. 1976. "Monosynaptic inputs to cuadate neurons identified by intracellular injection of horseradish peroxidase." *Brain Res.* **109**, 601–606.

Kitazawa, S., Kohno, T., and Uka, T. 1995. Effects of delayed visual information on the rate and amount of prism adaptation in the human. *The Journal of Neuroscience*, **15(11)**, 7644–7652.

Kojima, S., and Goldman-Rakic, P. S. 1984. "Functional analysis of spatially discriminative neurons in prefrontal cortex of rhesus monkey." *Brain Res.* **291**, 229–240.

Konen, W., and Vorbrüggen, J. C. 1993. Applying dynamic link matching to object recognition in real world images. In *Proceedings of the International Conference on Artificial Neural Networks,* ed. S. Gielen, and B. Kappen, ICANN, pages 982–985, London. Springer-Verlag.

König, P., and Engel, A. K. 1995. Correlated firing in sensory-motor systems. *Current Opinion in Neurobiology* **5**, 511–519.

Lades, M. 1995. Invariant Object Recognition with Dynamical Links, Robust to Variations in Illumination. PhD thesis, Fakultät für Physik und Astronomie, Ruhr-Universität Bochum, D-44780 Bochum.

Lades, M., Vorbrüggen, J. C., Buhmann, J., Lange, J., von der Malsburg, C., Würtz, R. P., and Konen, W. 1993. Distortion invariant object recognition in the dynamic link architecture. *IEEE Transactions on Computers* **42(3)**, 300–311.

Lee, Y. B. 1986. *A Neural Network Model of Frog Retina: A Discrete Time-Space Approach*. Ph.D. Dissertation, Department of Computer and Information Science, University of Massachusetts at Amherst.

Lee, H. B. 1994. *A Neural Network and Schematic modeling of anuran visuomotor coordination in Detour Behavior*. Ph. D. Thesis. University of Southern California.

Linsker, R. 1986. From basic network principles to neural architecture. (Three papers). *Proc. Natl. Acad. Sci. USA*. **83**, 7508–7512, 8390–8394, 8779–8783.

Linsker, R. 1990. Perceptual neural organization: Some approaches based on networks models and information theory. *Annu. Rev. Neurosci*. **13**, 257–281.

Lynch, J. C., Graybiel, A. M., and Lobeck, L. J. 1985. The differential projection of two cytoarchitectonic subregions of the inferior parietal lobule of macaque upon the deep layers of the superior colliculus. *J. Comp. Neurol.* **235**, 241–254

Marr, D. 1969. A theory of cerebellar cortex. *Journal of Physiology* **202**, 437–470.

Martin, T., Keating, J., Goodkin, H., Bastian, A. J., and Thach, W. T. 1995. Throwing at visual targets: Acquisition and specificity of eye-hand coordination and its dependency on the olivocerebellar system.

Mason, C., and Kandel, E. R. 1991. Central Visual Pathways. *Principles of Neural Science*. New York, Elsevier.

Maturana, H. R., Lettvin, J. Y., McCulloch, W. S., and Pitts, W. H. 1960. Anatomy and physiology of vision in the frog (Rana pipiens). *Journal of General Physiology* **43**, (Suppl.), 129–175.

Mays, L. E., and Sparks, D. L. 1980. Dissociation of Visual and Saccade Related Responses in Superior Colliculus Neurons. *J. Neurophysiol.* **43**, 207–232

McCulloch, W. S., and Pitts, W. H. 1943. A Logical Calculus of the Ideas Immanent in Nervous Activity. *Bull. Math. Biophys.* **5**, 115–133.

McEntee, W. J., Biber, M. P., Perl, D. P., and Benson, D. F. 1976. "Diencephalic amnesia: A reappraisal." *J. Neurol. Neurosurg. Psychiatry* **39**, 436–441.

Miller, K. J., Keller, J. B., and Stryker, M. P. 1989. Ocular dominance columnar development: Analysis and simulation. *Science* **245**, 605–615.

Mitz, A. R., Godshalk, M., and Wise, S. P. 1991. Learning-dependent Neuronal Activity in the Premotor Cortex. *Journal of Neuroscience* **11(6)**, 1855–72.

Moore, J. W., Desmond, J. E., and Berthier, N. E. 1989. Adaptively timed conditioned responses and the cerebellum: A neural network approach. *Biological Cybernetics* **62**, 17–28.

Munoz, D. P., and Wurtz, R. H. 1993a. "Fixation cells in monkey superior colliculus. I. Characteristics of cell discharge." *J. Neurophysiol.* **70**, 559–570.

Munoz, D. P., and Wurtz, R. H. 1993b. "Fixation cells in monkey superior colliculus. II. Reversible activation and deactivation." *J. Neurphyusiol.* **70**, 576–589.

Munoz, D. P., and Wurtz, R. H. 1993c. "Interactions between fixation and saccade neurons in primate superior colliculus." *Soc. Neurosci. Abstr.* **19**, 787.

Murre, J. 1995. Neurosimulators. In *Handbook of Brain Theory and Neural Networks*, ed. M. Arbib. The MIT Press.

Optican, L. M. 1994. Control of saccadic trajectory by the superior colliculus. Contemporary Ocular Motor and Vestibular Research: A Tribute to David A. Robinson. Stuttgart, Thieme.

Orban, G. A. 1984. *Studies on Brain Function. Neuronal Operations in the Visual Cortex*. Springer-Verlag, Berlin.

Ousterhout, J. 1994. Tcl and the Tk Toolkit, Addison-Wesley.

Parent, A., Mackey, A., and De Bellefeuille, L. 1983. "The subcortical afferents to caudate nucleus and putamen in primate: a florescence retrograde double-labeling study." *Neurosci.* **10**, 1137–1150.

Petrides, M., and Pandya, D. N. 1984 Projections to frontal cortex from the posterior parietal region in the rhesus monkey. *J. Comp. Neurol.* **228**, 105–116.

Rall, W. 1959. Branching dendritic trees and motoneuron membrane resistivity, *Exp. Neurol.* **2**, 503–532.

Robinson, D. A. 1970. Oculomotor unit behavior in the monkey. *J. Neurophysiol.* **33**, 393–404.

Robinson, D. A. 1972. Eye Movement Evoked By Collicular Stimulation In The Alert Monkey. *Vision Res.* **12**, 1795–1808

Rosenblatt, F. 1961. Principles of Neurodynamics: Perceptrons and the Theory of Brain Mechanisms. Spartan Books, Washington, D.C.

Rumelhart, D. E., Hinton, G. E., and Williams, R. J. 1986. Learning internal representations by error propagation, in *Parallel Distributed Processing: Explorations in the Microstructure of Cognition,* ed. D. E. Rumelhart, J. L. McClelland, and PDP Research Group, vol. 1, *Foundations*, Cambridge, MA: The MIT Press, pp. 318–362.

Rumelhart, D. E., and Zipser, D. 1986. Feature Discovery by Competitive Learning. In *Parallel Distributed Processing: Explorations in the Microstructure of Cognition Volume 1: Foundations,* ed. J. L. McClelland and D. E. Rumelhart, pp. 151–193. Bradford Books/The MIT Press.

Sadikot, A. F., Parent, A., Smith, Y., and Bolam, J. P. 1992. "Efferent connections of the centromedian and parafascicular thalamic nuclei in the squirrel monkey: A light and electron microscopic study of the thalamostriatal projection in relation to striatal heterogeneity." *J. Comp. Neurol.* **320**, 228–242.

Sawaguchi, T., and Goldman-Rakic, P. S. 1991. "D1 dopamine receptors in prefrontal cortex: Involvement in working memory." *Science* **251**, 947–950.

Sawaguchi, T., and Goldman-Rakic, P. S. 1994. "The role of D1-dopamine receptor in working memory: Local injections of dopamine antagonists into the prefrontal cortex of rhesus monkeys performing an oculomotor delayed-response task." *J. Neurophysiol.* **71(2)**, 515–528.

Schiller, P. H., and Sandell, J. H. 1983. Interactions between visually and electrically elicited saccades before and after superior colliculus and frontal eye field ablations in the rhesus monkey. *Exp. Brain Res.* **49**, 381–392.

Schürg-Pfeiffer, E., and Ewert, J.-P. 1981. Investigation of neurons involved in the analysis of gestalt prey features in the frog, "Rana temporaria." *Journal of Comparative Physiology* **141**, 139–152.

Scudder, C. A. 1988. A New Local Feedback Model of the Saccadic Burst Generator. *J. Neurophysiol.* **59**, 1455–1475.

Segraves, M., Goldberg, M. E. 1987. Functional Properties of Corticotectal Neurons in the Monkey's Frontal Eye Field. *J. Neurophysiol.* **58**, 1387–1419.

Singer, W. 1987. Activity-dependent self-organization of synaptic connections as a substrate of learning. In *The Neural and Molecular Basis of Learning,* ed. J.-P. Changeaux and M. Konishi, pp. 239–262. Dahlem Konferenzen. Chichester: John Wiley & Sons Ltd.

Smith, M. 1993. "Neural Networks for Statistical Modeling," Van Nostrand Reinhold.

Sparks, D. L. 1986. Translation of Sensory Signals Into Commands for Control of Saccadic Eye Movements: Role of Primate Superior Colliculus. Physiol Rev 66: 118–171.

Sparks, D. A., Mays, L. E. 1983. Spatial Localization of Saccade Targets I. Compensation for Stimulation-Induced Perturbations in Eye Position. *J. Neurophysiol.* **46**, 45–63.

Squire, L. R., and Moore, R. Y. 1979. "Dorsal thalamic lesion in a noted case of human memory dysfunction." *Ann. Neurol.* **6**, 503–506.

Stirling, R. V., and Merrill, E. G. 1987. Functional morphology of frog retinal ganglion cells and their central projections: The dimming detectors. *Journal of Comparative Neurology* **258**, 477–495.

Stryker, M. P. 1986. The role of neural activity in rearranging connections in the central visual system. In *The Biology of Change in Otorrino-laryngology,* ed. R. Ruben, et al. Elsevier Science Publisher, B. V., pp. 211–224.

Subramaniam, S., Biederman, I., Kalocsai, P., and Madigan, S. R. 1995. Accurate identification, but chance forced-choice recognition for rsvp pictures. In *Proceedings of the Association for Research in Vision and Ophtalmology,* ARVO, Ft. Lauderdale, Florida.

Teeters, J. L., and Arbib, M. A. 1991. A model of anuran retina relating interneurons to ganglion cell responses, *Biol. Cybern.* **64**, 197–207.

Teeters, J. L., Arbib, M. A., Corbacho, F., and Lee, H. B. 1993. Quantitative modeling of responses of anuran retina: Stimulus shape and size dependency. *Vision Research* **33**, 2361–2379.

Tootell, R. B., Silverman, M. S., and de Valois, R. L. 1981. Spatial frequency columns in primary visual cortex. *Science* **214**, 813–815.

von der Malsburg, C. 1973. Self-organizing of Orientation Sensitive Cells in the Striate Cortex. *Kybernetik,* **14**, 85–100.

von der Malsburg, C. 1981. The correlation theory of brain function. Internal report, 81–2, Max-Planck-Institut für Biophysikalische Chemie, Postfach 2841, 3400 Göttingen, FRG. Reprinted in *Models of Neural Networks II,* ed. E. Domany, J. L. van Hemmen, and K. Schulten, chapter 2, pages 95–119. Springer, Berlin, 1994.

von der Malsburg, C. 1987. Synaptic plasticity as basis of brain self-organization. In *The Neural and Molecular Basis of Learning,* ed. J.-P. Changeaux and M. Konishi, pp. 411–431. Dahlem Konferenzen. Chichester: John Wiley & Sons Ltd.

von der Malsburg, C. 1990. Network self-organization. In *An Introduction to Neural and Electronic Networks,* ed. S. F. Zornetzer, J. L. Davis, and C. Lau, Academic Press, pp. 421–432.

von der Malsburg, C., and Buhmann, J. 1992. Sensory segmentation with coupled neural oscillators. *Biol. Cybern.* **67(3)**, 233–242.

von der Malsburg, C., and Reiser, K. 1995. Pose invariant object recognition in a neural system. In *Proceedings of the International Conference on Artificial Neural Networks ICANN '95,* pages 127–132, Paris. EC2 & Cie.

von der Malsburg, C., and Singer, W. 1988. Principles of cortical network organization. In *Neurobiology of Neocortex,* ed. P. Rakic and W. Singer, p. 69–99.

Vorbrüggen, J. C. 1995. Data-driven segmentation of grey-level images with coupled nonlinear oscillators. In *Proceedings of the International Conference on Artificial Neural Networks ICANN '95,* pages 297–302, Paris. EC2 & Cie.

Wasserman, P. D. 1989. Neural Computing: Theory and Practice, 127–149, Van Norstrand Reinhold.

Weitzenfeld, A.. 1993. ASL: Hierarchy, Composition, Heterogeneity, and MultiGranularity in Concurrent Object-Oriented Programming, *Proceedings of the Workshop on Neural Architectures and Distributed AI: From Schema Assemblages to Neural Networks,* USC, October 19–20.

Weitzenfeld, A., and Arbib, M. 1991. A Concurrent Object-Oriented Framework for the Simulation of Neural Networks, *Proceedings of ECOOP/OOPSLA '90 Workshop on Object-Based Concurrent Programming, OOPS Messenger* **2(2)**, 120–124, April.

Werbos, P. J. 1974. Beyond Regression: New Tools for Prediction and Analysis in the Behavioral Sciences, Master Thesis, Harvard University.

Wilson, C. J., Chang, H. T., and Kitai, S. T. 1983. "Origins of postsynaptic potentials evoked in spiny neostriatal projection neurons by thalamic stimulation in the rat." *Exp. Brain Res.* **51**, 217–226.

Wiskott, L. 1995. Labeled Graphs and Dynamic Link Matching for Face Recognition and Scene Analysis, volume 53 of Reihe Physik. Verlag Harri Deutsch, Thun, Frankfurt am Main, Germany. (PhD thesis).

Wiskott, L., Fellous, J.-M., Krüger, N., and von der Malsburg, C. 1997. Face recognition by elastic bunch graph matching. *IEEE Transactions on Pattern Analysis and Machine Intelligence* **19(7)**, 775–779.

Wiskott, L., and von der Malsburg, C. 1993. A neural system for the recognition of partially occluded objects in cluttered scenes. *Int. J. of Pattern Recognition and Artificial Intelligence* **7(4)**, 935–948.

Yonezawa, A., and Tokoro, M. 1987. Object-Oriented Concurrent Programming. The MIT Press.

Zucker, R. S. 1989. Short-term synaptic plasticity. *Ann. Rev. Neuroscience* **12**, 13–31.

Index

control window, 61
Convergence, 52, 58, 155
Conversions, 108, 113, 116
convolution, 44, 159, 164, 177, 178, 190, 191, 247, 322, 340, 341, 358
convolution operation, 44
copy, 85, 86, 113, 118, 310, 315, 341, 348, 350, 351
cortical, 7, 230, 231, 235, 253, 254, 257, 260, 270, 272, 276, 286, 333, 370
create a library, 85
create icons, 63
credit-assessment, i
crosstalk, 26
cue interaction model, 162
curly brackets, 21, 27, 33, 35, 37, 129

dart, 282, 283
data ports, 34, 102
data structure, 41, 55, 67, 150, 333
data types, 41, 81, 102, 104
decision box, 202
declaration, 36, 41, 105, 110, 111, 113, 125, 128
Declarations, 105, 110
defining a path, 104
delete, 93, 359
Deleting a Canvas, 93
delta rule, 204
dendritic tree, 172, 230, 369
Depolarizing, 170, 171, 176
depth computation, 155
depth map, 157, 162, 289
depth perception, ii, 155, 157, 162, 168, 287, 367
DepthModel, 159, 166, 167
descend, 46, 61
Deselecting, 93
detouring, 287, 288, 292, 301
development environment, i
DevModel, 159
differential equations, 2, 5, 16, 18, 41, 122, 144, 166, 176, 186, 190, 192, 309, 322, 323, 324, 326, 327, 333
diffusion of synaptic activity, 185
dimension, 35, 36, 51, 67, 70, 97, 105, 109, 110, 111, 112, 113, 114, 116, 129, 131, 132, 133, 139, 148, 157, 242, 320, 321, 323, 325, 327, 331, 336, 337, 339, 340, 343, 345, 350, 351, 358, 360
direct programming, i, 44

direction, 27, 67, 68, 69, 74, 75, 140, 141, 142, 155, 162, 173, 196, 197, 198, 201, 203, 207, 208, 231, 241, 247, 251, 270, 275, 277, 279, 282, 283, 285, 286, 288, 290, 291, 292, 303, 304, 334
directory, 11, 13, 20, 23, 63, 85, 105, 130, 137, 357
discrete binary models, 1
discrete-event, 16
discrete-time, 16, 22, 24, 27
Display Delta, 96, 97, 98, 99, 347
Display Menu, 88
displaypath, 139
distributed computing, 2
distributed simulation, ii, 118
documentation, i, 10, 11, 12, 85
dopamine, 7, 262, 276, 369
doRunEpochTimes, 136
DoRunEpochTimes, 88
dot plot, 96
doTrainEpochTimes, 135
DoTrainEpochTimes, 87
double, 13, 22, 36, 40, 46, 65, 78, 101, 105, 106, 107, 108, 109, 110, 112, 121, 129, 130, 141, 142, 198, 231, 232, 235, 238, 239, 246, 250, 251, 252, 260, 265, 266, 270, 273, 274, 275, 276, 279, 280, 282, 283, 310, 335, 336, 339, 341, 345, 347, 348, 349, 350, 351, 353, 360
double buffer, 40, 65, 125, 126, 338
double clicking, 13, 46
double saccade experiment, 235, 250, 252, 274, 276
do-while statement., 108
download, i, ii, 364
drawcolor, 141, 142
drawing area, 16, 89, 93
drawstyle, 141, 142
duplicateData, 348
duplicateThis, 348
dynamic equations, 146, 154, 159, 165
dynamic link matching, 309, 368
dynamic memory, 60, 236, 320, 337
Dynamic Memory algorithm, 237
Dynamic Memory Allocation, 337
dynamic remapping, 231, 235, 239, 247

edge effects, 44
edit, 62, 64, 330
Edit Menu, 86
editing, 15, 64